THEOLOGY AND LIFE SERIES

Volume 39

BIOETHICS

ier Book published by The Liturgical Press

Ann Blattner

ael Cunningham
gineering) translated by Caroline M. White
ston

a
linas, Madrid, Spain
1994 St Pauls, Slough, United Kingdom.
his edition for the United States of America an
e Liturgical Press, Collegeville, Minnesota 5632
rinted in the United Kingdom.

BIOETH

Francisco Javier E

A Michael Glaz

Cover design by

The Scripture quo
dard Version of t
tian Education of
United States of Ar

Translated by Mic
Ch. 12 (Genetic En
Edited by Roger Ru

Original title: *Bioéti*
© 1991 Ediciones Pau
English translation ©
All rights reserved. T
Canada published by T
ISBN 0-8146-5503-3. P

Contents

PART II
THE ORIGIN AND EARLY PHASES OF
HUMAN LIFE

PART III:
THE FINAL PHASE OF LIFE

PART IV:
THE DOCTOR-PATIENT RELATIONSHIP

PART V:
MEDICAL TREATMENT AND RESEARCH

12

Editor's Introduction

In editing Fr Elizari's book for an English-language readership a number of changes have been made to the original, with the author's agreement. These changes are mostly of three kinds: the replacement of some Spanish sources (e.g., statements of bishop's conferences) with English-language ones; the addition of material on some topics (e.g., fertility treatment) that have undergone significant development since the publication of the Spanish edition, especially in Britain or other English-speaking countries; brief information on the legal situation in regard to some topics (e.g., abortion) in Britain and other countries. The latter includes a summary of recent changes in Dutch law relating to euthanasia, which is of general interest. Apart from the omission of some material which has little relevance to a non-Spanish readership, the translation of Fr Elizari's text has been left intact, and additions are in the form of 'editor's notes'. The Spanish edition includes extensive bibliographical notes, especially at the end of each chapter. Fr Elizari's extremely wide reading on most topics has ensured a good representation of English-language sources in many of these notes. However some additional bibliographical material has been added to important chapters, and some Spanish and other non-English references have been omitted where these are unlikely to be traceable by English-speaking readers.

Preface

Anyone writing about bioethics in the early 1990s has to take account of a much wider range of ideas than was available 30 or 40 years ago. Another problem is that more modern approaches to bioethics vary considerably between Third World countries and the developed world. This book is aimed at the latter.

It was my intention that the inspiration of this book should be Catholic. Whether this is so will be determined by several unavoidable elements such as the author's personal characteristics, the world in which we live, and the situation that the Church currently finds itself in.

Given the multiplicity and variety of issues to be found in this area of moral thinking, it is not easy to set them out in a logical, orderly way. The themes overlap enormously, and for this reason they could be dealt with at several different stages. I am therefore fully aware that the structure I have chosen is only one of many.

The 31 chapters cover five main areas, the first of which deals with general themes while the other four examine particular issues. The basic structure of the book is therefore as follows:

Part I: General issues
Part II: The origin and early phases of human life
Part III: The final phase of life
Part IV: The doctor-patient relationship
Part V: Medical treatment and research

I have not entered the field of general morality, and have instead confined myself to a limited number of bioethical issues.

Abbreviations

AAS	Acta Apostolicae Sedis
ACl	L'Ami du Clergé
AetF	Amour et Famille
Ang	Angelicum
AS	Aggiornamenti Sociali
BMJ	British Medical Journal
CARS	Cahiers de l'Actualité Religieuse et Sociale
CC	La Civiltà Cattolica
CFT	Conceptos Fundamentales de Teologia
CIS	Cahiers Internationaux de Sociologie
CMAJ	Canadian Medical Association Journal
CMQ	Catholic Medical Quarterly
COF	Cuadernos de Orientacion Familiar
COggi	Credere Oggi
CRS	Cuadernos de Realidades Sociales
DC	La Documentation Catholique
DETM	Diccionario Enciclopédico de Teologia Moral
DH	Dolentium Hominum
Div	Divinitas
DT	Divus Thomas
EB	Encyclopedia of Bioethics
EE	Estudios Eclesiásticos
EgT	Eglise et Théologie
ESM	Ethics in Science and Medicine
ETL	Ephemerides Theologicae Lovanienses
EVedat	Escritos del Vedat
EVic	Esprit et Vie
EvT	Evangelische Theologie
FC	Familia Cristiana
FH	Folia Humanistica
HCR	Hastings Center Report
HK	Herder Korrespondenz
ITQ	Irish Theological Quarterly
IV	Iglesia Viva
JAMA	Journal of the American Medical Association
JME	Journal of Medical Ethics
JMPh	Journal of Medicine and Philosophy
JRE	Journal of Religious Ethics

LH	Labor Hospitalaria
LQ	Linacre Quarterly
LTP	Laval Théologique et Philosophique
LV	Lumière et Vie
LVitae	Lumen Vitae
ManM	Man and Medicine
MC	Miscelanea Comillas
MH	Médecine de l'homme
Mhyg	Médecine et Hygiène
MM	Medicina e Morale
MSR	Mélanges de Science Religieuse
NEJM	New England Journal of Medicine
NPM	Nouvelle Presse Médicale
NRT	Nouvelle Revue Théologique
PRMCL	Periodica de Re Morali, Canonica et Liturgica
PSFU	Problemi di Sessualità e Fecondità Umana
QVC	Questions de Vida Cristiana
RCIC	Revista Católica Internacional Communio
RDC	Revista de Derecho Canónico
REB	Revista Eclesiastica Brasileira
REDC	Revista Española de Derecho Canónico
RET	Revista Española de Teologia
RF	Razón y Fe
RFS	Revista de Fomento Social
RMM	Revue de Métaphysique et de Morale
RN	Revue Neurologique
RO	Revista de Occidente
RPL	Revue de Philosophie de Louvain
RSPT	Revue des Sciences Philosophiques et Théologiques
RSR	Revue des Sciences Religieuses
RSReview	Religious Studies Review
RT	Review Rivista di Teologia
RTeol	Rassegna di Teologia
RTh	Revue Thomiste
RTL	Revue Théologique de Louvain
RTM	Rivista di Teologia Morale
RTP	Revue de Théologie et de Philosophie
Sal	Salesianum
SC	Social Compass
ScC	La Scuola Cattolica
ScEc	Science Ecclésiastique
SM	Studia Moralia
Spec Supp	Special Supplement
SSM	Social Science and Medicine
ST	Sal Terrae
STeol	Selecciones de Teología
STh	Studia Theologica
StP	Studia Patavina

Supp	Supplément
SZ	Stimmen der Zeit
ThGl	Theologie und Glaube
ThRundschau	Theologische Rundschau
TS	Theological Studies
TX	Theologica Xaveriana
VieC	Vie Chrétienne
VN	Vida Nueva
VV	Verdad y Vida
ZEE	Zeitschrift für Evangelische Ethik

PART I

General issues

Chapter 1

Moral thinking on bioethics

1.1 A new interest in bioethics

At the present time, the developed world is showing great interest
in moral issues related to medicine and biology.[1] This 'boom'
manifests itself in a wide variety of ways. To start with, since the
1970s, there has been a dramatic increase in the number of serious
journals devoted to the subject (a list of these publications
appears at page 31). However, discussion on bioethics is not
confined to specialized magazines. Articles on moral themes appear in all the major medical reviews, and there are also many
bibliographies and books on the subject.

  Another indicator of the interest that is aroused by bioethics is
the increase in the number of well-established courses on medical
ethics that are provided for university medical students. A new
sensitivity is now developing, together with a new approach to
moral discourse. Another pointer to the renewed interest in
bioethics is the number of conferences and symposia specifically
devoted to the subject, and of conferences which contain a
bioethical dimension.

  The establishment of bioethics centres or departments not only
reflects one of the anxieties of our times; it also significantly
stimulates interest in the subject itself. In addition, there are
ethical commissions of all kinds being set up in many different
fields: these include hospital ethical committees, and committees
to evaluate research and experimentation protocols; there are also
standing national ethical committees as in France, Germany and
Denmark, and occasional ones in the United States, to advise the
President and legislative body. What is more, public authorities
are drawing up documents and laws at national and supranational
levels to deal with medical issues which incorporate a moral
component. Lastly, the media have done much to publicize

the various views that have been exchanged between doctors, scientists and ordinary people.

Several factors have led to the growing interest in the role that ethics has been playing in biology and medicine. Scientific and technical advances have given doctors increasing powers to intervene in people's lives and destinies, but these techniques are double-edged in that they hold out wonderful promises for humanity, but at the same time present serious threats to the humanizing status of some individuals. Alarm bells have frequently rung about actions which appeared to be abuses on the part of doctors and, despite occasional successes, the indications are that people's respect for the person generally leaves a lot to be desired. General sensitivity to the rights of the individual has now moved into the ambit of health, albeit somewhat late in the day, and the social and political aspects of health care have helped to stimulate interest in moral problems of a less individualistic type.

It is in this climate that the word 'bioethics' has come into existence, and it is around this new discipline that a substantial proportion of current moral studies is concentrated.

1.2 Bioethics[2]

The word 'bioethics' is new. It was originally coined in the USA, but it is now widely used. The cancer researcher, Van Rensselaer Potter, claims to have invented the word in a book entitled *Bioethics: Bridge to the Future*.[3] What is not disputed is that the word derives from *bios*, meaning 'life', and the word 'ethics'.

There is some disagreement as to whether bioethics is an independent discipline, or simply a branch of ethics like economic, sexual or political morality. There are some who insist that it is a new discipline, and not a sub-division or sub-discipline of ethics; they do so despite claims that bioethics is not yet fully established. Others believe that bioethics is a component of ethics, although they fully acknowledge the new context and elements that have been added on to old-style medical ethics.

There is also disagreement as to where it should be taught, and which people should be responsible for doing the teaching.[4] Proposals for venues include medical schools, law schools, public administration courses and philosophy courses. Such controversy highlights the fact that certain aspects of bioethics are of more interest to some doctors than to others; it also underlines the open, non-compartmentalized direction that study takes when it affects humanity at its most profound levels. Health professionals are also somewhat suspicious of moralists and ethical philosophers, on the grounds that the latter pay too much attention to principles and shy away from practice. Others, by contrast, distrust doctors and health workers for their excessive preoccupation with concrete matters. Bioethics attempts to deal with such exclusiveness and distrust by integrating all the various approaches, thereby avoiding one-sided versions of what is a richly varied subject.

There is still much confusion over what bioethics actually means; some people merely identify it with advances such as new techniques of assisted reproduction and genetic engineering. Like W.T. Reich, we might call it a systematic study of human behaviour in the fields of life sciences and health care, in so far as this behaviour is examined in the light of moral values and principles.[5]

Such a description provides us with a number of useful definitions for the study that we are undertaking. The object of this book is human behaviour in two specific areas, life sciences (biology) and health care, which behaviour is systematically studied from a very specific angle – that of moral values and principles.

The above definition does not, however, explain bioethics in its entirety. If we confine ourselves strictly to what the definition says, we might conclude that everything to do with human nature is to do with bioethics in one way or another. We would then run the risk of turning bioethics into a vast, heterogeneous subject – one lacking any consistency, and so immense that it could never be properly tackled. I have no wish to deny the unity of human reality – not to mention the vast horizons that have been correctly opened up for, and by, bioethics – but we do need to have some form of agreement as we go about organizing this knowledge into our society. When all is said and done, ways of organizing this knowledge are less important than finding a way of focusing on what actually goes on in our lives.

There are debates taking place on a whole range of issues;

some of them are of little relevance, but all of them present at least a reasonably clear picture of what bioethics is about.

Some people wonder whether this moral debate should be more practical or more theoretical in tone. Others insist on a primary orientation, that is to say it should be helping doctors, scientists and politicians to take the right decisions. And then there are those who believe that it is simply a question of illuminating knowledge that we already have, and has nothing to do with translating these principles into action to deal with specific cases. Nowadays, this alleged separation between two dimensions of life is not at all simple; however, if that is what takes place, the ideas involved have little value.[6]

Bioethics began to be discussed in the 1960s at a time when such phrases as 'medical ethics' and 'biomedical ethics' were in fashion. The change in terminology may have been partly a question of arbitrary convention, but it was the opinion of many that the new term underlined major differences between bioethics and the earlier medical ethics. Others felt that the old term 'medical ethics' was sufficient to incorporate the new areas of debate. In my view, the whole business of names is of secondary importance. What really matter are the differences between what was going on in the past and what is happening now.

Bioethics does not deal solely with the doctor-patient relationship from a moral standpoint, but also involves concern for 'allied' professions such as mental health. It also extends into biomedical research and research into human behaviour, whether or not there are any therapeutic aims involved. The study of bioethics also incorporates a wide range of social issues such as public health, the working environment and demography. Sometimes, it even goes beyond human life and health, and involves itself in animal and plant life.

Leaving to one side these disagreements about what bioethics means, what we really need to do is to turn the spotlight on bioethics in terms of what it is based on, its methodology and its numerous options, all of which are closely linked. The issues of fundamental principles and methodology bring us back to basic questions of the study of moral issues, something which I do not propose to deal with here.[7]

1.3 Involvement of the Church[8]

The Church's interest in medical ethics has been well documented down through the centuries, but what the Church has
actually said has changed as medicine itself has evolved. This has
been in line with social changes, the Church's understanding of
itself and development of morality. However, side by side with
this area of debate, there is another field of activity which is to do
with caring for the sick, especially the handicapped, although
such work is somewhat dominated by a spiritual dimension.

For a long time, the Church's thinking on sickness was dominated by religion. Sickness was associated with faith, and was
therefore interpreted both in terms of its origin and the therapy
needed to cure it.

From a moral point of view, one of the contributions made by
the Church's teachings is the support given to the ethical tradition, itself linked to certain aspects of the Hippocratic Oath. The
basis of the therapeutic relationship is not love of nature – or even
love of universal nature – but a Christian love of one's neighbour.
This follows the example of Christ, whom Christian literature
frequently presents as a doctor.[9] New developments which stem
from Christianity include equal treatment for all, medical care
free of all payment, and a refusal to attach limits to treatment even
when the sickness is terminal or incurable. Medical ethics is
following in the footsteps of medicine, and is slowly but surely
becoming more consistent.[10]

The Catholic Church's position on medical ethics has been of
great importance since World War II, and has been greatly stimulated by the many interventions of Pope Pius XII. At the present
time, the input of Catholics around the world is not as great as it
has been, but Catholic influence is certainly significant if we take
papal interventions into account. Much more documentation is
now being produced by various Bishops' Conferences around the
world than in the past, and it is usually of considerable relevance
to the various problems that arise. There continues to be a large
number of publications brought out by Catholics, but they do not
offer the homogeneous model of a few decades ago. The variety
of documentation that exists in our society as a whole finds its
reflection in the Church.

The spread of bioethics in the Western world has opened it up

to religious interpretations outside Catholicism.[11] In dialogue with
these and with secular schools of bioethics, the Church is continuing to provide a valuable service to humankind through the inspiration of the gospels.

The Bible presents us with a religious view of human beings
and, according to current exegetic studies, there is little likelihood that it will produce answers to the complex problems thrown
up by bioethics. However, this religious view may well be able
to provide us with clear guidelines that will enable us to discriminate between the many interpretations that currently abound.

The life and experiences of past Christian communities are a
source of knowledge for today's Christians. The memory of this
past, however, needs to steer clear of two dangers: one is the
possibility that it is nothing more than an anachronistic hango-
ver that lacks any sparkle of relevance in today's world; the
other is that it could be interpreted as a definitive point of departure that ignores its historical context.

In the past, Christian morality has paid close heed to what
was going on in the world, although the Christian interpretation
of morality – in a world that was much more stable than ours
and less benumbed by the unparalleled impact of technology –
was powerfully influenced by an excessively static model of
nature and natural law. A thorough knowledge of everything
that goes on in our lives is decisive if we are to adopt positions
concerning the various problems posed by bioethics. Faithful
observation of reality is a basic ethical attitude, whether it con-
firms or denies our personal preferences. We all confront reality
in a non-neutral way with our own preconceptions. However,
there is a big difference between doing so with blinkered views,
and being prepared to accept the challenges and any subsequent
correction. Dialogue has to be an essential component of moral
experience; if this does not happen, the experience will count
for very little.

The role of teaching in this context has been, and continues to
be, both substantial and illuminating.

1.4 Bibliograhy

1. BIBLIOGRAPHICAL WORKS

Bibliography of Bioethics. Published every year since 1975 for the Kennedy Institute of Ethics, Georgetown University. Editors include Leroy Walters and Tamar Joy Kahn.

Ethics in Nursing. Bibliography with notes on the ethics of nursing. Published by the National League for Nursing (USA), editor Terry Pence; second edition 1986.

Bioethics: A Guide to Information Sources, Doris M. Goldstein, Gale Research, Detroit 1982.

The Hastings Center's Bibliography of Ethics, Biomedicine and Professional Responsibility, compilation under the aegis of The Hastings Center team.

New Titles in Bioethics. Monthly since 1975 under the aegis of the National Reference Center for Bioethics Literature, at the Kennedy Institute of Ethics, Georgetown University. Marlene Fine is the overall editor.

Biolaw. Formerly known as *Bioethics Reporter.* The publication is edited by James Childress and Ruth D. Gaare. Started in 1983, it is annual. It provides a summary of articles and legal documents concerning legal-ethical issues in medicine, administration of health care, and experiments on human beings. It also includes the text of important legal decisions.

Bioethicsline. This is a databank prepared by the Kennedy Institute of Ethics, for the National Library of Medicine.

2. REVIEWS

Anime e Corpi, Catholic in inspiration, bimonthly, covers themes of pastoral involvement in the field of public health; Italy.

Artz und Christ, quarterly journal for Catholic doctors in Germany, Austria and Switzerland.

Bioethics, quarterly journal published in Britain since January 1987.

Cahiers de bioéthique, annual publication from Laval University (Canada); each number is a monograph.

Dolentium hominum, published since 1986 by the Papal Commission for clergy working for health organizations.

Ethics in Science and Medicine, quarterly, it appeared with this title between 1973 and 1980. Before that, it bore the title *Science, Medicine and Man*. Since 1981 this excellent journal has no longer been published separately but has been incorporated into *Social Science and Medicine* as 'Part F: Medical and Social Ethics'.

Hastings Center Report, bimonthly journal, of high quality, published in the USA by the Institute of Society, Ethics and the Life Sciences. During the years 1973-74 the same centre published *Hastings Center Studies*.

Journal of Medical Ethics, quarterly, excellent journal published by the Institute of Medical Ethics, London.

Journal of Medical Humanities and Bioethics, USA.

Journal of Medicine and Philosophy, quarterly, University of Chicago; each issue is normally in monograph.

Journal of Religion and Health, quarterly, issues are approached from diverse religious perspectives.

Labor Hospitalaria, published by the Brothers of San Juan de Dios, Barcelona.

Laennec, bimonthly.

Man and Medicine, quarterly, dedicated to the values and ethics of high quality health care, USA.

Médicine de l'homme, bimonthly, journal of the Catholic Centre of French Doctors.

Medicina e Morale, quarterly, clearly Catholic in its views, published by the Catholic University of the Sacred Heart, Italy.

Res Medicae, monthly journal published in Rome; all the issues normally contain a section on moral medicine.

Saint-Luc mèdical – Saint-Lucas Tijdschrift, journal of the Belgian Association of Catholic Doctors.

Two types of journal references could usefully be added to this list:

Major journals of a general nature which often deal with medical ethics: *British Medical Journal*; *Canadian Medical Association Journal*; *Journal of the American Medical Association*; *Lancet*; *Médicine et Hygiène*; *New England Journal of Medicine*.

Non-medical journals dealing with moral issues: *Business and Professional Ethics Journal; Environmental Ethics; Ethics; Ethos; Journal of Moral Education; Journal of Value Enquiry; Journal of Religious Ethics; Morale et Enseignement; Moralia; Pentecostes; Réseaux; Revue de Métaphysique et de Morale; Rivista di Teologia Morale; Zeitschrift für Evangelische Ethik.* Several journals which do not deal only with moral issues but are of interest with regard to medical ethics: *Supplément* (France); *Theological Studies* (USA); *Concilium* (many countries).

3. MAJOR WORKS ADDRESSING BIOETHICS

B.M. Ashley and K.D. O'Rourke, *Health Care Ethics: A Theological Analysis,* Catholic Association of the U.S., St Louis 1982.

T.L. Beauchamp and J.F. Childress, *Principles of Biomedical Ethics,* Oxford University Press, 3rd edn. 1989.

T.L. Beauchamp and Leroy Walters (eds.), *Contemporary Issues in Bioethics,* Wadsworth Publ. Co., Belmont 3rd edn. 1982.

B.E. Brody (ed.), *Moral Theory and Moral Judgements in Medical Ethics,* Kluwer, Dordrecht 1987.

James T. Burtchael, *The Giving and Taking of Life,* Notre Dame 1989.

A.S. Duncan, G.R. Dunstan and R.B. Welbourn (eds.), *Dictionary of Medical Ethics,* DLT, London 1977; Crossroad, New York 1981.

H.T. Engelhardt, *The Foundations of Bioethics,* Oxford University Press, New York 1986.

J. Gafo (ed.), *Dilemas éticos de la medicina actual,* Univ. Pont. Comillas, Madrid 1986.

R. Gillon, *Philosophical Medical Ethics,* John Wiley & Sons, London and New York 1986.

S. Gorovitz et al. (eds.), *Moral Problems in Medicine,* Prentice Hall, Englewood Cliffs 1983.

D. Gracia, *Fundamentos de bioetica,* Eudema-Universidad, Madrid 1989.

B. Häring, *Medical Ethics,* St Paul Publications, Slough 1972 (third edition 1991).

S. Hauerwas, *Suffering Presence,* Notre Dame University Press 1986.

34 GENERAL ISSUES

A.R. Jonsen, *Clinical Ethics: A Practical Approach to Ethical Decisions in Clinical Medicine*, MacMillan, New York 1986.

L. Kass, *Toward a More Natural Science: Biology and Human Affairs*, Free Press, New York 1985.

G.H. Kieffer, *Bioética*, Alhambra, Madrid 1983.

S.E. Lammers and A. Verhey (eds.), *On Moral Medicine*, Eerdmans, Grand Rapids, Mich. 1987.

C. Levine, *Taking Sides: Clashing Views on Controversial Bioethical Issues*, Dushkin Publ. Group, Guildford 1987.

E. López Azitarte, *Ética y vida. Desfíos actuales*, Paulinas, Madrid 1990.

S.J. Loringer, *Human Values in Critical Medicine*, Praeger Publ., New York 1986.

Th.A. Mappes and J.S. Zembaty, *Biomedical Ethics*, McGraw Hill, New York 1986.

John Mahoney, *Bioethics and Belief*, Sheed and Ward, London 1984.

J.K. Mason and R.A. McCall-Smith, *Law and Medical Ethics*, Butterworth, London 3rd edn. 1991.

R.A. McCormick, *Health and Medicine in the Catholic Tradition*, Crossroad, New York 1984; *How Brave a New World?* Georgetown University Press, Washington, DC 1985.

J.F. Monagle and D.C. Thomasma (eds.), *Medical Ethics. A Guide for Health Professionals*, Aspen Publ., Rockville 1988.

E.D. Pellegrino and D.C. Thomasma, *A Philosophical Basis of Medical Practice: Toward a Philosophy and Ethic of the Healing Professions*, Oxford University Press, New York 1981.

G. Perico, *Problemi di etica sanitaria*, Ancora, Milan 1985.

J. Rachels, *The Elements of Moral Philosophy*, Temple University Press, Philadelphia 1986.

Paul Ramsey, *Patient as Person: Exploration in Medical Ethics*, Yale University Press, New Haven 1970.

W.T. Reich, *Encyclopedia of Bioethics*, 4 vols, MacMillan-Free Press, New York 1978.

E. Sgreccia, *Manuale di bioetica*, Vita e pensiero, Milan 1988.

Thomas A. Shannon (ed.), *Bioethics*, 1987, Paulist Press, New Jersey 3rd edn. 1987.

E.E. Shelp (ed.), *Theology and Bioethics: Exploring the Foundations and Frontiers*, Kluwer Academic, Hinham 1985.

P. Sporken, *Medicina y ética en discusión*, Verbo Divino, Estella 1974.

D. Tettamanzi, *Chiesa e bioetica*, Massimo, Milan 1988.

I.E. Thompson, K.M. Melia and K.M. Boyd, *Nursing Ethics*, Churchill Livingstone, London, 2nd edn. 1988.

A.C. Varga, *Bioética. Principales problemas*, Paulinas, Bogota 1988.

R.M. Veatch, *A Theory of Medical Ethics*, Basic Books, New York 1981.

M. Vidal, *Bioética. Estudios de bioética racional*, Tecnos, Madrid 1989.

John Wilkinson, *Christian Ethics in Health Care*, The Handsel Press, London 1988.

R. Wright, *Human Values in Health Care: The Practice of Ethics*, McGraw-Hill Book Company, New York 1987.

1.5 Bioethics centres

There are many organizations, particularly in the United States, which concern themselves with bioethics. For the best and most up-to-date information, the most useful publication is the *International Directory of Bioethics Organizations*, published by Kennedy Institute of Ethics, Georgetown University. The numbers continue to grow, but here is a selected list:

Kennedy Institute of Ethics, since 1979 called the Joseph and Rose Kennedy Institute for the Study of Human Reproduction and Bioethics; founded in 1972, University of Georgetown, Washington.

The Hastings Center, or Institute of Society, Ethics and Life Sciences; organizer of many workshops and with several different publications, in particular, *The Hastings Center Report*.

The Linacre Centre for Health Care Ethics, London.

Ian Ramsey Centre, Oxford.

Society for Health and Human Values, McLean, Va.

Institute of Medical Ethics, London.

King's College, London.

Institut de recherches cliniques, Montreal.

Institut Borja de Bioética, Sant Cugat, Barcelona.

Centre d'Études Bioéthiques, Catholic University of Louvain.

Instituut voor Gezondheidsethiek, Maastricht, Netherlands.

Laboratoire de médicine légale, Lyons, France.

Centre d'Éthique médicale, Lille, France.

Centre for Bioethics, Faculty of Medicine and Surgery of the Catholic University of the Sacred Heart, Rome.

Inserm, Centre de Documentation et d'Information d'Éthique des Sciences de la vie et de la santé, Paris.

Département d'Éthique biomédicale, Centre Sèvres, Paris.

Centre de sociologie de l'éthique, Paris.

Group for the Study of Medical Ethics, Athens.

Dipartimento di Bioetica della Fondazione Internazionale Fatebene-fratelli, Rome.

Commission d'éthique de L'Académie suisse des sciences médicales, Basle.

Delegation for Medical Ethics of the Swedish Society of Medicine, Stockholm.

NOTES

1. VV.AA., 'International Perspectives on Biomedical Ethics', in *HCR* 18 (1988) Spec. Supp., no. 4; VV.AA., 'Biomedical Ethics: A Multi-National View', in *HCR* 17 (1987) no. 3, Spec. Supp., 27-36; E. Feldman, 'Medical Ethics the Japanese Way', in *HCR* 15 (1985) no. 5, 21-24; VV.AA., 'Biomedical Ethics around the World', in *HCR* 14 (1984) no. 6, 14-27; F. Regnier and J.-M. Rouzioux, 'Contemporary Aspects of Medical Ethics in France', in *JME* 9 (1983) 170-174; H.T. Engelhardt, Jr., 'Bioethics in the People's Republic of China', in *HCR* 10 (1980) no. 2, 7-10; R. Gillon, 'Britain: the Public Gets Involved', in *HCR* 14 (1984) no. 6, 16-17; R.M. Veatch, 'Medical Ethics in the Soviet Union', in *HCR* 19 (1989) no. 2, 11-14; Medicine, 'Morality and Culture: International Bioethics', in *HCR* 19 (1989) no. 4, Spec. Supp.; D. Gracia. 'The Intellectual Basis of Bioethics in Southern European Countries', in *JME* 7 (1993) 97-107.
2. L.R. Churchill, 'Reviving a Distinctive Medical Ethics', in *HCR* 19 (1989) no. 3, 28-34; F. Böckle, 'Biotechnology and Human Dignity. Theological and Ethical Dimensions of Biotechniques', in *LH* 214 (1989) 320-324; R.M. Veatch, 'Comparative Medical Ethics: An Introduction', in *JMPh* 13 (1988) 225-229; H.T. Engelhardt, 'The Foundations of Bioethics: the Attempt to Legitimate Biomedical Decisions and Health Care Policy', in *RMM* 92

(1987) 387-399; VV.AA., 'Philosophy and Medicine: A Decade Later', in *JMPh* 11 (1986) no. 1; L.B. McCullough, 'Methodological Concerns in Bioethics', in *JMPh* 11 (1986) 85-91; J. Mahoney, 'La démarche morale. A propos de la bioéthique', in *Études* 363 (1985) 233-246; F. Abel, 'Bioética: un nuevo concepto y una nueva responsabilidad', in *LH* 196 (1985) 101-111; M. Vidal, 'La medicina en las nuevas dimensiones éticas', in *LH* 16 (1984) 169-172; F.J. Elizari, 'Pasado y presente de la ética médica', in *LH* 16 (1984) 109-116; N. Siegler, 'Bioethics. A Critical Consideration', in *EgT* 13 (1982) 295-310; D.C. Thomasma, 'The Possibility of a Normative Medical Ethics', in *JMPh* 5 (1980) 249-259; T.F. Ackerman, 'What Bioethics Should Be', in *JMPh* 5 (1980) 260-275; S. Tovlmin, 'How Medicine Saved the Life of Ethics', in J.P. De Marco and R.M. Fox (eds.), *New Directions in Ethics*, RUP, London 1986, 265-281.

3. Van Rensselaer Potter, *Bioethics: Bridge to the Future*, Prentice Hall, Englewood Cliffs, New Jersey 1971.

4. L.W. Osborne and C.M. Martin, 'The Importance of Listening to Students' Experiences when Teaching Them Medical Ethics', in *JME* 15 (1989) 35-38; W.T. Teel, 'Five Ethical Doctrines for Medical Education', in *JME* 8 (1982) 37-39; VV.AA., 'Teaching Clinical Medical Ethics. A Model Programme for Primary Care Residency', in *JME* 14 (1988) 91-96; VV.AA., 'Multidisciplinary Teaching in a Formal Medical Ethics Course for Clinical Students', in *JME* 14 (1988) 125-128; VV.AA., 'Teaching Medical Ethics Symposium', in *JME* 13 (1987) 127-151; R. Gillon, 'Medical Ethics Education', in *JME* 13 (1987) 115-116; VV.AA., 'GMC: Medical Ethics Education Conference', in *JME* 11 (1985) 5-41; A.J. Johnson, 'Teaching Medical Ethics as a Practical Subject: Observations from Experience', in *JME* 9 (1983) 5-7; D. Belgum, 'Medical Ethics Education: A Professor of Religion Investigates', in *JME* 9 (1983) 8-11; J.P. Ruane, 'Clinical Experience of Teaching Medical Ethics', in *LQ* 42 (1981) 33-39; R.B. Wellbourn, 'A Model for Teaching Medical Ethics', in *JME* 11 (1985) 29-31.

5. W.T. Reich (ed.), *Encyclopedia of Bioethics* I, The Free Press, New York 1978, XIX.

6. Ibid.

7. T.L. Beauchamp and J.F.Childress, *Principles of Biomedical Ethics*, OUP, Oxford, 3rd edition 1989.

8. D. Hollinger, 'Can Bioethics be Evangelical?', in *JRE* 17 (1989) 161-179; B. Kiely, 'Bioethics: The Catholic Tradition, New Technology and the Question of Method', in *Seminarium* 28 (1988) 478-488; J. Fuchs, 'Gibt es eine katholische medizinische Moral?', in *SZ* 206 (1988) 103-111; D. de Marco, 'Bioethics and the Church Teaching', in *LQ* 54 (1987) no. 3, 52-58; Card. Lustiger, 'Médecine, éthique et foie chrétienne', in *MH* 167 (1987) 4-7; R.A. McCormick, 'Health and Medicine in the Catholic Tradition', in *LQ* 53 (1986) 85-91; C.E. Curran, 'Moral Theology in Dialogue with Biomedicine and Bioethics', in *SM* 23 (1985) 57-79; D.F. Kelly, 'Roman Catholic Medical Ethics and the Ethos of Modern Medicine', in *ETL* 59 (1983) 170-174; R.A. McCormick, 'Theology and Biomedical Ethics', in *EgT* 13 (1982) 311-332; F.I.A.M.C., 'Ethical Recommendations for Catholic Doctors', in *CMQ* 38 (1987) 74-76; A. Dumas, 'Fondements bibliques d'une bioéthique', in *Supplément* 142 (1982) 353-368.

9. Cf S. Spinsanti, *Medico*, in VV.AA., *Nuovo Dizionario di Teologia Morale*,
     Edizioni Paoline, Milan 1990, 740-743.
10. Cf P. Laín Entralgo, 'History of the Relationship', in VV.AA., *EB* 1651-
     1657.
11. P. Ratanakul, 'Bioethics in Thailand: The Struggle for Buddhist Solutions',
     in *JMPh* 13 (1988) 301-312; A.A. Nanji, 'Medical Ethics and the Islamic
     Tradition', in *JMPh* 13 (1988) 257-275; VV.AA., 'Medical Ethics from the
     Jewish Perspective', in *JMPh* 8 (1983) no. 3; P. Goldberg, 'Positions
     rabbiniques sur les problémes de pratique médicale', in *MH* 146-147 (1983)
     26-29; D. Nowak, 'Judaism and Contemporary Bioethics', in *JMPh* 4 (1979)
     347-366; J. Gereboff, 'Jewish Bioethics Redefining the Field', in *RS Review*
     8 (1982) 316-324.

Chapter 2

Principles and general moral criteria

2.1 Respect for life

Christianity is faithful to a God who creates and loves life. It has taught, and still teaches, human awareness of a growing respect for life.[1]

a. Dignity of life in itself – not solely a gift from God

Within the Christian tradition, there is a corpus of thought that is frequently employed to underline the dignity of human beings. This includes the notions of life as a gift from God, of men and women created in the image and likeness of God, and the presence of a spiritual soul infused by God. We must bear in mind that, in the Old Testament, what we call physical life is not discussed as such, but integrated into the total unity that is humankind created in the image and likeness of God. Life is received from God, is lived in his presence and returns to him. A further confirmation of the value of all human life comes from the Incarnate Word, who assumes our nature and our history: faith in Christ the man strengthens and consecrates all human beings.[2]

The Christian who accepts these realities existentially cannot fail to respect all human life with a special urgency. Because of our faith in God the creator and Christ the man, human life appears surrounded by God's love, and carries with it a divine vocation.

However, this religious basis must be presented simply, in a way that does not give rise to any equivocation. Human life, irrespective of any religious focus, has a value in itself and for itself. It is the foundation on which any other human value can

develop in a personal and social context. For this reason, the
dignity of life itself must not suffer when we make an appeal to
God. An assumption of Christian faith – it is, after all, an idea
firmly anchored in human consciousness – is that life is a basic
value to be promoted because of what it intrinsically contains. If
we take this as our starting point, we will avoid the impression
given by some Christians that those who live without believing
in God are somehow at the mercy of the elements. It is important
to affirm the gift of God, but without undervaluing the dignity
that is inherent in every human life.

b. A committed life

The inviolability of life has been so forcefully integrated into
Christian morality that another aspect of the Christian mystery
has been obscured. This is the example of Christ, who gives his
life for love. Works of spirituality and devotion used to try and
develop this evangelical inspiration even further; if Christian
ethics had developed along these lines more energetically, I think
that views on the radical disposition of one's life might well have
been different from those commonly held today.

Life is a very precious gift that should arouse in men and
women a sense of gratitude and appreciation; however, the example of Christ integrates yet another dimension. He is the good
shepherd who lays down his life for the sheep (Jn 10:11). 'We
know love by this, that he laid down his life for us – and we ought
to lay down our lives for one another' (1 Jn 3:16). The example of
Christ must inspire similar attitudes in those who follow him: 'No
one has greater love than this, to lay down one's life for one's
friends' (Jn 15:13).

Although life is an important, fundamental value, it is not an
absolute value in itself. The example of Christ clearly demonstrates to us that respect for life – a vital, ethical demand – must
not adopt idolatrous forms that are an end in themselves. The
gospel teaches us that faith and following Christ, in addition to
certain human values, are worthy of any kind of sacrifice. That
includes one's own life: 'For those who want to save their life
will lose it, and those who lose their life for my sake, and for the
sake of the gospel, will save it' (Mk 8:35). The possibility of

sacrificing one's life seems sufficiently clear from Christ's example, and it has also been legitimated by morality from other perspectives.

If the situations in which humankind had to operate were pure – that is to say, if values were only promoted in each action and none were sacrificed – the ethical options would be very obvious. However, reality is more confused and more complicated than that. In a given action, both values and counter-values are frequently, although not always, involved. In this way, we can go along with Böckle and accept that, when all is said and done, all ethical norms relating to behaviour between human beings are based on a judgement of preferences.[3]

None-the-less, human life can come into conflict with moral and non-moral values – the latter include health, pleasure, happiness, technical advances, art, knowledge and so on. The possession of these values does not make men and women morally good; nor does their absence make them immoral. Moral values are all to do with a correctly formed conscience. If life comes into conflict with a moral value, the latter takes ethical priority over the former. In the case of Christ, the realization of God's design had precedence over the preservation of his own life. When the conflict is between life and a non-moral value, the correct decision will depend on a comparison of all the values involved. The choice that is made will be moral in so far as it protects the affirmation of the value or values which, from a global standpoint and in a particular situation, are considered to be a priority by the formed conscience.

So the Christian is confronted by a double demand. On the one hand, there is the task of becoming ever more aware of the dignity of all human life; this growing awareness must translate into a generous welcome for everything that favours life, and a rejection of any move in the opposite direction. On the other hand, it is also a question of avoiding an idolatrous worship of life. These two demands nip two opposed abuses in the bud, but they are common in this society of ours which is permeated by so many contradictions. However, alone these guidelines do not give us a clear solution to the many problems, and particularly the more controversial ones, which arise in this area. For this reason, it is necessary to bear in mind what I will be saying in due course on the right of men and women to make up their minds about their lives in respect of 'ordinary and extraordinary means': suicide, euthanasia and so on.

2.2 The mediation of principles and general criteria

Christian morality has never contented itself with general statements on the duty to protect human life and health. Clearer and clearer formulations have been crystallized down through the centuries, and we now have hard and fast rules of conduct. If life is not an absolute value, it is sometimes neither obligatory nor legitimate to defend it at all costs. There has, however, been a need to define as accurately as possible the frontier separating the legitimate from the illegitimate in actions aimed at supporting life, in attacks on life itself, and at times when it is decided not to defend life. Given that life is something so basic, it is hardly surprising that there should be so much enthusiasm for leaving no stone unturned.

The principles and ideas that have been used to define morality in relation to life and health are legion. Some of them will now be analysed in this chapter.

According to one first principle, it is related to a basic belief shared by all Christians – the sovereignty of God. All created beings live under God's absolute sovereignty. God, the absolute lord of life, can authorize and order actions against life.

When this divine authorization is not to hand, other considerations intervene to indicate which concrete actions are permitted and which are forbidden. At this point, three dual relationships emerge. The first refers to the person, or the victim of an attack on his/her life: here, the major moral issue is the distinction between innocent and guilty. The second focuses on the perpetrator of the attack, be it a public authority or a private individual. The third deals with the way in which the aggression is produced – whether it is produced directly or indirectly. The innocent party is much more untouchable than the guilty one; furthermore, the public authority is allowed to make certain interventions that are forbidden to private individuals. Lastly, directly aggressive actions are much more difficult to accept than indirect ones.

Certain other principles also come into play; they include the principle of totality, the distinction between ordinary and extraordinary means, the distinction between action and omission, the quality of life, double effect, and conflict of values.

2.3 Is everything legitimate if God authorizes it?

Traditional morality has not totally excluded the idea of human beings taking the most radical decisions affecting their own and other people's lives. However, it has always been on one condition: that the action was an act of obedience to God. Through God's order, authorization, command, permission or inspiration, any action against one's own or another's life is legitimate, whether the persons involved are innocent or wrongdoers, or whether the action is directly or indirectly performed by a public authority or a private individual. On the other hand, when no such inspiration or order exists, an attempt on somebody else's life is circumscribed by fundamental restrictions.

To be fair to those who have defended the validity of this distinction for so many centuries, we need to try and understand its genesis. The point of departure is those extraordinary Biblical events whose authenticity was never in doubt – and for which an explanation had to be found. The Bible contains many stories describing suicides and murders apparently carried out with divine approval. The order given to Abraham, 'Take your son, your only son Isaac, whom you love, and go to the land of Moriah, and offer him there as a burnt offering on one of the mountains that I shall show you' (Gen 22:2), was interpreted literally. Cases of suicide which appear to have been carried out with divine authorization include those of Samson (Judg 16:27-30), Eleazar, called Avaran (1 Macc 6:43-46) and Razis (2 Macc 14:37-46). As for instructions attributed to God, and apparently inviting the indiscriminate killing of innocent and guilty alike, Francisco de Vitoria's explanation is that they were carried out by a special order of God; the example adduced from the Scriptures (Deut 20), de Vitoria says, was carried out by a special order of God, but it was a special decree of God, not a general law.

In addition to these Biblical texts, there are other events attributed to the early Christians that present similar problems. These concern women who took their own lives rather than surrender to assaults on their faith or their chastity. In St Augustine's view, these events, far from attracting moral condemnation, are acts of obedience to God. St Thomas Aquinas agrees with St Augustine on this, and also says that 'not even Samson is to be excused that he crushed himself together with his enemies under the ruins of the house, except the Holy Ghost, Who ... had secretly commanded him to do this'.

This was a society which had a powerful concept of God's sovereignty, and a rather uneven idea of the autonomy of humankind. It also lacked the interpretative resources of the Bible which are available to us today. Their solution, which they applied to events that did not initially square with morality, is hardly surprising.

This doctrine, as it was formulated, may be explained by the circumstances in which it developed, but it is still extraordinarily shocking and incomprehensible for believers and non-believers alike. At first sight, it even appears to suggest a picture of God as an absolutist and arbitrary monarch.

This distinction is of virtually no importance in that the existence of orders, divine inspiration and the like is only vindicated for specific events in the past; their applicability to our world is hardly considered. Symbolically, however, its meaning is important in so far as it contains a particular interpretation of God's power and a special view of humankind.

2.4 Culpable – Non-culpable

The distinction drawn between innocent people and wrongdoers always sparks off spontaneous reactions among peoples and individuals; it is a feeling that encourages us to protect ourselves from those who are thought to be a threat to others. This distinction is applicable both in respect of an individual's 'legitimate defence' and in the context of war. Another field where it is particularly relevant is that of criminal law. The distinction between innocent and guilty parties is fundamental if a person is to avoid punishment which might include the death penalty. However, I want to concentrate exclusively on the distinction between innocent and guilty in the sense that someone's life may depend on it. On the face of it, this distinction does not appear to throw up major problems, in that it reflects a feeling which permeates everyone's consciousness. However, it does contain a number of ambiguities. Moralists have given support to some of the consequences of this distinction; today, though, having assimilated the conclusions of social science, we can see the need to clarify the concept of innocent and guilty parties, and of criminal and wrongdoer.

Society cannot be denied the right to characterize certain modes of behaviour in this way, but a few questions will serve to underline the value of the distinction. Who determines which particular form of behaviour is to be considered criminal and which not? Which criteria and interests does the distinction really serve? What percentage of criminality is down to the perpetrator and how much to social conditioning? It has been said, for instance, that the penalty that criminals have to pay is a simple form of exorcism which lets society off the hook and allows people to duck their responsibility for the cause of the crime. Then, there are those who believe that harsh actions simply camouflage society's cruelty, vengeance, laziness and inability to cope. Finally, some continue to see those actions as a necessary part of social self-defence.

2.5 Public authority – Private individual

Public authorities have been endowed with great powers to act against people's lives; these range from deciding who is innocent and who is guilty to the waging of wars. As far as warfare is concerned, prerogatives granted to public authorities have been excessively generous. In practice, the people who once wielded this power were those who decided whether a war was just or not, and, despite claims to the contrary, there was very little legitimate space for either legal or moral dissent. Nowadays, the right to dissent, once jealously guarded by public authorities, is being exercised with increasing zeal, not only because conscientious objection is now legally recognized in many countries, but because it is acknowledged that there is also a moral dimension to be considered in war. This situation has been partly brought about by research into the phenomenon of war; this has served to uncover the shameful interests and ambitions that so often lurk behind calls to justice.

I do not mean to undermine the basis of criminal law. What I am trying to do is to highlight the ambiguities and injustices that have crept into the law, following pressure from interest groups that have little connection with justice. This demonstrates that defending justice by violent means still ends up with innocent people being killed, even when it is done in the name of the public authorities. It is a very poor way of encouraging respect for the value of life.

2.6 Direct-indirect[4]

The distinction between direct and indirect has been of great importance in many areas of the history of morality, including actions that are related to human life and health. It only emerged in the context of morality after several centuries.

According to this distinction, such things as indirect abortion, indirect suicide and the indirect killing of innocent people are legitimate, whereas direct suicide and direct killing (this would include direct euthanasia and direct abortion) are unacceptable. To decide whether an effect can be imputed or not in the case of an action with various effects, we make use of the so-called 'double effect' principle. This principle has been formulated in several ways.

If we insist that the good effect does not come from the evil effect, but that the two of them both proceed from an action at least with the same immediacy, an objective norm has been established. In this way, giving such decisive importance to the physical way in which effects are produced prevents the introduction of subjective assessments which could give rise to arbitrary evaluations. The great positive contribution of this principle would lie in the intended objectivity for important decisions that affect life and health.

All in all, moralists' criticism of this principle in its most rigid formulation is so well-founded that it is not thought to be of much help in seeking a solution to conflicts. It has also been accused of being minimalist and incapable of responding to change. I will make only two points.

The first derives from the difficulty of defining the concept of action. What do we call an action, and what do we consider the effect of an action? Any action, even the simplest, can be divided up into a number of actions, or alternatively integrated into a broader, more global, action. Thus, what is effect for one person may be an integral part of the action for another. In this way, we can see the obscurity, even the ineffectiveness, of the principle when we attempt a moral clarification of behaviour.

However, the main accusation levelled at this approach is that of physicism. It attaches too much importance to the physical nature of the action at the point at which a decision is being taken on morality; moreover, the way in which cause and effect are physically connected determines whether the action is good or bad. Fundamentally, this principle reveals an attitude that is very common in traditional morality – respect for physical nature as a moral criterion. I think that respect for nature has a part to play, but it seems to be an exaggeration to make it into a moral arbiter, because that leaves out the spiritual faculties with which men and women perceive and give meaning to things.

These days, there is a preference for an approach that takes the form of comparing the values that are involved. This system of moral approximation incorporates a number of things. In the first place, very honest analysis is needed to detect the values, and it is not only immediate values that have to be borne in mind but also a perspective of the future. It is self-evident that, generally speaking, the more immediate values will be perceived more easily, but this does not make it legitimate for us to settle for short-term solutions which make a nonsense of reality. At the same time, there is no need to begin searching obsessively for the more remote, distant and problematic values, as they will do nothing but paralyse action completely.

When personal awareness has before it the full range of values involved in a given action, there is then a second step to be taken. This is to compare them in the light of the hierarchy of values, in order to decide on which route to follow, and to opt for those values which genuinely appear to be most imperative at a given moment.

The hierarchy of values is the fruit of many factors such as the training that one has received, the community in which one lives, historical influences, faithfulness to one's conscience, and personal character. However, for a Christian's conscience to be correctly directed, the hierarchy of values needs to be open to the scrutiny and influence of the Christian community in the light of the Church's teaching.

2.7 The principle of totality[5]

The principle of totality in its most general form states that the good of the part may be sacrificed for the good of the whole. It is now claiming that it is the moral arbiter which justifies approval of certain actions and condemnation of others. St Thomas Aquinas relied on it, for example, to justify capital punishment for criminals[6] and to prevent suicides.[7] Nowadays the principle of totality is also used by some to provide legitimacy for artificial methods of birth control, although the encyclical *Humanae Vitae* (14) expressly excludes its use in this context.

The use of this principle for such a wide range of purposes emphasizes the fact that its basis is unusually complex. We apply the concepts of the part and the whole to a wide range of contexts. There is no doubt that there is something common to all these parts and wholes – the need of the whole to help the parts, and the collaboration of each one of the parts for the good of the whole. As long as we stay on this general level, there are no problems. The difficulty arises when we confront an option where we have to choose between the part and the whole. It is never an easy answer, because the relationship between a part and a whole, and between a whole and a part, varies according to the circumstances. The human body is a whole, and the organs, functions and limbs are part of it; the reproductive life of a couple is a whole, a totality, while each sex act is part of this whole; human society, the nation, the local council, the church, the religious institution, the company we work for are wholes, while the people who are members are parts of these wholes. When all is said and done, the most important thing is how the relationship between a concrete part and a concrete whole is conceived, but this is not to say that the formulations of the principle of totality are useless. Pius XII formulated it well when he said that the principle 'affirms that the part exists for the whole and that therefore the good of the part remains subordinated to the good of the whole; that the whole determines the part and may make use of it for its own interests; that the principle derives from the essence of notions and things, and must therefore have an absolute value.'⁸ However, Pius XII's attempts to provide a solution are not really so obvious if we look at the different conclusions that are reached. It is a useful principle, but it is not capable of solving concrete examples for us. There are other matters that the solution needs to take on board. That is why I think it is more interesting to move on to possible situations in which might include implications relating to the principle of totality.

a. Situations involving one person

It is perfectly obvious that all organs and organic functions, parts of the body and tissue and so on, are ordered for the good of the whole. However, in order to satisfy the whole's needs or requirements, the removal of organs and the elimination of organic functions is quite legitimate. If this were not so, we would fall victim to the tyranny in which parts might ruin the whole.

The problem of the legitimacy of subordinating physical functions to the good of the spirit was placed within a moral code, and this code may have drawn too sharp a line between body and spirit. There have been formulations of the principle of totality that appeared to place obstacles in the way of a direct subordination of this type, for instance when Pius XI spoke of the use of parts of the body for their natural ends and functions.⁹ Pius XI's words may have been ambiguous, but Pius XII unequivocally removed all doubts on the subject when he stated that there is not only subordination of individual organs to the body and the body's purpose, but also subordination of the body to the person's spiritual purpose.¹⁰

b. Situations involving two persons

What I am talking about here is removing a healthy organ from one person and transplanting it into a sick person. Pius XII seemed to condemn such behaviour as immoral, although what he might have been trying to do was demonstrate the difference between the human body and society from the point of view of its capacity for forming a whole:

In order to demonstrate that the removal of organs necessary for a transplant from one person to another conforms with nature and is legitimate, it should be placed on the same plane as the removal of a given physical organ for the benefit of a total physical organism... It is argued that, if it is allowed in a case of need to sacrifice a particular part of the body (a hand, a foot, an eye, an ear, a kidney or a sexual organ) for the good of the 'human's' body, it would be equally legitimate to sacrifice a part for 'humanity's' body (in the person of one of its sick, painful, parts). The objective of this line of approach – remedying someone's illness, or at least mitigating it – is understandable and laudable, but the proposed method and the evidence on which it is based are wrong... As far as their physical beings are concerned, individuals are in no way dependent on one another or on humanity.[11]

Here we have an indication of the curious consequences that would prevail if we did not follow Christ's example. The Christian message of charity and solidarity, illuminated by the example of Christ, was more than sufficient to justify donating parts of the body to another human being. However, an abstract principle like that of totality could lead to situations that are completely at odds with the Christian message of charity. Catholic moralists gradually came to realize that these transplants between living people could be perfectly legitimate from a moral perspective.

2.8 The principle of double effect[12]

The very words 'double effect' tell us something about this principle. The principle is used to weigh up an action which produces two (or more) effects, both good and bad. The question then is whether the action is legitimate or not.

The principle of double effect attempts to establish when such an action is morally legitimate – even if it is followed by effects that are bad – and when it is not. For such an action to be morally legitimate, it must fulfil four conditions which are not always formulated in the same way:

- the morally good or indifferent nature of the action;

   – the doer's good intentions (i.e. seeking to do good and avoid evil);

   – a causal connection between the good effect and the action, or at least a connection that is as immediate as that of the bad effect;

   – an equally important reason to allow the production of the bad effect.

If these conditions are fulfilled, the bad effect is described as indirectly willed. This principle has been applied in the notorious case of the removal of a cancerous uterus from a pregnant woman, in actions connected with killing people, and in the performance of sexual functions.

There is much discussion at the present time on the extent to which this principle is able to mark a dividing line between what is legitimate and what is illegitimate.

2.9 The sanctity and quality of life[13]

a. Quality of life

This phrase is now widely used in developed countries where it has been appropriated by politicians, advertising executives and scientists, and even occurs in everyday language. Its uses are so disparate, and its definitions so numerous, that it is easy to conclude that it means whatever the speaker wants it to mean. Advertisements appeal to the quality of life in the context of whatever object they are trying to sell, whether it be a car, a perfume, or whatever. Meanwhile, in everyday language, quality of life is regularly used as a synonym for well-being, happiness or simply a pleasant life. What is more, the phrase often acquires a financial connotation, although it should not be confused with 'standard of living'. Sociology offers us two schools of thought; the objectivists who seek to define quality of life on the basis of objective criteria, and the subjectivists who prioritize the subjective elements of personal satisfaction. It is the latter group that has been holding sway in recent years. From the subjectivists' perspective, it is clearer how quality of life is a concept that varies from one to person to the next, and even

varies in a given person at different times and in different situations depending, for instance, on his/her health. It is extremely
difficult to determine exactly what quality of life is. This also
goes for the meanings of the words 'quality' and 'life', as
well as the elements that form the background to it – in other
words, an image of the human being and his/her needs and
aspirations.

If we consider medicine, there have been many indicators of
quality of life that have come from the field of health; these
include the age to which people live, attempts to prolong life, and
the general standard of health and medical care. In terms of
bioethics, the idea of quality of life is used to help solve a wide
range of problems; these include abortion, euthanasia, antenatal
tests, the prevention of life by contraception or sterilization, modi-
fying nature through genetic engineering, defective newly-born
children, public health, environmental health, population, and
decisions whether or not to prolong a person's life. The concept
of quality of life varies according to the situation in which it is
applied. For example, the quality of life of a nearly terminal
cancer patient does not raise the same issues and demands that
would be relevant to someone with a physical handicap. The most
complicated of all situations occurs when a decision is taken on
whether or not to prolong someone's life. In such a case, quality
of life is sometimes opposed to sanctity of life, an issue that will
be examined shortly.

There is an inescapable moral requirement to deal with quality
of life, if what we mean is any kind of action that seeks to create
favourable conditions for the broadening and development of
human beings. Quality of life must never be thought of as a
bourgeois luxury or a concern for those whose basic material
needs have been sorted out.

Quality of life is sometimes understood to be basically an
economic issue. This is a very partial interpretation, given that
sobriety and austerity can also be major components of people's
lives. To achieve true quality of life, spiritual aspects of being
are more important than physical ones. Affective factors such as
accepting one another, being accepted, friendship and love also
play a major role. It has been said that our society probably
contains perverse mechanisms that impede the pursuit of real
quality of life. On the other hand, quality of life is not solely the

result of individual action; there are also the public and political dimensions to consider.

b. Sanctity of life

Although the expression 'sanctity of life' belongs originally to religious discourse it also has a secular interpretation. Just because all life is sacred, this does not mean to say that it necessarily has a religious basis; this characteristic emerges from life itself. The sacred character of life, according to those who support this position, is the most important of all experiences. If life is not sacred, nothing is sacred. In theory, establishing a common basis for the sanctity of life that is independent of religious beliefs could be used for dialogue within a pluralistic world. However, there are questions about the validity of experience said to affirm the sacred character of life. Furthermore, many people do not like this kind of language and prefer to use the language of rights.

There is another interpretation of the sanctity of life: the doctrine of the creation, of human beings in the image of God, the alliance of God with his people, and their redemption in Christ.

Like quality of life, the theme of the sanctity of life or life's sacred character is raised both inside the field of medicine and outside it.

In principle, an appeal to the sacredness of life appears to offer a more secure guarantee of protection for life, and it attempts to eliminate from these decisions the role played by tastes, customs and human laws.

c. Quality and sanctity of life

Let us now try and link the two concepts. Some people look upon them as counterposed when they are used to deal with decisions about whether or not to prolong a new or terminal life. It is generally felt, however, that the differences between the two positions lie in whether or not to sustain the sacred character of human life or physical life, the absolute character of the norm, and a choice between the quality and length of life.

However, the differences between the two positions – at least as they are understood by many moralists – should not encourage us to see them as mutually exclusive, or to opt for one and totally forget about the other. In an article entitled 'Feeding Policy Protects Patients' Rights, Decisions', Fr Dennis Brodeur says, 'If terms like "quality of life" and "sanctity of life" are used correctly, they need not be perceived as polar opposites. One can maintain the sacredness and avoid arbitrary and false judgements while also considering the quality of a person's life as he or she pursues the ends or goals of life.'[14]

We may ask with some justification whether the different choices about prolonging a life that relate to the sanctity and quality of life really refer to these ideas, or whether they really refer to certain tenets of a religious culture or belief which people take on board in different measures.

In conclusion, we should mention ordinary and extraordinary means, to be discussed in chapter 14.4.

NOTES

1. D.M. Holley, 'Voluntary Death, Property Rights, and the Gift of Life', in *JRE* 17 (1989) 103-121; Ch. Hennau-Hublet, 'Le droit de disposer de soi-même', in *MH* 177 (1988) 409-420; J. McMahan, 'Death and the Value of Life', in *Ethics* 99 (1988) 32-61; J. Fuchs, 'Christian Faith and the Disposing of Human Life', in *TS* 46 (1985) 645-684; C. Bernardin, 'La recherche d'une éthique cohérente de la vie', in *DC* 83 (1986) 569-572; F.J. Elizari, '¿Es la vida humana un valor absoluto?', in *Moralia* 1 (1979) 21-39.
2. Gen 1:26; 2:7; 5:1; 9:6; Wis 2:23; Ps 8:6. On Man as the Image of God, cf Th. Camelot, 'La théologie de l'image de Dieu', in *RSPT* 40 (1956) 443-471; C. Spicq, *Dieu et l'homme selon le Nouveau Testament*, Du Cerf, Paris 1961; G.B. Fernagren *'The imago Dei* and the sanctity of Life: the origins of an idea', in McMillan, Englehardt and Spicker, *Euthanasia and the Newborn*, 23ff.
3. F. Böckle, 'Faith and conduct', in *Concilium* 138-bis (1978) 262.
4. J. Langan, 'Direct and Indirect. Some Recent Exchanges between Paul Ramsey and Richard McCormick', in *RSR* 5 (1979) 95-101; A. Regan, 'The Accidental Effect in Moral Discourse', in *SM* 16 (1978) 99-127; A.R. di Ianni, 'The Direct/Indirect Distinctions in Morals', in *Thomist* 41 (1977) 350-381; L. Rossi, '"Direct" and "indirect" in moral theology', in *RTM* 3 (1971) 37-65.
5. M. Zalba, 'The Meaning of the Principle of Totality in the Doctrine of Pius XI and Pius XII and Its Application to Cases of Sexual Violence', in *LQ* 52

(1985) 218-237; A.M. Hamelin, 'The Principle of Totality and personal free will', in *Concilium* 15 (1966) 98-112; G. Kelly, 'Pope Pius XII and the Principle of Totality', in *TS* 16 (1955) 373-396.

6. 'Everything is part of the whole just as the imperfect and the perfect form part of the whole, and thus everything is naturally a part of the whole ... Therefore, each individual makes up part of the whole community; and by extension, if a man is a danger to society and corrupts it by committing sin, it is right and proper to take away his life in order to preserve the common good' (II-II, q. 64, a. 2, Resp.).

7. 'Every part, in so far as it is a part, can be such only if and when it forms part of a whole. A man, whosoever he may be, is part of the community, and therefore all that he is belongs to the society; hence he who takes his own life damages the community' (II-II, q. 64, a. 5, Resp.).

8. Pius XII, in *AAS* 44 (1952) 787.

9. Pius XI, in *AAS* 32 (1930) 565.

10. Pius XII, in *AAS* 50 (1958) 693-694.

11. Pius XII, in *AAS* 48 (1956) 461.

12. R. Barry, 'Stones and Street Cars. A Clarification of the Doctrine of the Double Effect', in *ITQ* 48 (1981) 127-136; J.M. Boyle, 'Toward Understanding the Principle of Double Effect', in *Ethics* 90 (1980) 527-538; R.A. McCormick, 'The Principle of Double Effect', in *Concilium* 120 (1976) 564-582.

13. A. Shaw, 'Quality of Life Revisited', in *NCR* 18 (1988) 2, 10-12; H. Kuhse, *The Sanctity Doctrine of Life in Medicine. A Critique*, Clarendon Press, Oxford 1987; L.S. Cahill, 'Sanctity of Life, Quality of Life, and Social Justice', in *TS* 48 (1987) 105-123; J.R. Connery, 'Quality of Life', in *LQ* 53 (1986) no. 1, 26-33; J.M. Mardones, 'Health, quality of life and salvation', in *IV* 119 (1985) 469-487; B.V. Johnstone, 'The Sanctity of Life, the Quality of Life and the New "Baby Doe" Rule', in *LQ* 52 (1985) 258-270; K.C. Calman, 'Quality of Life in Cancer Patients, An Hypothesis', in *JME* 10 (1984) 124-127; A. Cribb, 'Quality of Life. A Response to K.C. Calman', in *JME* 11 (1985) 142-145; C.B. Cohen, '"Quality of Life" and the Analogy with the Nazis', in *JMPh* 8 (1983) 113-135; H. Shipper, 'Why Measure Quality of Life', in *CMAS* 128 (1983) 1367-1370; R.A. McCormick, 'The Quality of Life, the Sanctity of Life', in *HCR* 8 (1978) no. 1, 30-36; D.H. Smith, 'The Sanctity of Social Life: Physicians and the Critically Ill', in *HCR* 6 (1976) no. 3, 31-34.

14. D. Brodeur, 'Feeding Policy Protects Patients' Rights, Decisions', in *Health Progress* 166 (1985), no. 6, 43. Cf analogous affirmations in R.A. McCormick, *op.cit.*, 637.

Chapter 3
Medical codes of ethics[1]

Medical ethics has been expressed in a variety of ways at different stages of history, ranging from prayers, oaths and deontological codes to directives, guidelines, and declarations issued by medical conferences. Together, they manage to express a variety of global and partial approaches, systematic approaches, religious and secular inspiration, general and detailed examinations and so on. This chapter is restricted by limitations of space to no more than a rapid survey of the subject.

As their name suggests, prayers of religious inspiration express gratitude to God for blessings received and ask for divine assistance in the correct performance of medical duties. An example is the daily doctor's prayer, once attributed to Moses Maimonides (1135-1204) but now thought more likely to be the work of a Jewish doctor of the eighteenth century, Marcus Herz.

For centuries, the most important formula for passing on bioethics has been the oath. The oath was a common way of expressing ethical concepts in the ancient world. It incorporated the notion that an alliance with the gods was essential if a patient was to be treated successfully. It also sought protection for those treating the patient, and punishment for those who broke their word. The most famous of all oaths is the Hippocratic Oath. It is of immense importance to medical ethics; it forms part of the essential hub of Western spiritual heritage, and has attracted respect from many parts of the world including the Christian, Jewish, Muslim and civil traditions.

The Hippocratic Oath has an introduction containing the formula of the oath, and a conclusion which requests blessings and curses. Otherwise, it is in two parts, the first referring to relations between doctors, and the second to relations with patients.

Its origin is shrouded in obscurity. It appears in the collection of Hippocrates' writings catalogued and published by librarians in Alexandria, and the oldest surviving copies date from a time after the coming of Christ. It has been suggested that it could have been the work of many people, and it is even thought that some of it could have been written by Pythagoras, as it bears similarities to some of the latter's teachings that date from the fourth century BC.

Another question turns on whether the ethics referred to in the oath were commonly practised by Greek doctors. History provides insufficient evidence as to whether medical practice of the day was in fact at odds with the oath or not.

The Christian tradition had no difficulty accepting the Hippocratic Oath, although a number of amendments have been made to ensure that it harmonizes better with Christian ideals and norms. One example of this involves turning the reference to Greek gods into an invocation to the Trinity; another is the way that the 'alliance' within the medical profession gives its services for nothing and is increasingly interested in its teaching role.

In line with traditions that originated in the Middle Ages, medical schools incorporate some of Hippocrates' ideas in oaths taken on graduating, and sometimes the whole text is reproduced. It has been common practice for much of the twentieth century to take the Hippocratic Oath on graduating, although this died out after World War II. It has now been adapted in a number of ways to make it applicable to culturally mixed societies and to the practice of medicine in the modern world.

Opinion is divided about the use of the Hippocratic Oath and its meaning. Many believe it is still the Magna Carta of medical ethics and commands profound respect. Others accord it a more symbolic role, saying that it seems to have more to do with the mythical foundation of a group or the consecration of a caste, even conferring a noble title or a title of quasi-apostolic succession.

Clearly, it would be wrong to confuse the undoubtedly important historic significance of the oath with the meaning it may have in our present-day society and in the practice of specified forms of medicine. It is pilloried by some for favouring an ideal of religious, undemocratic, paternalistic medicine that ignores social and political realities. However, if such criticism is to become dominant, it needs to take on board the historical context in which something like an oath appears and survives. This is a quite different matter from the social and medical circumstances of the present day.

The most developed and systematic codification of medical ethics is to be found in the professional codes of doctors, and to a lesser extent, the House of nursing (deontological codes). In today's world, doctors are not happy about spiritually inspired texts, and are becoming increasingly dissatisfied with oaths. They now want a more complete and systematic codification of how a doctor is supposed to behave towards his/her patients and other colleagues.

Medical Ethics by Thomas Percival (1740-1804) was written in 1794 and published in 1803. It was the prototype of the deontological codes that have proliferated particularly in the twentieth century, and was the first comprehensive outline of professional conduct to serve as a model for the American Medical Association's first code in 1847.

Since the 1940s, there has been a plethora of national, and even international, medical codes. In North America, not only do doctors have a code for themselves, but various medical specialists – including surgeons, gynaecologists, psychiatrists, cardiologists, health workers and experts in legal claims for occupational injury – also have theirs.

Deontological codes consist of a variety of texts containing lists of specific duties which the members of the profession must observe. These duties are distinct from those imposed by the law, and they do not necessarily coincide with an individual's personal ethics. They neither exclusively nor predominantly deal with morality. They contain norms of behaviour, etiquette and good relations, and serve the interests of the group directly and those of the users indirectly. The rules are considered to be essential for the correct performance of a doctor's duties. Their function is to safeguard the dignity of professional practice and thereby win the patient's confidence. They are much more than regulations; they are more like a way of thinking. Interest in regulations of this type has declined considerably, and the codes that survive are strongly reminiscent of texts that were popular decades ago.

In the current world of social and moral pluralism – and we should not forget the situation that the medical professions are in at the present time – there is a trend towards less detailed, and more general, regulations. By contrast, legislation, which was

once practically non-existent in the field of medicine, has proliferated on issues like abortion, contraception, new techniques of
human reproduction, problems related to dying, confidentiality
and informed consent.

Those who are still in favour of these ethical codifications see
in them a way of promoting, stimulating and preserving a medical
ethos, a guarantee of a unified model of behaviour, and the
possibility of exercising control more effectively over the conduct of fellow doctors. The assistance of professional ethics committees is certainly needed if the latter objective is to be achieved.

From certain professional and political points of view, there is
support for marginal, even hostile, views of deontological codes.
Some consider them to be useless on the grounds that there is
already ample and varied guidance for correct behaviour to be
found in laws and customs, and within professional bodies and
trade unions; there is also the moral sense in one's own conscience. Sometimes, the codes are also criticized for supporting
the interests of the profession in a rather underhand way, instead
of promoting the social good or the benefit of the patients. Codes
that confine themselves to general statements are thought to be
useless; if, on the other hand, they adopt more concrete positions,
they are accused of providing a framework that is too rigid and
strict for the pluralistic society we live in. Furthermore, the criticism runs, they stifle all sense of personal responsibility, and
appear to betoken distrust of the younger generation by giving
them a rigid structure of behaviour. They are also censured for
being a bastion of liberal medicine and lacking sensitivity for the
doctor's social duties.

It is clear from the above that codes are going through a
process of intellectual ferment, social transformation and ethical
re-definition.

Nowadays, there are new ways for doctors to express their
opinions on medical matters. Declarations put out by various
international medical assemblies and other bodies are vested with
particular authority, particularly as these meetings frequently produce monographs on issues of current interest, e.g., the BMA
report on euthanasia (1988). The advantages of these declarations
are obvious, one of them being that they do not try to tackle the
enormous number of questions that are dealt with in deontological
codes. Moreover, the production of these documents and the

processes of correcting behaviour are both speedy and to the point. Declarations of this type also usually reflect an inter-disciplinary and pluralistic style, one that is well able to deal with all sides of the question. Deontological codes, in short, seem to be somewhat in eclipse.

Finally, of all the ethical statements, I would like to draw attention to the so-called declarations of the rights of patients and of other people suffering from certain illnesses, e.g., AIDS. I shall be looking at declarations of this type later in this book.

NOTE

1. L. Edelstein, *The Hippocratic Oath*, The Johns Hopkins Press, Baltimore 1943; C. Calhoun, *Annotated Bibliography of Medical Oaths, Codes and Prayers*, Kennedy Institute, Washington D.C. 1975; C.L., 'AMA, Updates Its "Current Opinions" on Medical Ethics', in *HCR* 14 (1984) no. 4, 5-6; D.E. Cunningham, 'Moral Codes in Human Care', in *Journal of Religion and Health*, 7 (1968) 299-310; M.B. Etzioni, *The Physician's Creed*, C.C. Thomas Publisher, Springfield 1973; D.A. Frenkel, 'Human Experimentation: Codes of Ethics', in *Legal Medical Quarterly* 1 (1977) 7-14; R.S. Gass, 'Codes of the Health-Care Professions', in *EB*, IV, 1725-1730; D. Konold, 'Codes of Medical Ethics', in *EB*, I, 162-171; R.M. Veatch, 'Codes of Medical Ethics, Ethical Analysis', in *EB*, I, 172-180; R. Gillon, 'Medical Oaths, Declarations and Codes', in *BMJ* 290 (1985) 1194-1196; A. Heijder and H. van Geuns, *Codes of Professional Ethics*, Amnesty International, London 1976; J. Kultgen, 'The Ideological Use of Professional Codes', in *Business and Professional Ethics Journal* 1 (1982) no. 3, 53-69; A. Verhey, 'The Doctor's Oath and a Christian Swearing It', in *LQ* 51 (1984) 139-157; *International Code of Medical Ethics*, reprinted as Appendix C in J.K. Mason and R.A. McCall-Smith, *Law and Medical Ethics*, 1991, 441-2.

PART II

The origin and early phases of human life

Chapter 4

The techniques
of assisted reproduction

Until very recently, infertile married couples simply had to accept the fact that they were not going to have children. Either that, or they had to adopt. Science and technology had no way of helping them overcome the hostility of nature and thereby have children. The only solutions were popular remedies – usually religious and magic practices – that had survived in various cultures. Today, scientific and technological advances offer these couples some hope, although there are no guarantees.

4.1 Scientific and technical considerations[1]

There are currently three basic techniques: artificial insemination (AI), *in vitro* fertilization and embryo transplant (IVF/ET), and gamete inter-fallopian transfer (GIFT). There are also auxiliary techniques for storing semen, ova and embryos.

a. Artificial insemination

Strictly speaking, artificial insemination (AI) consists of artificially placing human semen into the woman's vagina and not by means of intercourse. Then, as soon as fertilization has taken place, the whole of the rest of the process happens quite naturally. This is the simplest of the techniques; it is also the oldest and the one which has been the subject of most experimentation. It has to be preceded by a number of steps.

Before a couple move to this (or any other) technique, they must be examined to see if the reasons for the infertility can be ascertained.

For artificial insemination to take place, fresh or stored human semen must be available. We must not forget that this semen is provided through masturbation, and this in itself raises moral problems. The semen can come from the male partner (artificial insemination by the husband [AIH] or artificial insemination within marriage) or from a donor (artificial insemination by donor [AID]).

Before the semen is placed in the woman's body, it has to be carefully prepared in the laboratory, and this process makes different demands on the people involved, according to the circumstances. One condition that is vital for the success of the operation is knowing the precise moment when ovulation is about to take place. Once these preparatory phases have been completed, the semen is placed in the vagina, cervix or uterus according to medical indications. Artificial insemination does not require an anaesthetic.

The main medical indications for artificial insemination within marriage are as follows: it is impossible to place the semen naturally at the top of the vagina or in any other part of it because of the man's impotence or because of some congenital deformity of the man's or woman's sexual organs; there are no indications of fertile sperm (e.g. a small number of spermatozoa, or lack of vitality or motility), although this can be rectified under laboratory conditions; alterations in the mucus at the neck of the cervix (for example due to scarcity, dryness or infection); immunological rejection of the semen in the vagina or at the neck of the uterus; and idiopathic sterility, that is to say when examination of the infertile couple reveals no abnormality and yet the woman does not become pregnant.

A donor's semen is used mainly in the following circumstances: the man is sterile; the man suffers from chromosomal or genetic abnormalities which, although they do not impede fertilization, cause numerous abortions in the first three months; and the man has genetic diseases or serious genetic infections which can be passed on to his children.

Artificial insemination is very successful, but it does depend on certain factors such as the use of fresh or stored semen and the presence of highly skilled medical staff; other conditions include a knowledge of the causes of infertility, and how many inseminations have already taken place. The incidence of abortion, death and perinatal morbidity is in line with rates for normal confinements.

The first known case of artificial insemination within marriage took place in 1779. It is credited to Hunter. Over a century later, in the United States, Dickinson carried out the first artificial insemination using a donor's semen (1899). After World War II, the practice began to spread in the United States, a country that has always been a pioneer in the field. According to some estimates, around a quarter of a million inseminations have been performed in the USA, and since 1959 they have been carried out with stored (or frozen) semen.

b. In vitro *fertilization and embryo transplant*

As the name suggests, the technique of *in vitro* fertilization and embryo transplant (IVF/ET) is divided into two parts. The first is the process of fertilization in a test tube and not in the woman's body, and the second is the transfer of the embryo or embryos to the uterus.

This technique involves several stages. In the first place, there need to be human gametes, that is to say sperm and ova. In order to obtain sperm, the same procedure is followed here as for artificial insemination. The ova have to be extracted from the ovaries, and modern scientific and technical advances not only tell us exactly when ovulation is imminent, but also enable us to stimulate multiple ovulation by hormonal stimulation.

When the sperm and ova have been correctly prepared, they are placed in a glass dish; if cellular cleavage is observed, that is a sign that fertilization has taken place. The fertilized ova are kept in a medium culture until the optimum moment for transfer to the uterus; at that point, they are introduced through the cervix. There are minor differences of opinion among doctors about the moment when the ova should be transferred. It is generally agreed that this should take place 24-48 hours after fertilization, as early contact with the cervical mucus increases the likelihood of success. It is also considered advisable to use three embryos as the chances of succeeding seem to be better than with two or one.

Like artificial insemination, IVF/ET can be performed using the gametes of the couple or of donors. The main indications for this technique are as follows:

- the woman is sterile: she has no ovaries or they are not functioning (in other words, donors are needed), absence or abnormality of the fallopian tubes;
- endometriosis: the presence of endometrium (mucous lining of the uterus) in places other than the uterus;
- the man is sterile: azoospermia, impotence, severe abnormality of the semen;
- both partners are sterile: for instance, build-up of antibodies in the woman which are hostile to spermatozoa, or immunological incompatibility between the semen and the cervical mucus;
- the prevention of congenital diseases;
- idiopathic sterility, (i.e. when medical examinations reveal nothing abnormal but the woman does not get pregnant).

It is very difficult to make a confident evaluation of this technique as the available data do not always use the same criteria: for example, some refer to successful pregnancies, while others refer to births. Effectiveness is heavily dependent on the skills of the medical team, the number of transferred embryos and so on; this is more true of IVF/ET than it is of artificial insemination. While some centres boast very good success rates, the average for a pioneering country like Australia in 1988 was about 6-7 per cent; this is likely to improve in time.

IVF/ET began to be developed in 1950, and was first used on human beings in 1969. The first completely successful operation took place in 1978 when Louise Brown was born in Britain on 25 July. The first child was born following ovum donation in March 1984 in Los Angeles.

c. Gamete inter-fallopian transfer

The technique of gamete inter-fallopian transfer (GIFT) is the newest and least developed of the three. It involves putting the ova and spermatozoa in contact with each other inside the fallopian tubes; while this is being done, the ova are removed from the ovary by means of a puncturing technique or by aspiration of the follicle.

As with artificial insemination and IVF/ET, fresh or stored

semen is essential and, as is the case with IVF/ET, the ova have to be removed just as they are on the point of ripening. It is claimed that this technique gives the gametes a more appropriate environment than the laboratory; the main danger seems to be ectopic pregnancy.

The main indications for using this technique are as follows: male sterility (e.g. impotence or changes in the semen), female sterility (e.g. insufficient mucus for the spermatozoa to pass through the cervix, or immunological rejection on the part of the woman), the failure of artificial insemination, and idiopathic sterility.

d. Storage techniques[2]

The use of storage techniques (freezing and unfreezing) has helped to make procedures of assisted reproduction much easier. It is now possible to freeze semen, ova and embryos.

The freezing of semen is the oldest, the simplest and the most widespread of all freezing techniques. It was first proposed by Montegazza in 1886, but the basis for the technique was only properly established in 1949 when Polge and his team demonstrated the cryopreservative action of gossypol (a substance obtained from cottonseed oil) on the sperm of various mammals. Bunge and Sherman carried out the first successful pregnancies with frozen semen in 1953. This technique developed rapidly during the 1970s, and subsequent advances, although less significant, have had an impact on minor details of the procedures. The storage of ova that can be used for human reproduction is the newest technique of the three. Australia has been in the vanguard of this work, although it is still not widely used as many of the stored ova are damaged and therefore unusable for human reproduction. The first pregnancies using stored human ova occurred in Australia at the end of 1985.

The storage of embryos pre-dates that of ova and, on the face of it, presents fewer problems. The first known pregnancy using a frozen embryo took place in Australia on 2 May 1983, but the experiment was unsuccessful. The first human being conceived with a frozen embryo was born on 28 March 1984; it was a girl and she was called Zoe, the Greek word for 'life'. The number of frozen embryos almost trebled between 1985 and 1986, going from 289 to 824. In 1988, it was estimated that there had been 10 live births in the United States and 60 throughout the world. There have been many more since then.

Stored semen retains its fertility for a long time, even years, although the quality is inferior to that of fresh semen. Stored ova, however, frequently suffer from the passage of time to the extent that very few can be used for human reproduction. However, technical progress and the improving skills of medical teams are bringing better results with even the most complicated storage techniques. In addition to medical considerations, there are human and social issues that need to be addressed;[3] these draw a clear distinction between the storage of gametes and that of embryos. Some people are concerned that storage might influence the physical and mental characteristics of individuals conceived with frozen ova and embryos. However, given that any ova or embryos that are unsuitable for freezing are thrown away, there do not appear to be any serious grounds to justify these fears.

4.2 Psychological issues

There is a danger that successful applications of these techniques over the last few years, and the sometimes unjustified hopes that people have of them, will cause us to forget the psychological and related matters. For this reason, the problem has been addressed by medical teams that are aware of the importance of these issues, and in recommendations contained in expert reports presented to governments and legal bodies. They have demanded that counselling and support services should be made available to people who wish to make use of these techniques. The psychological effects can be examined under a number of headings.

Couples wishing to have children, but unable to do so using normal means, are often troubled by their infertility in several ways. For instance, their self-image can deteriorate sharply, and their whole relationship can also be very negatively affected. Social expectations placed upon the couple in certain family settings can also contribute to increased tension. We therefore need to think carefully how such couples should deal with their infertility.

Throughout the investigation into the causes of their infertility and the subsequent treatment, there are all manner of analyses and tests that bring doctors and the couple very close together. Understandably, the man and the woman concentrate more on fertility than on their relationship during this period.

If recourse to techniques of assisted reproduction results in failure, this can make life particularly difficult for the couple, and at this time they may experience great frustration as they realize that this last resort has come to nothing.

It is equally important to deal with the problem from a psychological point of view. There is no question that the donation of semen, even if it is anonymous, can have psychological repercussions. Furthermore, it is important to bear in mind the impact on a child conceived by one of these techniques. It would be wrong to exaggerate people's fears, but equally we should not lose sight of the possibility that problems can arise. As long as proper counselling and support services are available, any negative psychological effect can be adequately dealt with.

One last point which needs to be examined is the psychological characteristics of the donors.

4.3 Legal issues[4]

The techniques of assisted reproduction are both new and socially complex. Despite the innumerable recommendations that committees of experts submit to governments and legal bodies, there is little current legislation at world level. That does not prevent these techniques being used without any major problems for the most part, and there are very few difficult cases that end up in court.

As far as the law goes, there are matters of administrative law (the authorization of centres to carry out these techniques, confidentiality/anonymity, the holding of data, a policy on obtaining gametes, information and so on), civil law (contracts, maternity, paternity, filiation, rights of succession) and penal law.

This is a very specific aspect of these techniques, but I am going to confine myself to the most important trends in the few laws that exist, and in the many expert reports and recommendations.

There are no problems of principle about the legal acceptability of all these techniques (i.e. artificial insemination, IVF/ET, and the storage of semen, ova and embryos). The only minor reservations refer to the storage of ova, but that is only because of the poor results achieved so far and the technique's generally experimental character.

As for people who have legal access to these procedures, there are no problems for married couples and for men and women in stable heterosexual relationships. Generally speaking, the door also appears to be open to single people (e.g. widows, and unmarried, divorced or separated women) who want it. It has to be said, however, that opinions are divided on this point.

The donation of ova, semen and embryos does not present any important problems either. Emphasis needs to be placed on the circumstances of the donors, and the condition of what they donate, to ensure that the donation takes place in as humane a manner as possible. To this end, it is important that all information is made freely available; otherwise, there can be conflict arising from issues such as the woman being paid, irreversibility, a limit on the number of children, anonymity, informed consent, and health. Surrogate motherhood, particularly on a commercial basis, meets with widespread, although not total, disapproval.

When there has been no donation of semen, the father/mother/ child link poses few difficulties on the whole. Even when it has been donated, the situation remains quite clear as long as the principle of irreversibility has been established. All rights and obligations revert to the receivers of the donation and not to the donors.

There is a wide range of procedures relating to research into, and experimentation on, embryos. The least complex situation involves non-viable embryos, and then there is no disagreement. Opinions are divided, however, on the issue of viable embryos that are left over following *in vitro* fertilization. Some people believe that embryos are created in laboratories exclusively for the purposes of research and experiments.

[*Editor's note*: As an example of legislation on this issue, the UK Human Fertilization and Embryology Act may be cited. AID is not discouraged by the Act, but is declared illegal without a licence unless it is a mutual treatment between the man and the woman (i.e. the donor is not anonymous). Moreover, the Act is uneasy about AID for single women or unmarried couples (including lesbian couples), declaring that 'A woman shall not be provided with treatment services unless account has been taken of the welfare of any child who may be born as a result of the treatment (including the need of that child for a father)' (13.5). The problem of illegitimacy and paternity claims is avoided by the rule that, given she has been inseminated with the sperm of a man other than her husband by a person licensed to do so and provided that her husband has consented, it is he – and no other man – who will be treated as the father of the child. This also gives to the donor freedom from any parental responsibility. There is a similar provision in the matter of egg donation and IVF: a woman who carries a child as a result of the placing in her of an embryo or of sperm and eggs – and no other woman – is to be treated as the mother of the child.]

4.4 The morality of these techniques: introduction[5]

Here we find ourselves face to face with a new issue. It is one that seems to be urging a certain degree of caution, suggesting that we might forgo the possibility of temporary aims, but on no account give up the search for absolute certainties. On the other hand, given the impact that these techniques have on human life, not to mention their rapid advance and expansion, it is desirable that we should be as clear about everything at as early a stage as possible. It is no secret that, in our pluralistic society, there are now different moral ideas being heard simultaneously within the Church. It is a subject on which the magisterium has laid down teaching that has well-defined, clear stages.[6]

In an attempt to set out some moral indications on this question, I thought of a number of different frameworks in which I could place them.[7] In this way, our point of departure might have been the rights and interests of the various individuals affected, in other words the people who owe their existences to these techniques, people who want to have the child through these procedures, and finally donors and health professionals. There are also the interests of society to be born in mind. Another focus could have looked at the values involved – sterility, fertility, fertility

control, the dignity of human reproduction, the dignity of the
child, marriage as an appropriate framework for procreation, and
various social implications.

In fact, I have gone for a third option. I have decided to take
concrete situations as my basis, despite the fact that this unavoid-
ably causes repetition. I am also going to start with the simplest
technique, artificial insemination.

4.5 Artificial insemination: morality[8]

A wide variety of situations is possible through the use of this
procedure: artificial insemination within marriage, artificial insemination of an unmarried woman or of a widow, artificial
insemination with or without a donor, and the use of fresh or
stored semen. I will keep to those situations that are of most
interest, and I will leave the donation of semen till later.

a. Artificial insemination within marriage

This is clearly the least complicated situation of all from a
technical, social, legal and moral point of view. The technique is
used with a married couple, and fertilization takes place in the
woman's body with semen and ova provided by the same two
people. The only new aspect compared with totally natural reproduction is that the semen is introduced artificially and not by the
conjugal act.

Our society takes a very broad view of this, and sees no
particular problems. By contrast, the position taken by the Congregation for the Doctrine of the Faith is clear and emphatic:
'Homologous artificial insemination within marriage cannot be
admitted except for those cases in which the technical means is
not a substitute for the conjugal act but serves to facilitate and to
help so that the act attains its natural purpose'.[9] The moral issue in
this document depends on whether or not the technique replaces
the conjugal act by helping or facilitating. From a purely medical
point of view, the curious notion of doctors helping or facilitating
the sex act is difficult to follow; it also raises a number of
questions, and stimulates some imaginative hypothetical replies.

This doctrine is not new, having been stated clearly by Pius XII on many occasions.[10] Nor is it based on contingent, historical circumstances, but on the Church's teaching on the connection between the married state and procreation, and on the personal nature of the conjugal act and procreation.

Artificial insemination within marriage is not condemned out of hand simply because semen is obtained by masturbation, as is sometimes claimed. The real reason is that, even if the semen were obtained differently and legitimately, the Congregation's moral rejection would still be absolute because a scientific technique is replacing the conjugal act as the origin of human life. Masturbation, both in these circumstances and in a more normal setting, introduces an additional element of immorality. 'Masturbation, through which the sperm is normally obtained, is another sign of this dissociation: even when it is done for the purpose of procreation, the act remains deprived of its unitive meaning.'[11]

It is important to examine how this idea is justified. The reasons will be equally valid for the rejection of other techniques which are even more artificial than AI. To that end, I offer three matters for consideration.[12]

1. The first is based on the inseparable union desired by God between the uniting and procreative meanings of the conjugal act, a union that human beings cannot break on their own. According to the Congregation for the Doctrine of the Faith, this principle is based on the nature of marriage and on the intimate connection of its goods. This doctrine has long been used to condemn contraception (the conjugal act removed from procreation); it is now put forward to reject all techniques of assisted reproduction (procreation removed from the conjugal act).

2. Secondly, the unity of the human being composed of a body and a spiritual soul. This principle is accepted in Christian anthropology; what it is now important to establish is how it provides support for the notion that artificial insemination within marriage is immoral. Just as a human being is made up of a body and spirit, so the conjugal act has to be at once physical and spiritual. It is obvious that if the conjugal act is reduced to a merely physical union, it becomes impoverished and adulterated, even though it can still lead to procreation. 'In order to respect the language of their bodies and their natural generosity, the conjugal

union must take place with respect for its openness to procreation; and the procreation of a person must be the fruit and the result of married love.'[13]

3. The third issue is based on the personal nature of human procreation, or, to put it in another way, on the dignity of the origin of all human beings. The Vatican instruction is based on a self-evident proposition that we could summarize thus: every child has the same dignity as his/her parents, and can never be an object for manipulation, or reduced to the level of a mere object or product. 'In his unique and irrepeatable origin, the child must be respected and recognized as equal in personal dignity to those who give him life.'[14]

A human being, the Instruction goes on to say,

> cannot be desired or conceived as the product of an interven-
> tion of medical or biological techniques; that would be equiva-
> lent to reducing him to an object of scientific technology. No
> one may subject the coming of a child into the world to
> conditions of technical efficiency which are to be evaluated
> according to standards of control and dominion.[15]

This third issue raised in *Donum Vitae* was probably inspired by a document produced by the British Catholic Bishops' Joint Committee on Bioethical Issues of 2 March 1983. There is only one difference: the British document seems to refer to IVF/ET and not to artificial insemination, although some of the ideas could be extended to include it. The Vatican instruction makes similar points on these issues, including artificial insemination within marriage.

> Thus the IVF child comes into existence, not as a gift super-
> vening on an act expressive of marital union, and so not in the
> manner of a new partner in the common life so vividly ex-
> pressed by that act, but rather in the manner of a product of a
> making ..., as the end-product of a process managed and car-
> ried out by persons other than his parents. ... To choose to have
> a child by IVF is to choose to have a child as the product of a
> making. But the relationship of product to maker is a relation-
> ship of radical inequality, of profound subordination.[16]

If a child who is conceived by these techniques is objectively a product, if s/he is the result of a relationship of manipulative control, and finds him/herself in a situation of fundamental sub-ordination and not of equality, there can be no escaping the inhuman and immoral character of artificial insemination – let alone other techniques – within marriage.

b. Posthumous insemination[17]

The fact that artificial insemination within marriage is not a morally acceptable option, according to the Vatican in-struction, does not prevent us from making a moral assessment of other, more complex, situations with specific characteristics.

I discuss some of these situations elsewhere in this book – artificial insemination with a donor's semen (see the section dealing with donations), using stored semen (which I shall exam-ine when I make a moral evaluation of storage), and artificial insemination of an unmarried woman (this is covered when I look at the overall framework of these techniques). There is, however, one situation which I want to discuss now, and that is artificial insemination within marriage using the deceased husband's fro-zen semen. Although there have been very few cases of this process, the issue has been given plenty of publicity by the media, and has inspired lively debates on related moral, legal and psy-chological issues.

In 1984, a French episcopal commission published a docu-ment which dealt with several questions related to birth and death, but also examined posthumous insemination on the basis of the varied social response which a case in France had stimulated during the summer of that year. As I do not propose to go over again what I have said above about artificial insemination within marriage, I would now like to concentrate on the new element in this situation.

From the outset, the bishops acknowledged the positive side of a widow's wish to have a child by her dead husband. It was noted elsewhere what a wonderful thing it was to want to prolong one's husband's life in a way, by conceiving a child by him after his death. Why turn down the opportunity if there are no minor details standing in the way?[18]

A proper understanding of what was happening should not be mindlessly obscured by sentiments which are in themselves noble. If we look at the global consequences of these practices, reality simply seems to be that little bit more complex. The negative effects and the undesirable consequences for the child and the couple are legion.[19]

When a child's arrival as an orphan is intentional and planned, it means that his or her interests are not being acknowledged. It was pointed out at the time of this case in France that a child who has been conceived an orphan, so to speak, comes into the world with the misfortune of never being able to have a father – although that role might be filled quite soon by someone else. Will the father's image in the mother's heart and words be enough to enable the child to settle down? In practice, the poor child not only has to work out how to deal with his mother; s/he also has to come to terms with the father-mother-child triangle – something which specialists agree is so important for the maturation of personality.[20]

In the bishops' view, the high number of single parent families, of children who have only a mother or only a father, is not an argument in favour of tolerating this practice. The 'accidental' existence of such families (e.g. resulting from the death of one of the partners or separation) does not legitimate the intentional, planned creation of a situation which, in the opinion of numerous child psychologists and psychiatrists, will not help the child to grow up in a balanced way.

4.6 In vitro fertilization and embryo transplantation: moral considerations[21]

As with artificial insemination, there is a wide range of situations covered by IVF/ET. This is equally true of users (married couples, stable heterosexual couples, and women on their own – widows and unmarried, separated and divorced women) and of the ova, semen or embryos used (e.g. the couple's own semen and ova, one from the couple and one from a donor, both from donors, or a donated embryo). The most important of these situations have already been dealt with under artificial insemination or will be examined later on.

For the moment, I am more interested in examining the new moral issues that this technique brings to artificial insemination, irrespective of the users' circumstances and the origin of the gametes and embryos.

What is new about *in vitro* fertilization is that it does not work simply with gametes, but with embryos. It works with a human life that has started off its existence outside the woman's body, in the laboratory, and it follows that the attendant dangers are legion. IVF obliges us to have respect for human life from its very earliest stages, and there is persuasive, reliable evidence that few of these lives last for long. In most cases, there is no intention of cutting short the vital process that has been initiated; we are talking here of accidents that occur for various reasons, not unlike the sad losses that occur when conception has been natural. Besides these accidents, there are cases when surplus embryos that have resulted from multiple fertilization in the laboratory are deliberately eliminated. In theory, there are many things that can be done with surplus embryos: they can be stored for later use with the same woman in the event of earlier attempts failing, they can be given to another woman (this is not really viable, and anyway it is very rare), they can be destroyed, and they can be used for research or experiments (in which case they would have to be destroyed very soon indeed). The creation of embryos in laboratories solely for the purpose of research, and the subsequent destruction of any surplus ones, are two of the most criminal attacks on respect for early human life. In this context, *Donum Vitae* sees a certain analogy with abortion and a usurping of God's place, with human beings making themselves arbiters of the destinies of others.[22]

Apart from these dangers to human life, the Vatican instruction points to other anxieties around the issue of IVF/ET.[23]

4.7 Gamete inter-fallopian transfer (GIFT): moral considerations[24]

This technique is not referred to in *Donum Vitae*. At all events, it does not have the disadvantages of *in vitro* fertilization and embryo transplantation which are referred to above, as it works solely with human gametes. However, given the way in which

GIFT is performed these days, it would appear that the views expressed on the subject of artificial insemination are equally valid for this technique.

4.8 Storage: moral considerations

Scientific and technical data on the use of storage techniques in assisted reproduction are set out above. I now want to make a moral assessment, and for this purpose it is useful to draw a distinction between the storage of gametes (i.e. semen and ova) and of embryos.

a. Storage of semen[25]

There does not appear to be any moral problem about the storage of semen in itself. This technique moved on from the experimental stage a long time ago. Stored semen retains excellent fertility for many years, and there is no danger of children being born handicapped in any way after being conceived with it.

The only issues of any moral significance for the Church's traditional doctrine are the way in which the semen has been obtained (see the section on artificial insemination) and its possible use for fertilizing purposes outside the natural process.

b. Storage of ova

This question has hardly ever aroused any moral interest, and this may be because the technique is new and ova are obtained differently from semen.

It is still an experimental technique. Many ova deteriorate as a result of being stored, and they are not suitable for human reproduction because there is an understandable fear that children could be born with abnormalities and deformities.

I am not aware of any moral reservations being expressed on the surgical methods used to obtain ova, by comparison with the difficulties raised by masturbation. The only fears concern the operation – it is performed under a general anaesthetic – and the possible stimulation of ova which could result in multiple ovulation. Otherwise, storing ova does not seem to present any particular moral problems.

c. Storage of embryos[26]

If the purpose of storing surplus embryos is to use them later in experiments and further study, it shows no respect for the dignity of life. The thirst for progress – and, of course, I accept it could one day well contribute to therapeutic interventions carried out on other people – means that these lives do nothing more than serve alien interests.

When embryos are frozen in order to extend these lives beyond their normal term, it is unacceptable according to *Donum Vitae*:

> The freezing of embryos, even when carried out in order to preserve the life of an embryo – cryopreservation – constitutes an offence against the respect due to human beings by exposing them to grave risks of death or harm to their physical integrity and depriving them, at least temporarily, of maternal shelter and gestation, thus placing them in a situation in which further offences and manipulation are possible.[27]

[*Editor's note*: As an example of legislation in this area, the UK Human Fertilization and Embryology Act 1990 may be cited: the creation, storage and destruction of surplus embryos is permitted, but strict conditions are laid down. Having granted in principle that embryos may be manipulated and discarded in the course of treatment, the law seeks to avoid what it sees as practices unacceptable to public morality: i.e. the creation of hybrids, open-ended experimentation for purposes other than infertility treatment, and a traffic in embryos. Embryos may not be kept after the appearance of the primitive streak (14 days). There is a limit of five years on the storage of embryos (10 years for gametes). The Act establishes a strict licensing regime and seeks to avoid the use of embryos for anything other than the specific reason for which the licence was granted, which can include specified research. Moreover, any production, use or disposal of an embryo brought about *in vitro* depends on the common consent of the persons whose gametes were used to make it and can only be done by persons licensed by the Authority for strictly-defined purposes. There is no general freedom to make human embryos *in vitro* for the purposes of experiment.]

4.9 Recipients outside marriage

Earlier sections have looked at the various techniques of assisted reproduction. Here, we examine a variety of situations which are not relevant technically speaking, but are highly important from a moral, legal and psychiatric point of view. Of the many situations that could be studied, two are particularly interesting from a moral standpoint. One deals with the recipients of these techniques. Should they be confined to married couples? And what about relationships outside marriage? Should they include stable heterosexual couples, or only men or only women? And what about gay men and lesbians? Assuming that the recipients are married to one another, this gives rise to yet another question: must the semen, ova and embryos used automatically come from the couple in question, or can we think in terms of donations? These issues are dealt with in Chapters 9 and 11.

The Catholic Church believes that marriage is the only morally acceptable framework for human reproduction. 'The tradition of the Church and anthropological reflection recognise in marriage and in its indissoluble unity the only setting worthy of truly responsible procreation.'[28]

This position relies on the specific characteristics of the human race which demand respect for the personal dignity of parents and children. It is also based on the needs of the common good. 'The vitality and stability of society require that children come into the world within a family and that the family be firmly based on marriage.'[29]

4.10 Donation: moral aspects

Even where the user or the recipient of these techniques is married, the origin of the semen, ova and embryos used presents us with two situations which have possible implications of a legal, psychological and moral nature, and other implications for the relationship itself. If everything originates within the married couple (and that includes the recipient), it is much less complex than if outside donors are involved.

Donations can consist of either ova or semen, or of both, or of an embryo; surrogate motherhood, which is dealt with in the next section, might also come under the heading of 'donations'. The donation of semen is older and more common; the donation of ova and embryos began in the mid-1980s and is still rare.

In the light of what I have said above about the morality of the various techniques, I now want to concentrate exclusively on the newer aspects of donation, and proceed to a moral assessment.

Donum Vitae states clearly that there are several negative aspects about any type of donation: for example, it is an attack on the institution of marriage, it is contrary to the dignity of the married couple, it harms the child's rights, and it prejudices the true interests of society.

The issue that *Donum Vitae* most forcibly and repeatedly raises relates to marriage. The point is made from a number of different angles including the following: donation is opposed to the unity that is demanded of a married couple, it is a violation of both the bond of conjugal fidelity that unites them, and of the reciprocal promise that they have made; it is unsupportive of the couple's rights and is opposed to the objective and inalienable proprieties of marriage; it signifies a break in the common calling of motherhood and fatherhood; and it alters personal relations.[30]

On the subject of the damage that donations of this type cause to the rights of the child, *Donum Vitae* is much more restrained, but no less clear: a donation, the instruction states, deprives the child of a relationship with his/her real parents, it runs counter to a child's right to be conceived and brought into the world within marriage and by the married couple of that marriage, and it can lead to difficulties in personal development.[31]

The negative effects for society – I mean the discords, confusions and injustices thrown up by social life – are viewed by *Donum Vitae* as a consequence of altering the relationships within the family.[32]

A document on the family produced by French bishops includes a list of questions on the most frequent form of donation, that of semen. First, the French bishops make the point that the donation of sperm is said to be a generous act. That may be so, they point out, in the spirit of the father, but what kind of generosity is it that has already washed its hands of all responsibility for the child's future upbringing? Is donation of human sperm comparable to the donation of blood, for example? Semen contains information, a genetic heritage that performs a decisive role in a child whose father wants to have nothing to do with it.[33]

4.11 Surrogate motherhood[34]

Surrogate motherhood involves using the services of a woman to bear a child. Then, immediately after the birth, she hands the child over to the person who has fathered it.

Surrogate motherhood can take a variety of forms. The most extreme fragmentation of the father-mother-child link occurs when there are three 'mothers' and two 'fathers'. These are the 'social' or 'rearing' parents who take responsibility for bringing the child up after s/he has been born, the genetic parents who donated the ova and sperm, and the woman carrying the baby whose job consists of no more than giving birth to the child.

Donum Vitae dismisses this approach succinctly, saying it is

> contrary to the unity of marriage and to the dignity of the procreation of the human person. Surrogate motherhood represents an objective failure to meet the obligations of maternal love, of conjugal fidelity and of responsible motherhood; it offends the dignity and the right of the child to be conceived, carried in the womb, brought into the world and brought up by his own parents; it sets up, to the detriment of families, a division between the physical, psychological and moral elements which constitute those families.[35]

The experience of bearing a child establishes a profound relationship between mother and child. It is from the mother that the child receives food to eat and air to breathe, but that is not all: the two of them also develop close bonds of love which are very difficult to break after birth. In surrogate motherhood, pregnancy seems to be reduced to a simple function of manufacture that knows nothing of this intimacy. In all probability, the woman carrying the baby sees herself as no more than a means or 'incubator' for processing the pregnancy.

Even feminist groups have argued against surrogate motherhood on the grounds that there can be commercial exploitation. They cite as proof of this the appearance of a new profession of mothers who offer a form of intra-uterine hospitality service in exchange for money. This may be exaggerating things somewhat, but these groups even claim that we might be moving towards a stage where privileged rich women can find liberation on the backs of a caste of child-bearers. Such predictions may be overpessimistic, but there is no denying the possibility of commercial exploitation. When the issue was debated in the British Houses of Parliament, an MP referred to the danger of capitalist gangsterism and, as a way of avoiding this, made the curious suggestion that surrogate motherhood should be paid for out of Social Security.

The fact that there are women who will bear children for no payment at all eliminates some of the more disgraceful connotations, but it does not assuage all our anxieties. Women who do this sort of thing may well have the best of intentions – but they may also be concealing from themselves other aspirations such as a yearning for power, an element of narcissism, and an egocentric satisfaction about giving pleasure to other people. Facilitating conception, and promptly separating the child from the woman who has carried him or her, does not respond to the child's interests in any way.

4.12 Applications unrelated to reproduction[36]

So far, we have looked at techniques of assisted reproduction in so far as they are a way of helping people who want to have children, but are unable to do so using natural means. I now want to look at other applications and possible developments of the same techniques which may result from research and experimentation. As long as such interventions are confined to human gametes, there do not appear to be any major ethical difficulties; the problem arises when a human embryo or foetus is used, but not to produce a human being.

A wide range of reports, proposals and suggestions on these techniques have been circulating in the scientific community and are published in some of the media. The questions that they elicit are numerous, and are sometimes more profound than the original issues. Some of the time, the published material deals with ideas that are technically possible. Otherwise, technical feasibility still seems a long way off: at best, it is medium-term, if not long-term. In fact, some of the ideas border on science fiction. If we then pass from the purely technical field to more human, moral matters, we sometimes have the impression that we are peering into a bizarre new world which is in many ways opposed to all basic human sensitivity. Wherever one looks, one can only hope that good moral sense will prevail over the seductive fascination of new techniques which apparently claim they are capable of anything. For the time being, statute laws, draft laws and the recommendations of expert commissions are generally saying very little about many of the ideas put forward in this field.

a. Applications

In this section, I will do no more than comment briefly on applications and developments that can be predicted, or have simply been suggested, in connection with the techniques of assisted reproduction.

Creation of hybrids. The creation of hybrid beings, a mixture of human being and animal, has haunted the human imagination since time immemorial. Although there is a general trend to oppose such experiments, there have been reports of attempts to fertilize monkeys with human semen, but some of these ideas are difficult to credit. On the other hand, hamster tests are now being performed with appropriate authorizations and within the law. When a couple's infertility is being investigated, an attempt is sometimes made to fertilize a hamster's ovum with human sperm. If this fertilization is successful – this is established if the ovum cell multiplies and there is cleavage into two cells – it is concluded that the man's sperm is capable of fertilizing his wife. If a small hybrid is formed, further development is prevented as it is essential to interrupt the process of hybridization at the two-cell phase.

Parthenogenesis. Parthenogenesis, or virgin birth, is the development of the ovum in a human being without being fertilized by semen. This technique exists in nature – in plants and in some invertebrates. Among humans, it is not possible at present, and does not appear to be feasible in the foreseeable future.

Ectogenesis. This application consists of creating an artificial environment, similar to the uterus and placenta, which can sustain an entire pregnancy; it thus does away with what is still the irreplaceable role of the mother.

Gestation of human embryos/foetuses in the uterus of another species. This is a strange idea that offends everyone's sensitivity. Its chances of success are remote, but that does not stop people from trying to make it work.

Gestation of animal embryos/foetuses in a human uterus. See my comments in the paragraph above.

Embryo biopsy. After *in vitro* fertilization, but before transferring the embryo to the uterus, one or two cells are removed without compromising the development of the embryo, so as to analyse them and see if it is normal, find out the sex and so on. The embryo is frozen while these analyses are being carried out. Then, depending on the results of the tests, it is then destroyed if it is not considered acceptable for reproduction or transfer to the uterus to perform its former and natural function.

Chorionic biopsy. This technique, which is apparently now practised with reasonable success, consists of taking samples of the chorionic membranes and analysing them in the laboratory to find out certain things about the embryo/foetus. Such information would include sex and chromosomal abnormalities. This technique also makes it possible to carry out a diagnosis of the foetus round about the tenth week of pregnancy, and a long time before amniocentesis takes place.

Testing new medicines. One of the most important tests that new medicines now have to pass relates to any harm they might cause to pregnant women. It has been suggested in many quarters that the human race could benefit substantially if these tests could be performed on human embryos in laboratories. This would avoid risks for women who are already pregnant, and the checks that a new medicine is obliged to undergo would be quicker and cheaper.

Scientific knowledge of the first stages of the embryo's devel-

opment. If embryos could be studied under laboratory conditions for, say, two weeks, it would obviously be possible to observe their development very carefully, and this information could well be of assistance to other people.

Supply of organs and tissue. This question is mentioned more frequently in connection with abortion, and I shall deal with it elsewhere. It involves the use of embryos/foetuses as donors of organs and foetal material, and it incorporates therapeutic objectives for other people.

b. Moral issues

The Catholic Church's teaching demands absolute respect for human life from the moment of conception. Although there is an element of uncertainty about whether we can talk of a person at this initial stage, the same teaching states that the basic capacity to be a person renders the embryo worthy of the maximum respect. On the basis of this fundamental view of the world, research and experiments are only admissible if they are for the benefit of that embryo or foetus. Experiments that are not directly therapeutic, and use either viable or non-viable embryos, cannot be justified by any other objective, irrespective of the impressive scientific advances or benefits that may accrue to other people or society in general. To quote *Donum Vitae*, '... all research, even when limited to the simple observation of the embryo, would become illicit were it to involve risk to the embryo's physical integrity or life by reason of the methods used or the effects induced'.[37]

On the subject of procedures which seek to achieve fertilization between human and animal gametes, gestation of human embryos in an animal's uterus, and ectogenesis, *Donum Vitae* has this to say: 'These procedures are contrary to the human dignity proper to the embryo, and at the same time they are contrary to the right of every person to be conceived and to be born within marriage and from marriage'.[38] Equally, hypotheses and practical interventions relating to the production of a human being without the conjugal act (e.g. cloning, parthenogenesis or twin fission) 'are to be considered contrary to the moral law, since they are in opposition to the dignity both of human procreation and of the conjugal union'.[39]

For this reason, it is hardly surprising that nearly all these applications, whether they are still at the planning stage or have actually been carried out, are dismissed in expert reports and legal documents as an attack on human dignity.

4.13 Cloning[40]

As far as humans and species superior to animals are concerned, this procedure has potential – but no more. However, there are those who believe that human reproduction will be technically possible with the use of this technique by the end of the twentieth century.

The procedure, which has been successfully used on certain animals, consists of surgically removing the nucleus of an ovum, and then inserting the nucleus of a somatic cell which has a normal complement of chromosomes. If the ovum is grafted successfully and produces a new member of that species, there is said to be successful clonal reproduction. In principle, this process can be repeated an infinite number of times with the same person, and reproductions can be multiplied endlessly. We would then have a being that was as similar to him/herself as possible, having received his/her genetic inheritance from a single person.

From both a moral[41] and a legal point of view, this type of intervention is unacceptable.

[*Editorial Appendix – Some new developments*:

Since this book was written, there have been major developments in the field of fertility treatment, some of which have caused a great deal of public controversy. They include the treatment of women beyond normal child-bearing age and the use of eggs from aborted foetuses. While the latter is still in the proposal stage, the former is already practised, and a number of women in their late fifties and sixties have already given birth after treatment at fertility clinics in Italy and the USA. In this procedure, eggs from younger, fertile donors are fertilized *in vitro* and then placed in the older woman's uterus. Hormone replacement therapy makes her womb receptive to the eggs. The procedure has been declared illegal in several European countries, including

Germany, Sweden and France, which have banned *in vitro* fertilization using donated eggs. Although there is no age limit to fertility treatment in Britain, the licensing procedure and official discouragement would appear to prevent it. This discouragement arises from the central concern of the 1990 Human Fertilization and Embryology Act that the welfare of the children born from fertility treatment is always to be considered above the desires of the would-be parents. Opposition has also come from both the general public and from some IVF practitioners, who consider that a legitimate therapeutic procedure, designed to help infertile couples at considerable expense, is being used to subvert the natural biological event of menopause, which normally releases women for other, more mature activities. Needless to say, the Catholic Church, having ruled that fertility treatment must involve only the eggs and sperm from a married couple, would oppose this new development for that reason alone.

Far greater public disquiet was caused in 1993 and 1994 by the proposal to use egg tissue from aborted foetuses – a technique so far only practised on laboratory mice. The main reason for promoting it appears to be a chronic shortage of human donor eggs for IVF treatment. There have been a variety of opposing arguments from doctors, church people and the general public. Perhaps the most widespread is the fear that children born from such a procedure would have to cope with the fact that their biological mother had never been born. The child who manages to trace its true parentage could possibly accuse its biological grandmother, who had the abortion in the first instance, of murdering its mother. Moreover, the woman, on the verge of an abortion, would have to bring herself to agree to the donation of tissue that is not in any full sense 'hers' in order to create biological grandchildren. Any fertility legislation that takes as its main concern the well-being of the children should be hostile to this development. It at least has the merit of having concentrated public attention on the limits of the tolerable. This has led to popular demands in several countries for strict legal limits to what might be done in the pursuit of fertility.]

NOTES

1. For a good overall summary, see in M. Vidal, J. Elizari and M. Rubio, *El don de la vida*, PS, Madrid 1987, 7-37; J. Testart, *El embrión transparente*, Juan Granica, Barcelona1988; J.M. Furnon, 'Quelle est la proportion des couples stériles?', in *Laennec* 34 (1986) nos. 3-4, 7-8; O. França, 'Reproducción humana y manipulación genética. Vocabulario básico y datos históricos éticos', in *ST* 74 (1986) 507-518; R. Snowden and G.D. Mitchell, *The Artificial Family: A Consideration of Artificial Insemination by Donor*, Unwin, London 1983; J. Edwards et al., *Technologies of Procreation: Kinship in the Age of Assisted Conception*, 1993; P. Singer and D. Wells, *The Reproduction Revolution: New Ways of Making Babies*, OUP, Oxford 1984; A. Dyson, *The Ethics of In-Vitro Fertilization*, Geoffrey Chapman, London 1994.

2. A.L. Bonnicksen, 'Embryo Freezing: Ethical Issues in the Clinical Setting', in *HCR* 18 (1988) no. 6, 26-30; Ch. Chen, 'Pregnancy after Human Oocyte Cryopreservation', in *Lancet*, April 19 (1986) 884-886.

3. M.S. Frankel, 'Human-Semen Banking: Social and Public Policy Issues', in *ManM* 1 (1975-1976) 288-309.

4. J.K. Mason and R.A. McCall-Smith, *Law and Medical Ethics* (1991) Chapter 4, 'The Control of Fertility'; Episcopal Commission for the Doctrine of Faith, 'Note about the proposals for legislation on "Techniques for assisted reproduction", and "Use of embryos and human fetuses or cells, tissues or organs"', in *Ecclesia* 2365 (2-4-1988) 31-34; C. Labrusse-Riou, 'L'homme à vif: droit et biotechnologie', in *Esprit* 156 (1989) 60-70; L.R. Walters, 'Ethics and Reproductive Technologies: An International Review of Committee Statements', in *HCR* 17 (1987) no. 3, Sp. Supp., 3-9 .

5. M. Vidal, J. Elizari and M. Rubio, *El don de la vida*, PS, Madrid 1987; I. Inglesias, '*In Vitro* Fertilization: The Major Issues', *JME* 10 (1984) 32; G.R. Dunstan, 'The Moral Status of the Human Embryo', *JME* 10 (1984) 38.

6. M. Vidal, J. Elizari and M. Rubio, *"El don de la vida": Comentarios teológico-morales a la instrucción de la Santa Sede*, PS, Madrid 1987 (included in this work is the Latin text of the Instruction *Donum Vitae* and other ecclesial documents); 'L'autorité doctrinale de l'Instruction *Donum Vitae*', in *DC* 86 (1989) 114-116; Vatican Congregation for the Doctrine of the Faith, *Instruction on Respect for Human Life in its Origins and on the Dignity of Procreation: Replies to Certain Questions of the Day (Donum Vitae)*, Vatican City & CTS, London 1987; J.C. Harvey, 'Speculations Regarding the History of *Donum Vitae*', in *JMPh* 14 (1989); B.V. Johnstone, 'The Instruction *Donum Vitae* and the Reception', in *SM* 26 (1988) 209-229.

7. 'Infertility and the New Reproductive Technologies', in *JMPh* 14 (1989) no. 5; L.S. Cahill, 'Moral Traditions, Ethical Language, and Reproductive Technologies', in *JMPh* 14 (1989) 497-522; O. O'Donovan, *Begotten or Made?*, OUP, Oxford 1984; J. Mahoney, *Bioethics and Belief*, Sheed & Ward, London 1984; M.A. Farley, 'Feminist Theology and Bioethics', in Earl E. Shelp (ed.), *Theology and Bioethics*, D. Reidel 1988, 163-185; J.D. McDowell, 'Ethical Implications of In Vitro Fertilization', in S.E. Lammers and A. Verhey, *On Moral Medicine*, Eerdmans, Grand Rapids 1987, 335-339; P. Ramsey, 'In Vitro Fertilization', in S.E. Lammers and A. Verhey, *On Moral Medicine*, 339-345; R.A. McCormick, 'In Vitro Fertilization',

Contemporary OB/GYN, 20 November 1982, 227-232; A. Sutton, *Infertility and Assisted Conception: What You Should Know*, The Catholic Bishops Joint Committee on Bio-ethical Issues, 1983; D. Le Cunff, 'La procréation médicale. De l'interpellation de la dogmatique chrétienne', in *Supp.* 163 (1987) 93-104; H. Doucet, 'Technologies de réproduction et Églises chrétiennes', in *EgT* 18 (1987) 79-99.

8. C. Caffarra, 'The Moral Problem of Artificial Insemination', in *LQ* 55 (1988) 37-43; Sacred Congregation for the Doctrine of Faith, *Donum Vitae*, II, 6.

9. Sacred Congregation for the Doctrine of Faith, *Donum Vitae*, II, 6.

10. *AAS* 41 (1949) 557-561; 43 (1951) 835-854; 48 (1956) 467-474; 50 (1958) 732-740.

11. Sacred Congregation for the Doctrine of Faith, *Donum Vitae*, II, 6.

12. Ibid., II, 4.

13. Ibid., II, 4b.

14. Ibid., II, 4c.

15. Ibid.

16. Catholic Bishops' Joint Committe on Bio-Ethical Issues, *In vitro fertilization: morality and socio-political implications*, no. 24-25, in *MM* 33 (1983) 443-445.

17. French Bishops' Conference on the Family, 'Life and death to order', in *Ecclesia* 2201 (15-12-1984) 11-15.

18. P. Verspieren, 'L'insémination post-mortem', in *Études* 361 (1984) 193-196; D.J. Cusine, 'Artificial Insemination with the Husband's Semen after the Husband's Death', in *JME* 3 (1977) 163-165.

19. Ibid.

20. Ibid.

21. J.-L. Brugues, 'La F.I.V.E.T.E. au risque de l'éthique chrétienne', in *RTh* 88 (1988), 36-64 and 87 (1987) 45-83; J.-M. Hennaux, 'Fécondation in vitro et avortement', in *NRT* 108 (1986) 27-46; W.E. May, 'The Simple Case of In-Vitro Fertilization and Embryo Transfer', in *LQ* 55 (1988) 29-36; J.M. Hennaux, 'Fécondations *in vitro* et hôpitaux catholiques', in *VieC* 55 (1985) no. 2, 97-110.

22. Sacred Congregation for the Doctrine of Faith, *Donum Vitae*, I, 5.

23. Ibid., II, 5.

24. D. DeMarco, *Biotechnology and the Assault on Parenthood*, Ignatius Press, San Francisco 1991, chapter 8: 'Reproductive Technologies and Social Justice'; the same author, 'Catholic Moral Teaching and TOT/GIFT', in *Reproductive Technologies, Marriage and the Church*, The Pope John XXIII Medical-Moral Research and Education Center, Baintree, Mass 1988.

25. M.S. Frankel, 'Human-Semen Banking: Social and Public Policy Issues', in *ManM* 1 (1975-1976) 289-309.

26. A.L. Bonnicksen, 'Embryo Freezing: Ethical Issues in the Clinical Setting', in *HCR* 18 (1988) no. 6, 26-30; J.R. Connery, 'Orphan Embryos', in *LQ* 51 (1984) 310-314.

27. *Donum Vitae*, I, 6.

28. *Donum Vitae*, II, 1.

29. Ibid.

30. *Donum Vitae*, II, 2.

31. Ibid.

32. Ibid.
33. French Bishops' Conference's Committee on the Family, 'Life and death to order', in *Ecclesia* 2201 (15-12-1984) 13.
34. L.M. Whiteford and M.L. Polard, *New Approach to Human Reproduction*, Part 3: 'Ethical Implications of Family Formation by Surrogancy', Westview Press, London 1989; G.J. Annas, 'Death Without Dignity for Commercial Surrogacy: the Case of Baby M', in *HCR* 18 (1988) no. 2, 21-24; G. Higuera, 'Surrogate motherhood. What is it? Social, ethical, and legal implications', in *ST* 74 (1986) 551-562; Northern Ethical Committee, 'Surrogacy', in *CMQ* 37 (1986) 21-23; R. Barnet, 'Surrogate Parenting: Social, Legal and Ethical Implications', in *LQ* 54 (1987) 28-38; D. Brahams, 'The Hasty British Ban on Commercial Surrogacy', in *HCR* 17 (1987) no. 1, 16-19; I. Davies, 'Contracts to Bear Children', in *JME* II (1985), 61-65.
35 *Donum Vitae*, II, 3.
36. European Parliament, 'Ethical and judicial problems arising from genetic manipulation', in *AS* 40 (1989) 559-564; Assembly of the Council of Europe, 'Proposal 1100 on the Use of Human Embryos and Foetuses in Scientific Research', in *MM* 39 (1989) 397-404; J. Glover, *Ethics of New Reproduction Technologies: the Glove Report to the European Commission*, North Il. UP 1989; H. Caton, 'The Ethics of Human Embryo Experimentation', in *LQ* 54 (1987) 24-42; J.C. Fletcher and J. Schulman, 'Fetal Research: the State of the Question', in *HCR* 15 (1985) no. 2, 6-12; J. Brown, 'Research on Human Embryos. A Justification', in *JME* 12 (1986) 201-205.
37. *Donum Vitae*, I, 4.
38. *Donum Vitae*, I, 6.
39. Ibid.
40. L. Isaacs, 'The Once of the Future Clone', in *HCR* 8 (1978) no. 3, 44-46; A. Studdard, 'The Lone clone', in *ManM* 3 (1978) 109-114; L. Eisenberg, 'The Outcome as Cause: Predestination and Human Cloning', in *JMPh* 1 (1976-1977) 381-331; M. Labar, 'The Pros and Cons of Human Cloning', in *Thought* 59 (1984) 391-333.
41. *Donum Vitae*, I, 6.

Chapter 5

Population and birth control

Of the many issues related to population, there are three that I wish to examine in this chapter. They are demographic policies, responsible parenthood and methods of birth control.

5.1 Demographic policies

a. Population growth[1]

For many centuries, the population of the world grew very slowly. Throughout prehistory, the increase in the population is thought to have been in the region of 2 per cent every 100 years, whereas, by the mid-1950s, this had become the annual rate of growth. At the beginning of the Christian era, there were probably around 150-300 million people in the world, and the population took another 16 centuries to double. Two centuries later, in 1850, the population had doubled yet again to 1,300 million. By 1950, it had reached 2,500 million, and only 20 years later, in 1970, the figure topped 3,500 million. According to forecasts produced by the United Nations Population Fund, the world population will be somewhere between 6,100 and 6,500 million in the year 2000. The population goes up by 150 people every minute, 220,000 every day and 80 million every year, and by the end of the 1990s the annual rate of increase will probably be close to 90 million. Although growth rates are beginning to slow down, another 3,000 million will be added to the world's population between the years 1985 and 2025. It may be that there will be no slow-down in the next 100 years, during which time the population of the world may well pass 10,000 million.

These figures on their own say a lot, but they do not tell us all we need to know if we are to understand the population problem correctly. Population growth has certain unique characteristics. In the first place, it is distributed unequally in different areas and countries as the majority of births take place in developing countries. The total population of the industrialized world went from 800 million to 1,200 million during the period 1950-1985, but in developing countries it leapt from 1,700 to 3,700 million. Another feature of the population explosion is the age pyramid. Around 40 per cent of the people in developing countries are under the age of 15, whereas in developed countries it is the elderly that are rapidly increasing in number.

Population growth cannot be discussed in isolation, either. We also need to look at the various conditions which are necessary to give these people a decent standard of living. These include the amount of space that is available to them, together with food, energy, water, mineral and environmental resources. The availability of resources is closely linked both to the model of life that is defended as worthy of human beings and to world solidarity. Given the current level of food consumption in the United States, Colin Lark has estimated that the maximum population that the world can support is 35,000 million. Industrialized countries are home to 25 per cent of the world's inhabitants, but they consume 75 per cent of the energy, 85 per cent of the wood and 72 per cent of the steel. These and other statistics pose questions which the peoples of the developed countries cannot ignore if we are to focus on the population problem globally, and not concentrate exclusively on the statistics. This deserves our fullest attention, and we will be looking at it in the following pages.

b. Population policies

As M. Strassoldo has written, 'Population or demographic policy is the sum of legislative or administrative means with which governments hope to influence population growth in the light of the political or ideological advice which is given to them.'[2]

We must distinguish between quantitative demographic policies (which centre on the world-wide volume of the population and on growth rates) and qualitative policies (which seek to alter the composition of the population or its territorial distribution).

These policies are referred to as expansionist or populationist when they seek to increase the population, and restrictive when they favour a reduction.

The demographic situation is basically defined by the relationship between the birth-rate, the mortality rate and migrations. Within the last two, there is a small amount of room for manoeuvre as far as demographic policies are concerned. That is why policies are designed mainly to influence the birth-rate, and why this limited concept is what people frequently think population policies are all about.

There are four main ways for a government to act with the support of expansionist policies:

— favouring large families (tax relief, subsidies, pensions, family allowances and the like);
— favouring motherhood (jobs held open, substantial maternity leave, social welfare and nurseries);
— favouring marriage (including lowering the minimum legal age for getting married, financial assistance for new families);
— restrictions on information and on the distribution of contraceptive devices.

Restrictive policies have the effect of reducing the facilities referred to above, and above all favour the spread of family planning.

It may be that most countries do not have clearly detailed, well defined, systematic demographic policies. Just the same, there is no question that many legislative and administrative measures do have a real impact on the size of the population. On the other hand, sexuality and reproduction are both affected by numerous factors that can have anarchic and unpredictable consequences.

c. *Moral issues*

Society and public authorities have a legitimate interest in the subject of population, and in the profound social implications of human reproduction. In principle, interventions by the State aimed at influencing fertility trends should not be rejected as long as they observe certain principles and conditions.

These policies must incorporate respect for the freedom of individuals and of peoples. This freedom incorporates the following elements:

– the freedom of people to marry, to decide on how many children they want and on the methods they wish to adopt. Let us not forget that the freedom of individuals must be responsible, and there can be no thought of absolute or unrealistic freedom. Many measures taken by public authorities do not have a direct demographic objective, but none-the-less contribute to the social environment in which couples have to decide on the number of children they want. This does not necessarily add up to an atmosphere that abuses an individual's, or the couple's, independence;

– the freedom of peoples to act according to their own values.

It follows that we have to reject any coercive measures used to impose a particular fertility model on married couples – and that includes peoples of the Third World. Such measures might include sterilization, and making acceptance of it a condition of economic aid.

By contrast, the intervention of public authorities is to be welcomed if it means there will be sufficient information available to help couples to make up their minds about children in a free and responsible manner. However, this information is not enough on its own; steps must be taken to give couples the means to enable them to put their responsible decisions into practice.

Demographic policies need to steer well clear of ideological considerations such as matters associated with race or territorial expansion. The same goes for certain half-baked objectives. These include concentrating exclusively on the birth-rate, forgetting the need for solidarity which is so closely linked to population issues (sharing belongings, giving more freedom to migrations), covering up the fact that well-being can be just as easily threatened by consumption or pollution rates as by birth-rates, and adopting blinkered nationalist attitudes which conceal the fact that the problem is worldwide.

There are no theological bases on which to construct a policy for increasing or decreasing the birth-rate. Since the beginning of Christianity, there has been no reason to support the view that an undefined demographic increase answers the will of God.

5.2 Responsible parenthood[3]

Our western culture has peacefully and rapidly assimilated the idea of responsible parenthood, and the Church has incorporated it into its express teachings. When the Second Vatican Council spoke of the transmission of human life in which parents are 'cooperators with the love of God the Creator' and 'the interpreters of that love', it placed that noble mission under the sign of 'a human and Christian sense of responsibility'.[4]

At one time, the call for responsibility in human fertility was not a social concern and did not form part of the Church's teachings. For many reasons, the very idea of introducing the concept of responsible parenthood was unthinkable. There were many reasons for this: they included a theological and social insistence on the reproductive meaning of marriage, an absence of explicit awareness on the quality of life of individuals and couples, high infant mortality, a reverential sense of respect for nature, a shortage of contraceptive devices, general ignorance about sexuality, an esoteric interpretation of divine providence, and a variety of reasons for having a lot of children.

Parents' responsibility for their children continues for several years after they are born, and it takes many forms depending on the circumstances. From now on, I propose using the phrase 'responsible parenthood' in a much more restricted way. I also want to deal with decisions regarding fertility – in other words, whether to have children or not, whether to have more children and, if so, the most appropriate time at which to do so.

What I mean is that this highly intimate and important part of human life has to produce sensible, reasonable decisions within a climate of freedom and love. God has created human beings not only as his collaborators in the work of building the world, but also as free, responsible agents. Those areas of life which fall under the heading of a human being's free action need to be characterized by a clear sense of responsibility, and there is no reason why human reproduction should not be one of them. Indeed, it is a field where there are a large number of personal and social interests involved, and so a sense of responsibility is even more vital.

Responsible parenthood means that human reproduction must not be left to instinct, hazard or fate. Nor should it be left in the hands of nature, or of a misunderstood version of providence –

something very different from a trusting, hopeful attitude towards God. On the other hand, the introduction of a sense of responsibility is a way of avoiding not only fatalistic attitudes but arbitrary ones as well. In this way, responsible parenthood becomes rational, sensible and far-sighted as far as decisions relating to human fertility are concerned, but does not replace love, confidence and other noble sentiments.

a. *What* Humanae Vitae *has to say*[5]

According to the encyclical *Humanae Vitae*, a correct understanding of responsible parenthood includes certain ideas which are not universally accepted in circles outside the Church.

It involves a knowledge of, and respect for, the functions of biological processes in which human intelligence can discover laws. It also implies the ascendancy of reason and the will over instinct and passions, and due attention being paid to physical, economical, psychological and social conditions. Careful thought about these issues can lead in one of two directions: either a large family or a restricted one. However, responsible parenthood is not the same thing as the number of children the couple may have; we are not dealing with a quantitative concept, but a qualitative one. Responsibility – or the lack of it – can characterize a childless couple, just as it can a couple with a large or small number of children.

Lastly, *Humanae Vitae* emphasizes that morality is a vitally important element, in the sense that the decision is linked to an objective moral order that has been established by God and whose interpreter is the true conscience. I now wish to deal with certain details of responsible parenthood.

b. *The couple's decision*

Intentions concerning the reproduction of human life are a matter for the couple themselves. The decision is their right alone, and no one can take it away from them. What is more, it is a duty that they themselves have to perform; they cannot hand it over to someone else.

Ideally, the decision should be a joint one that is shared by the two partners; there should be as much agreement as possible and they should avoid imposing their own ideas on one another. Even when there is good exchange of ideas and a high degree of respect between the two people, complete agreement is not always possible, and here, as elsewhere, giving and taking is an essential part of the relationship.

This emphasis on the irreplaceable role of the couple does not mean to say that they have to make their decisions on their own. They are entitled to confide in those around them, and ask others for help so that the options can be examined with the maximum freedom and responsibility. It is society's job to try and guarantee these conditions through the availability of various services and personal skills.

Society will fulfil its function in providing the couple with support if it gives them the kind of information which can be the basis for them to reach a responsible decision. This will only be enough if the means and conditions are also made available to enable the couple both to decide freely and to carry out the decisions that they have taken freely and responsibly.

Interventions outside the couple's control, such as political groupings, multinational companies and health authorities, sometimes attempt to impose behaviour that does not respect individual wishes or a people's cultural values. These might include making contraception a condition for economic aid, or a job offer conditional on being sterilized. Such conduct is contrary to the dignity of individuals and of peoples. The Church has frequently denounced actual and potential instances of this 'contraceptive colonialism'.[6]

c. Reasonable decision

If the decision to have children or not – and even the moment when to have children – is to be clearly responsible, it has to be reasonable and based on sound reasoning. Many normal couples take these decisions quite spontaneously, without the need for complicated calculations and prolonged, careful thought.

The Second Vatican Council describes the criteria for a

responsible decision relating to a couple's wish to have children
thus:

> They will thoughtfully take into account both their own wel-
> fare and that of their children, those already born and those
> which may be foreseen. For this accounting they will reckon
> with both the material and the spiritual conditions of the times
> as well as of their state of life. Finally, they will consult the
> interests of the family group, of temporal society, and of the
> Church itself.[7]

We need to consider certain conditions that affect the couple.
They include the couple's health (both physical and psychological, and particularly the woman's), whether they are a stable
couple or whether there is a danger of them separating, and
whether the arrival of a new child will be accepted positively or
negatively by the children already born, and even by the parents
themselves. Consideration also has to be given to the kind of
future which the new child might reasonably expect. Obviously,
the most immediate elements within the framework of the family
are easier to assess than those related to the social conditions, as it
is more difficult to predict the way that social matters will develop. That is why a reasonable decision has nothing to do with a
neat, four-square formula with all points clearly defined. The
need for responsibility to be uppermost needs to be accompanied
by a sense of hope; there must also be a capacity to accept
surprises and the unexpected, and the couple must not alow themselves to be intimidated by the child – a feeling that appears to be
widespread in our society.

d. The decision to limit fertility

One way or another, married couples normally develop a
'policy' about limiting the number of children they are going to
have. In our society, this practice is now so widespread that it is
giving rise to political, economic and social anxieties. There is a
whole series of factors that are well established in our social
mentality which are contributing to this fertility crisis. Couples
living in a particular time and in a specific geographic environ-

ment are unconsciously incorporating these elements of our society into their own mentalities. A knowledge of the broad social
framework in which personal fertility options exist will help them
to reach decisions about having children with more foresight and
freedom.

The dramatic fall in child mortality and the results of improved hygiene, food and medicine, are decisive factors in the
declining birth-rate. There do not have to be so many births to
make up for the premature deaths of young children. An improvement in the standard of living has also raised people's aspirations,
sometimes beyond their economic means. A child can often appear to be a factor limiting the parents' will to maintain or raise
their standard of living and consumption. People in our society
are very aware of freedoms and of making their way in the world,
and a child can mean that independence is reduced and certain
associated pleasures are curtailed. Having a child also involves
giving up a way of life for a while, and free time in particular.
Additionally, for the woman there can be consequences for her
career as well as psychological and economic problems, despite
the improvements made through legislation.

Many married couples experience a vague anxiety about the
future, not only for themselves but also for their children. Having
a child is like taking a risky wager, and means assuming responsibility for leading him or her to adulthood, and to a better life if
possible. For the time being, the future looks uncertain, particularly with high youth unemployment.

In our society, with its high levels of consumption, spiritual
and other unselfish activities and important ideals are somewhat
in eclipse. People do not appear to believe that there is any sense
in sacrificing oneself for major causes. Sociological studies underline deep-rooted manifestations of egoism and of an absence
of solidarity, although there are occasionally examples of the
opposite. Generally speaking, we do not see in people any great
capacity for altering their ways of living by adopting a more
jointly-shared approach to life, and giving priority to realities
rather than to appearances.

There are many other factors that impact on a social mentality
that is clearly allergic to large families. These include the idea
that some countries are over-populated, ecological preoccupations, the threat of total destruction in a nuclear holocaust, new

ways of looking at sexuality which put more emphasis on quality of life and on relationships, feminism, and the decline of religious values. Some of these factors are orchestrated by the media, and in this way the collective subconscious in favour of reducing the birth-rate is strengthened.

All in all, no single factor supplies a complete, clear explanation. Decisions on fertility remain somewhat obscure both at a macrosocial level and at the level of each individual couple.

5.3 Methods of birth control: non-moral aspects[8]

In this section, I will be referring to scientific methods, not popular methods. There are several methods of classification. The distinction between natural and unnatural methods is very important for the Church from a moral standpoint, but not from all standpoints. I will here adopt the criterion of the moment at which the methods intervene in the process of human reproduction; I acknowledge, though, that some of these methods can operate at different moments, even though there is one moment that is all-important and critical. In order to give a complete picture, I will not confine myself to contraceptive methods; I will also deal with processes that interrupt gestation.

a. Methods that inhibit germ cells

These are methods that impede ovulation or spermatogenesis. As far as the latter is concerned, the prospects of discovering effective methods still seem a long way off. Despite intensive efforts, there is still no agent to control male fertility that has been subjected to extensive clinical tests. The only exception is gossypol and its derivatives, but its toxicity is such that it cannot be used as a contraceptive. Research is concentrating on preventing spermatogenesis, that is to say reducing the number of spermatozoa or affecting their motility.

As for pills that inhibit ovulation, the most common is a pill taken orally every day; this is followed by other ongoing treatments including subcutaneous injections and implants. There are numerous studies on the connection between oral contraceptives and the development of neoplasms in women, apart from changes in their metabolism. We must be careful not to extrapolate conclusions from some of these studies to other situations. For instance, there are studies on pills of a particular chemical composition which cannot be applied to other pills whose risk factors have declined. At the same time, though, there are other risk factors that can be analysed; these include age and the woman's general health and habits.

b. Methods of sperm transport

This group has the largest number of methods in existence. They are:

- coitus interruptus;
- barrier methods (condoms, diaphragms);
- spermicides normally used in conjunction with a condom, rather than being used on their own;
- sterilization (by cutting the fallopian tubes in the case of a woman, and by means of a vasectomy in the case of a man);
- the period (abstaining from having sex on those days when the woman is fertile). Infertile days can be worked out in a number of ways, including counting up days in a diary and calculating the duration of some of the woman's cycles. Some people prefer to rely on a variety of physiological changes that take place during the cycle, like body temperature and the presence or absence of cervical mucus.

c. Methods that prevent conception

- Taking a pill the following day;
- IUDs (intrauterine devices).

d. Methods that interrupt gestation

This is where we start looking at various types of abortion.

e. Miscellaneous information

Regarding the spread of contraceptive methods, figures vary enormously from one country to another. Trends in the developed world, after allowing for differences between individual countries, may be estimated on the basis of a recent study carried out in the United States.[9] Sterilization appears top of the list with 13,800,000 cases (8,100,000 women and 5,700,000 men), followed closely by oral contraception (13,200,000), and then condoms (6,900,000), spermicides (2,300,000), coitus interruptus (2,300,000), the diaphragm (1,700,000), the safe period (1,700,000) and IUDs (1,100,000). Although figures for male sterilization are still low, the incidence in western countries is rising rapidly.

Effectiveness. There are many reasons why it is not easy to determine the exact effectiveness of a given contraceptive method. For instance, a distinction is sometimes drawn between the effectiveness and failure of the method and between the effectiveness and failure of its use; the former distinction refers to whether the method is used correctly, while the latter distinction deals with the use of the method irrespective of whether it is correct or not.

Of the many factors influencing the effectiveness of contraceptive methods, the most important is frequently motivation. Natural methods are most influenced by motivation as far as their effectiveness is concerned, and the result is that only highly motivated couples can expect success to any degree. More or less the same can be said of coitus interruptus, and other methods related to coitus like the use of a condom. Other factors affecting effectiveness include age (barrier methods tend to be more effective for those over 30, and less effective for those under 25), socio-economic position and level of education.

Forecasts. Great efforts have been made since 1970 to find new ways of regulating the birth-rate. None-the-less, it is unlikely that any new important technique will emerge in the next decade, although there may be small gains as far as effectiveness and safety are concerned. It is also difficult to foresee any major advances in the control of male infertility in the medium term.

Criteria for a reasonable choice of method. I will leave the moral problem of methods until the next section. In the meantime, let me list a number of points that need to be considered if a couple wishing to control their fertility are to make a reasonable and sensible choice. No one method has only advantages or only disadvantages and, after all the pros and cons have been weighed up, the right choice will fall on the method that is the best or the least bad for a given couple at a particular moment in time. The points that must be born in mind when choosing are as follows:

- the age of the partners;
- their health;
- the importance of the couple's relationship;
- how easy or difficult it is to use the method;
- the need for training in how to use it correctly;
- the need for health departments to carry out control, administration and follow-up procedures;
- socio-cultural acceptance or resistance;
- moral acceptance or resistance;
- aesthetic acceptance or resistance;
- capacity for motivation on the part of the users;
- ease or difficulty of access to the method;
- reversibility or otherwise;
- cost;
- whether the method is natural or artificial;
- the pleasure angle;
- spontaneity of the sex act etc.

In the majority of cases, a reasonable choice is not complicated as long as the couple are quite clear about what they want in terms of fertility, have the relevant information, are sensitive to one another's needs and wishes, and have access to the right advice.

5.4 The morality of methods of birth control

a. Before Humanae Vitae[10]

The Church has been faithful to the doctrine of reproduction as the primary aim of marriage, and for many centuries has condemned actions that sought to deprive the conjugal act of its possible connection with the conception of children. This matter has come under particularly scrutiny since the nineteenth century. At that time, there was a plethora of reports on various issues sent to the Holy See, particularly from the French clergy, and various departments of the Holy See occasionally sent back replies. Most of the reports concentrated on coitus interruptus, which was normally called onanism. There were also references to sheaths and sexual abstinence when the woman was fertile.

As for onanism, there are two points which consistently appear in the Holy See's replies. They are the legitimacy or otherwise of the woman's co-operation, and the attitude of the confessor as to whether or not to ask about this behaviour. As far as the first question is concerned, cooperation is considered legitimate if the woman does not take the initiative; otherwise, the consequences for her could be serious. It is not clear whether the woman's request can be considered legitimate when there is good reason to believe that it is the husband who wants to practise coitus interruptus. On the subject of whether the confessor is obliged or not to inquire into these matters, no rigid standards are laid down. It is likely to depend on the confessor's view of the penitent's likely lifestyle.

The woman's co-operation in intercourse using a condom is held to be immoral.

Another question that arose concerned infertile periods and whether sexual relations may take place during this time. They were generally held to be acceptable. Some people cautiously speculate that this practice could be an alternative to onanism;[11] others say that it is permissible irrespective of the danger of onanism. There are also plenty of people who reject it out of hand on the grounds that it is contrary to the prime aim of marriage.[12] The argument that raged between moralists on this subject was resolved after a number of interventions by Pius XII. He laid down certain demands in the course of an address he gave in 1951. He said that there is no moral problem if the married couple *also* make use of infertile periods; on the other hand, for a couple to make use *only* of infertile periods could mean a breach of the Church's moral teaching under two headings depending on the circumstances. If such behaviour involves limiting or denying the other person's right to have children, it is not legitimate; if the intention is less radical, its legitimacy will depend on the reasons for avoiding having children in the first place.[13]

A new chapter in the history of this problem opened with the appearance of the 'pill' in the 1950s. It was immediately clear that this method had a positive side compared with onanism and the use of condoms, in that it did not interfere with the integrity and union of the conjugal act. Other commentators gave their approval to pills that inhibit ovulation as they believed that sterilization was thus achieved by a single act, and for acceptable reasons; by contrast, sterilization of the reproductive activity was seen as unacceptable.

In 1958, Pius XII condemned all types of direct sterilization and, in so doing, echoed a theme that was being hotly debated at the time between doctors and moralists. It was suggested that the pill could be used legitimately 'as a remedy to the exaggerated reactions of the uterus and body, even though such medication impeded ovulation and therefore made fertilization impossible'. If taking the pill turns into a form of 'necessary therapy', it is legitimate by virtue of the principle of double effect by causing only indirect sterilization. If the objective is to avoid conception by preventing ovulation, the practice is illegitimate.

Many moralists, some of them not noted for their innovative approach, introduced quite permissive ideas on the use of the pill, and based them on its therapeutic use as described by Pius XII.[14] They considered the use of the pill to be legitimate in certain circumstances; these included the correction of irregular cycles, while breast-feeding, when the woman is suffering from a neurotic fear of pregnancy, preventing the period from coinciding with stressful matters such as journeys, examinations and sporting activities, and as a defence against sexual attack.

Pope John XXIII set up a Commission for the Study of Problems of Population, Family and Birth; its remit included the question of whether birth control methods were moral. The Commission was broadened by Paul VI, and it was his personal decision during the Second Vatican Council to withdraw discussion on this subject from the Council's debates and hand it over to the Commission. The division that existed in the Commission was reflected in the large number of secret documents and reports that were sent to the Pope.

b. The Pope's teaching (Paul VI and John Paul II)

A decisive moment in this debate was the publication on 25 July 1968 by Pope Paul VI of the encyclical *Humanae Vitae*.[15] It gave decisive moral weight to the distinction between natural and unnatural methods. Many excellent things that were contained in *Humanae Vitae* have been eclipsed by the ruling on the morality of methods, and this itself gave further moral weight to this differentiation between natural and unnatural methods.

In view of the interest shown by Paul VI, and subsequently by John Paul II, in moving towards a clear position on this doctrinal issue, it is fascinating to analyse the basis of this doctrine. *Humanae Vitae* gave support for the doctrine under three headings: these were the earlier doctrine of the Church's teaching, demands made by nature and the aims of the conjugal act, and the likely outcome if unnatural methods were to be accepted.

The first argument is there for the benefit of Catholics; the other two are, in principle, aimed at circles outside the Catholic Church. The encyclical's efforts to generate a clear moral stance and a convinced moral position did not produce the results that had been hoped for. For that reason, it is not surprising that Pope John Paul II, already worried about extending the convinced acceptance of his predecessor's doctrine, took a particular interest in presenting the basis of this teaching with the help of new arguments. John Paul II has repeatedly referred to them. To my mind, the most important of them are the exhortation on the family,[16] a talk on 17 September 1983,[17] and the address to the Second International Congress on Moral Theology.[18]

The Pope puts forward two arguments, which he describes as theological and anthropological, in support of the Church's doctrine. At the origin of all human beings stands God's creative and loving inspiration, with which the man and woman are called to be his collaborators. It is from this assumption that the objectively atheist concept of contraception may be inferred: 'When, by means of contraception, the couple take away the potential for creation from the exercise of the marriage act, they attribute to themselves a task which belongs to God alone. That is the power to decide, in the final analysis, whether a human person comes into existence.' To defend the objective legitimacy of contraception 'is the same as defending the notion that situations can develop in human life in which it is legitimate not to recognise God as God.'[19]

In his Apostolic Exhortation on the family, the Pope developed an anthropological argument that sought to demonstrate the objective immorality of contraception. He said,

When couples, by means of recourse to contraception, separate these two meanings that God the Creator has inscribed in the being of man and woman and in the dynamism of their sexual communion, they act as 'arbiters' of the divine plan and 'manipulate' and degrade human sexuality – and with it themselves and their married partner – by altering its value of 'total' self-giving.[20]

In his address to the Second International Congress on Moral Theology, the Pope spoke of the advances in biblical anthropological thinking which have thrown light on the assumptions and meaning of the Church's teaching. Starting off from the premise that all Christian truth has a unitary and harmonious character, he concluded that questioning the moral norm of *Humanae Vitae* affected other fundamental truths of reason and faith. Such doubts offered a new concept of the conscience as the creator of the norm, thereby breaking the link of obedience to God. They are opposed to the Catholic doctrine on teaching, they question the very idea of the sanctity of God, and deprive Christ's cross and the mystery of humanity of all content.[21] It was this argument that gave rise to the so-called 'Cologne Declaration'.

In addition to this new light thrown on the subject by the Popes, there have been other attempts to strengthen the credibility and force of *Humanae Vitae*.[22] These have laid emphasis on the encyclical's lucid prediction of the negative consequences of contraception on a personal level, and the contraceptive colonialism inflicted on peoples of the Third World. It has been claimed that the doctrine of the encyclical, as distinct from the document itself, is infallible and should be believed compulsorily and unconditionally by all Catholics.[23]

c. The conscience as a guide to behaviour (Episcopal teaching)

The Catholic moral tradition has considered that the conscience contains the proximate norm of morality. This traditional and rather general teaching was recalled by the Congregation for the Clergy in relation to the subject under discussion here, and in the context of the so-called 'Washington case'. I would like to quote the following:

1. Conscience is the practical judgment or dictate of reason by which one judges what here and now is to be done as being good, or to be avoided as evil.

2. In the light of the above, the role of conscience is that of a practical dictate, not a teacher of doctrine.

3. Conscience is not a law unto itself and in forming one's conscience one must be guided by objective moral norms, including authentic Church teaching (cf *Gaudium et Spes*, 50).

4. Particular circumstances surrounding an objectively evil human act, while they cannot make it objectively virtuous, can make it inculpable, diminished in guilt or subjectively defensible (...).

5. In the final analysis, conscience is inviolable and no man is to be forced to act in a manner contrary to his conscience, as the moral tradition of the Church attests.[24]

Following *Humanae Vitae*, a number of meetings of bishops recalled the validity of precisely this traditional doctrine within the problem of the morality of birth control methods and the true teaching of the Church.[25] Of the many documents produced on the subject, I will quote only from the collective statement of the Scandinavian bishops:

When a person, for serious, well-considered reasons, is not convinced by the arguments of the Encyclical, s/he has the right to adopt a different opinion from that presented in a non-infallible document. May nobody, then, be considered a bad Catholic for such dissent! Anyone who, after examining his/her conscience, believes s/he has the right not to accept a teaching and not to carry it out must answer to God for his/her attitude and actions.[26]

It should not be forgotten that these bishops accept the doctrine of *Humanae Vitae*. By the same token, it must not be assumed that they have a low opinion of it, or even reject it; in accordance with the most traditional morality and in line with the Second Vatican Council, they recognize the rights of the conscience on a subjective plane and the dignity of an invincibly wrong conscience.[27]

That is not to say that any moral conscience possesses a moral quality in itself. It has to fulfil the requirements of an honest conscience. The bishops insist on a number of conditions:

– a healthy attitude towards the Church's magisterium. This implies a believing and grateful recognition of this service desired by Christ, and a spirit of receptivity. An attitude of fear, distrust and rejection conceals prejudices that are not compatible with a sincere conscience;

– love of the truth, which may be translated as taking all proportionate means to find it;

– sensitivity to the repercussions of one's attitude and conduct within the Church, since the conscience of a Christian is a conscience of the Church;

– an attitude of openness and inquiry together with a spirit of humility, and not retreating into fanatical attitudes.

Let us now look at some of the areas in which a conscience can legitimately reach subjectively honest convictions. The areas which I want to examine are all taken from documents produced by the Church's hierarchy.

Conflict of duties. Traditional Christian morality supports the so-called principle of the lesser evil in conflicts of duties or values. When a person finds s/he has to choose between various duties or values, and it will be impossible to fulfil them at the same time, his/her behaviour is morally good if s/he carries out the duty or duties which s/he deems most important, and leaves those which s/he considers to be lower down in the moral hierarchy.

Christian married couples can find themselves in situations of conflict when choosing how not to have a child. On the one hand, they must avoid having a child, because they have decided responsibly not to have one. On the other hand, they consider it a duty to obey the norm that respects the conjugal act as a way of giving life. Moreover, they believe they have a duty to watch over one another through their communion, through the stability of their marriage, and through their harmony and well-being. To quote from the proceedings of the French bishops,

In this context, let us simply remember the constant teaching on morality: when one is faced with a choice of duties and if, whichever decision is taken, it is not going to be possible to avoid evil, traditional wisdom teaches that we must choose before God which of the conflicting duties is the greater. Married couples will make their decision at the end of a period of joint reflection which they have undergone with all the assiduousness that is required by the greatness of their married vocation.[28]

Artificial methods as therapeutic remedies. This doctrine, first expounded by Pius XII, was picked up in *Humanae Vitae* and has been repeated by many meetings of bishops.[29] Apart from a small indication from the Austrian bishops, it has not been developed in any way.

Humanae Vitae comments as follows: 'But the Church in no way regards as unlawful therapeutic means considered necessary to cure organic diseases, even though they also have a contraceptive effect, and this is foreseen – provided that this contraceptive effect is not directly intended for any motive whatsoever.'[30]

If artificial methods are to be used legitimately, the encyclical states that certain conditions must be fulfilled. They are:

– that the objective of the method used must be therapeutic;
– that it is essential to use this method in order to achieve the therapeutic objective;
– that there must be no direct intention to prevent procreation.

Humanae Vitae confines itself to establishing a framework in which recourse to artificial methods may be legitimate.[31] It does not enumerate the cases in which the conditions must be checked. The various bishops' meetings have not yet shed much light on this issue, but there is a wide range of trends and interpretations to be found among moralists.

5.5 Sterilization

Sterilization is a contraceptive practice which is becoming increasingly widespread in our society; in the developed world, it is also becoming more and more acceptable inside marriage. In the not-too-distant past, this type of intervention was confined almost exclusively to women, but today the idea of male sterilization encounters much less resistance than it used to. In the Third

World and among less favoured groups, it is not infrequently a procedure that is imposed on the people dishonestly and through coercion.[32]

Sterilization has many applications, and has a large number of different objectives. For example, it is used as a curative therapy, and as a means of preventing certain illnesses or disorders by removing ovaries, the uterus and testicles; it can also be used with the eugenic aim of trying to avoid the possible reproduction of babies thought to be handicapped.

a. Introduction

In moral theology, sterilization comes under the heading of mutilation, and is usually punishable by the Fifth Commandment. This is undoubtedly due in part to the practice of castration which has survived since ancient times. The mutilation aspect is much less visible in vasectomy and in the cutting of the fallopian tubes; it has none-the-less remained an important item for moral consideration, despite the fact that such language is unknown in the medical world. At present, given that the contraceptive side of sterilization is dominant, it is correct to say that it is viewed as a method of birth control.

b. Moral considerations[33]

The Catholic Church has produced a large number of documents on the subject of sterilization.[34] These texts establish the general norm that direct sterilization is not legitimate, and this norm is applied to a variety of situations, particularly when sterilization has a directly contraceptive objective. On the basis of these documents and of more concrete statements issued by Catholic moralists, the Church's moral doctrine might be summed up as follows:

   – voluntary sterilization of a man or woman for the purpose of temporarily or permanently preventing conception is immoral;
   – voluntary eugenic sterilization is similarly unacceptable;
   – voluntary sterilization that is directly therapeutic and indirectly contraceptive is morally acceptable;

– sterilization directly imposed by the State or by other organizations or persons is unjustifiable as it runs counter to the dignity of the person, and cannot be legitimated by claims that it is for the common good.

As for penal sterilization, it does not appear to be excluded by any of the Church's teaching. Major theologians of the past have said it was legitimate, although according to a number of humane and Christian positions, it is usually looked upon as a degrading practice these days.

What I have written above about the morality of contraceptive methods applies equally to sterilization.[35] I should only add that there are certain characteristics of sterilization that need to be borne in mind. These are irreversibility, which is normal, and the possibility of psychological repercussions on the individual and on the relationship between the couple.

c. Sterilization of mentally handicapped people

Previous sections of this book have concentrated essentially on adults and on people capable of making conscious decisions. Now we tackle the problem of people who are mentally handicapped. The whole question of sterilizing mentally handicapped people arouses lively debate throughout our society. The people most directly affected are those who are mentally handicapped themselves, their families, and those responsible for bringing them up and looking after them in special schools and homes. Moreover, those who live particularly close to this problem are precisely those who are most sensitive to the rights of individuals marginalized by society. Legislators are very keen to safeguard the interests of the mentally handicapped, and society eagerly goes along with this, partly because of the abuses that the Nazis perpetrated on such people. There are many factors that cause the issue of sterilization of mentally handicapped people to be charged with high emotion, and this stands in the way of calm examination and social consensus.

The legal dimension. Many countries have regulated interventions[36] of this type by law, and there have been instances in which courts have actually handed down sentences.[37] Legislation in western countries is similar to laws that have been passed in Spain since 1989.

[*Editor's note*: The author cites an article of the Spanish Penal Code that allows the sterilization of mentally handicapped persons so long as certain conditions are fulfilled. In England there is no specific legislation and decisions involving mentally handicapped women continue to be made on a case by case basis, often with the intervention of the High Court and much publicity. Some urge a fundamental right to bear a child, while others argue from the 'best interests' of the woman and her right to the kind of treatment that competent persons could expect to receive in similar circumstances.[38]]

The moral aspect.[39] The sterilization of a mentally handicapped person is a very delicate matter. We need to approach the matter with love for the handicapped individuals themselves, and with a deep sensitivity for their rights, but this does not mean ignoring either the anxieties of parents and teachers or the legitimate interests of society.

The Church's official doctrine, as we have already seen, is opposed to all contraceptive methods including sterilization, and does not find the practice acceptable even in these circumstances. The teaching referred to above on the subjective legitimacy of contraceptive methods in certain circumstances[40] is still valid, but it still depends on the particular characteristics of the case in question.[41]

NOTES

1. Data from the UN on Population, in *MM* 38 (1988) 922-957; VV.AA., 'Population Ethics', in *EB* III, 1215-1316.
2. M. Strassoldo, 'Population', in VV.AA,. *Diccionario de sociologia*, Paulinas, Madrid 1986, 1307.
3. A.J. Maida, 'Responsible Parenthood in the Writings of Pope Paul VI, and John Paul II', in *LQ* 55 (1988) no. 4, 25-31.
4. *Gaudium et Spes*, 50.
5. *Humanae Vitae*, 10.
6. *Humanae Vitae*, 17.
7. *Gaudium et Spes*, 50.
8. D.R. Mishell, 'Contraception', in *NEJM* 320 (1989) 777-787.

9. J.D. Forrest and R.R. Fordyce, 'U.S. Women's Contraceptive Attitudes and Practice: How Have They Changed in the 1980's?', in *Family Planning Perspectives* 20 (1988) 112-118.
10. J.T. Noonan, *Contraception: A History of its Treatment by the Catholic Theologians and Canonists*, Harvard UP, Cambridge Mass. 1986.
11. Cf M. Zalba, 'Continentia periodica iam ab anno 1853 in Ecclesia probata fuerat', in *PRMCL* 70 (1981) 522-553.
12. *AAS* 43 (1951) 835-854.
13. *AAS* 50 (1958) 734-736.
14. In this respect see A. Valsecchi, *Regulación de los nacimientos. Diez años de reflexión teológica*, Sigueme, Salamanca 1968.
15. For a bibliography of the past ten years see G. Besutti, 'Contributo bibliografico sulla *Humanae Vitae'*, in *Lateranum* 44 (1978) 276-364. Writings on the moral perspectives of the issue declined; there was a resurgence in 1988 for the 20th anniversary of the *Humanae Vitae*, maintaining the extremely repetitive and scarcely original tone.
16. *Familiaris Consortio*, CTS, London 1982.
17. *Ecclesia* 2144 (1983) 8-9.
18. *Ecclesia* 2405-2406 (1989) 26-28.
19. *Ecclesia* 2144 (1983) 8.
20. *Familiaris Consortio* 32.
21. The text of the discourse may be found in *Ecclesia* 2405-2406 (1989) 26-28.
22. Cf F.J. Elizari, 'A los diez años de *Humanae Vitae'*, in *Moralia* 1 (1979) 235-253; M. Rhonheimer, 'Sexual Behaviour, and Natural Law. Philosophical Foundation of the Norm of *Humanae Vitae'*, in *LQ* 56 (1989) no. 2, 20-57; R. McEnerny, *'Humanae Vitae* and the Principle of Totality', in *LQ* 56 (1989) no. 2, 58-67; W.E. May, *'Humanae Vitae* Natural Law and Catholic Moral Thought', in *LQ* 56 (1989) no. 2, 61-87; C. Burke, 'The indivisibility of the bonding and procreative aspects of the conjugal act', in *STh* 21 (1989) 197-209; P. Coffey, *'Humane Vitae* and Contraception: A Forgotten Argument', in *LQ* 55 (1988) 27-30.
23. G.L. Hallett, 'Infallibility and Contraception: The Debate Continues', in *TS* 49 (1988) 517-528; G.L. Hallett, 'Contraception and Prescriptive Infallibility', in *TS* 43 (1982) 629-650; R.M. Schmitz, 'Contraception et infailibilité', in *Divinitas* 25 (1981) 320-323.
24. For information about this case and for the text of the Sacred Congregation's ruling see M. Vidal, 'Documents on the "Washington case" and the problem of *Humanae Vitae'*, in *Pentecosté* 11 (1973) 43-50.
25. Cf M. Zalba, *Las Conferencias episcopales ante la Humanae Vitae*, Cio, Madrid 1971; L. Sandri, *Humanae Vitae e magistero episcopale*, Dehoniane, Bologna 1969. The Statement of 33 hierarchies are printed in J. Horgan (ed.), *Humanae Vitae and the Bishops*, Irish University Press, Shannon 1972, including those of England and Wales (September 1968), Ireland (October 1968 and February 1969) and the United States (August and November 1968).
26. 'Lettre pastorale des évêques nordiques sur l'encyclique *Humanae Vitae'*, in *DC* 65 (1968) 2070. The complete text is in the columns 2067-2072.
27. *Gaudium et Spes*, 16.
28. *Document of the French Bishops' Conference*, no. 16, 2060.

29. 'Déclaration des évêques suisse sur l'encyclique *Humanae Vitae*', in *DC* 66 (1969) 18-21; 'Declaración del episcopado español sobre la encíclica *Humanae Vitae*', in *Ecclesia* 1418 (1968) 15-17.
30. *Humanae Vitae*, 15.
31. Ibid.
32. D. Callahan, 'Food Incentives for Sterilization; Can They be Just?', in *HCR* 3 (1973) no. 1, 10-12; 'American Indian Women Sterilized without Consent', in *HCR* 7 (1977) 420-422; D. Christiansen, 'Human Rights in India. Ethics and Compulsory Population Control', in *HCR* 7 (1977) no. 1, 30-33. Repeated denunciations in the Bishops' Synod were made about abuses in this area in 1980.
33. R.A. McCormick, 'Notes on Moral Theology: 1983', in *TS* 45 (1984) 110-115; F.J. Elizari, 'La esterilización', in *Pentecostés* 16 (1978) 233-249; E.F. Diamond, 'Sterilization in Catholic Hospitals', in *LQ* 55 (1988) 57-66.
34. For a list of the documents of the Holy See on the subject see, F.J. Elizari, *a.c.*, note 22. Here I would like to highlight the most comprehensive ones: Sacred Congregation for the Doctrine of Faith, 'Sterilization in Catholic Hospitals', in *Ecclesia* 1821 (1977) 7; a recent declaration of the Mexican Bishops' Conference, 'Documento sobre la esterilización', in *MM* 31 (1989) 771-780. For the text of declarations by the other Churches see F.J. Elizari, *op.cit.*
35. Cf pp. 104-111.
36. Law Reform Commission of Canada, 'Sterilizing the Mentally-Handicapped: Who Can Give Consent?', in *CMAJ* 122 (1980) 234-239; K.G. Evans, 'Sterilization of the Mentally Retarded. A Review', in *CMAJ* 123 (1980) 1066-1070; M. Bayles, 'Sterilization of the Retarded. The Legal Precedents', in *HCR* 8 (1978) no. 3, 37-41; 'Sterilization Rulings in the U.K.', *HCR* 17 (1987) no. 4, 48.
37. G.J. Annas, 'Sterilization of the Mentally Retarded: A Decision for the Courts', in *HCR* 11 (1981) no. 4, 18-19.
38. 'Sterilization of Mentally Retarded Minors' (editorial), in *BMJ* 281 (1980) 1025-1026. For a thorough discussion of the law in England see J.K. Mason and R.A. McCall-Smith, *Law and Medical Ethics*, 1991, 85-89.
39. 'Joint Ethico-Medical Committee', in *CMQ* 40 (1989) 143-144; R. Gillon, 'Sterilising Severely Mentally Handicapped People', in *JME* 13 (1987) 59-61; G.J. Annas, 'Sterilization of the Mentally Retarded', in *HCR* 11 (1981) no. 4, 18-19; A.J. Dyck, 'Mental Retardation as a Label: A Problem of Justice', in *LQ* 45 (1978) 111-115; R. Neville, 'Sterilization of the Retarded: The Philosophical Arguments', in *HCR* 8 (1978) no. 3, 33-37.
40. Cf pp. 108-111.
41. T. Thompson, 'Sterilization of the Retarded. The Behavioral Perspective', in *HCR* 8 (1978) no. 3, 29-32.

Chapter 6

Genetic counselling[1]

6.1 The scientific and human dimension

The phrase 'genetic counselling' means many things to many people. In practice, there are two main camps in genetic counselling, and the boundaries between them were drawn in the days when this type of counselling was first being developed. Put simply, there are those who give counselling before conception, and those who do it afterwards. In the former case, genetic counselling is done on the basis of selection and assessment of the parents-to-be; the purpose is to detect any genetic illness, and thereby predict how likely it is that they could conceive a child who was affected by it. The second type has been well described as 'antenatal diagnosis', and is carried out by means of an intra-uterine examination following conception, and includes a number of tests including ultrasound, amniocentesis and foetoscopy aimed at determining the state of the foetus.[2] A distinction can be drawn between these two types of diagnosis in terms of both the individuals who are diagnosed (potential parents, the embryo/foetus) and the objective of the diagnosis (decisions concerning reproduction and the couple or relating to the embryo/foetus). As antenatal tests are dealt with elsewhere, this section will look only at the first form of diagnosis.

The circumstances which precede genetic counselling are many and varied. These might include the birth of a child with a deformity of some kind, the existence of relatives who have hereditary diseases or of children affected by some abnormality of this sort, a history of spontaneous abortions possibly due to some genetic defect, a combination of infertility and a wish to have children, and the fact that caution has been advised for reasons of consanguinity, advanced age in the woman, or genetic disorders in the couple or their families.

If we are to make a serious study of the phenomenon, we will need to leave the issues which have to be examined for a moment. Let us briefly take a closer look at the psychological and social reactions that occur if one of the partners has serious genetic defects or already has children affected by them. Such abnormalities affect fundamental areas of the personality such as sexuality, fertility and family bonds; reactions vary according to the nature and seriousness of the genetic abnormality, family expectations and the sort of people the couple are.

If certain facts are established before marriage, this can affect the wish to get married in the first place and the choice of partner. The emotional reactions and style of behaviour that the diagnosis can bring about are varied. They include a sense of being punished, shame, confused guilt, anxiety, a sense of impotence leading to a fatalistic view of life, aggressiveness, religious rebellion, a deteriorating self-image, a deteriorating image of the partner, self-marginalization, confusion about whether one is the bringer of the illness or the sufferer, divorce, and an impulsive desire for sterilization. The likelihood of such conflicts means it is worth making a special effort to get to know the couple better; such circumstances call for humane support systems rather than reliance on medical examinations.

6.2 The moral context

If the medical examination reveals serious genetic abnormalities that will probably be handed down to the children, it means that there are several other issues that need to be considered at the same time.

One concerns the information that needs to be given to the affected party. In principle, the morally correct approach, and one that conforms most closely with the dignity of the person, involves notifying the results to all the people concerned – the individual him/herself, his/her partner or the two of them together. However, this information has its own attendant problems like scientific ignorance about the risks of the defect recurring, the impossibility of guaranteeing that children will be normal even though nothing abnormal has been discovered, the individual's capacity to understand, and his/her wish to be informed or not. When it is a question of passing information on to third parties such as a spouse, a fiancé(e), other members of the family or children, there is the additional problem of confidentiality and the legitimacy of giving the information in the first place.

Genetic examinations can sometimes reveal the existence of a serious illness for which there are not yet any symptoms, but which will get worse, possibly when the individual moves into his/her 40s or 50s. It is not easy to decide what to do in such circumstances. If a serious prognosis is revealed to the individual, s/he has to cope with a serious threat to his/her health; if nothing is said about the situation, it is possible that the individual will cease taking measures that could conceivably get rid of the visible signs of the illness. In situations like these, medical wisdom dictates that an attempt should be made to see if the doctor is entitled to make use of the 'therapeutic privilege' which overrides the otherwise basic necessity to tell the patient the whole story.

Medical professionals have several tasks over and above telling patients what is happening. They have to help the people affected to reach decisions in a responsible way, they must not impose their own opinions or manipulate them either openly or subtly, and they must respect the decision that is ultimately taken. It would also be wrong to treat someone in a discriminatory manner just because s/he has gone down a road that is different from the one recommended by the doctor.

People who suffer from grave physical abnormalities can find themselves having to take exceptionally difficult decisions. The same goes for their partners. Fertility and infertility must be considered very carefully, and must also be the subject of free choice. Responsible parenthood, the protection of the genetic heritage of humanity, and a sensitivity to the social situation in which the couple find themselves all indicate that every effort should be made to avoid conceiving children with serious physical or mental handicaps. A responsible search for these objectives is not moral by virtue of any of the procedures used, but correct behaviour involves a degree of honesty about the aims and methods used.

NOTES

1. J.P. Reilly, 'Genetic Counselling: The Sorrow and the Policy', in *HCR* 13
    (1983) no. 5, 40-42; M.J. Seller, 'Ethical Aspects of Genetic Counselling',
    in *JME* 8 (1982) 185-188; C. Forres and I. Markova, 'An International
    Survey of Genetic Counselling in Haemophilia', in *ESM* 6 (1979) 123-216;
    D. Bergsma, 'Social Effects of Genetic Counselling', in *BMJ* March (1973)
    724-726; C. Leonard and others, 'Genetic Counselling: A Consumer's View',
    in *NEJM* 287 (1972) 433-449; H. Gordon, 'Genetic Counselling: Considera-
    tions for Talking to Parents and Prospective Parents', in *JAMA* 217 (1971)
    1215-1225; M. Lappé, 'Genetic Counselling and Genetic Engineering', in
    HCR 1 (1971) n. 3, 13-14.
2. WMA, 'Genetic Counselling and Genetic Engineering (39 Meet, Madrid
    1987)', in *LH* 214 (1989) 339.

Chapter 7
Antenatal diagnosis[1]

At one time, no one in the medical world knew anything about the embryo and the foetus, but over the last three decades a series of new techniques has made it possible to explore this field for the first time. Although these procedures have enabled doctors to roll back the frontiers of knowledge as far as the embryo and the foetus are concerned, intra-uterine therapy is still a long way off.

7.1 Medical factors

The antenatal test is one that incorporates all interventions that seek to examine the embryo/foetus for any congenital defect, that it is to say for any abnormality in its morphological, structural, functional or molecular development. In industrialized countries, congenital malformations and hereditary diseases are among the major causes of children's illnesses and child mortality. Medical advances have made it possible for us to understand how many of these disorders come about, and antenatal tests allow us to find out about them before a child is born. When, as is usually the case, these tests confirm that the pregnancy will be normal, this gives much relief to families that have been anxious about the possibility of having handicapped children.

For the most part, the procedures used in antenatal tests concentrate on the embryo/foetus, although some focus on the mother. Procedures in the first group include amniocentesis, ultrasound, foetoscopy, the taking of foetal blood, chorionic biopsy, and other newer techniques that are not yet very widespread. Each one is distinctive and is appropriate in given circumstances, although it is also possible to use several of them for the same purpose. Furthermore, some of them are quite harmless, whereas others carry risks to a greater or lesser extent.

Amniocentesis, which consists of taking a small amount of amniotic fluid, makes it possible to investigate the karyotype (i.e., the chromosomal constitution of a cell). Using ultrasound and properly trained staff, this technique is now very safe, although accidents do occur. Apart from mishaps that occur when the needle aspiration technique causes a lot of blood to be lost, there is an abortion rate of about 1 per cent, in addition to other injuries and foetal infections. One of the drawbacks about this technique is that it is used round about the sixteenth week of the pregnancy, which is very late.

Ultrasound can be used as an independent technique or as a support for other techniques. It is the most harmless of them all, and the greatest danger lies in misinterpreting the pictures. It is most useful in diagnosing major congenital malformations.

Foetoscopy involves a direct visualization of the foetus by means of optical fibres placed in the abdomen. It is now being used more and more widely. The main interest in foetoscopy is its ability to detect external anatomical defects, and to facilitate the taking of foetal blood and some biopsies. The main risks are premature birth and foetal lesions, and it is another technique that is used in the later stages of pregnancy, in this case during the fourth, fifth and sixth months.

Foetal blood can be taken using a variety of procedures, and this is usually done as a way of confirming results that have been obtained by other procedures. It is never done in the first 20 weeks. This technique for taking a sample of foetal blood can also be used for therapeutic purposes, unlike others which have exclusively diagnostic objectives.

Chorionic biopsy involves removing chorionic material through the cervix or abdominal wall in order to detect any biochemical or chromosomal abnormalities. It is a new technique, but it has been well tested. One of its advantages is that it can be used as an early diagnosis between the eighth and twelfth week of pregnancy.

7.2 Moral issues

A very large number of moral issues need to be addressed here.

a. Antenatal tests used to find out what is wrong

There are no inherent moral problems about using antenatal tests as a way of finding out the state of the embryo/foetus *in utero*. Any reservations are likely to derive from shortcomings in areas such as the right training, skill and sense of responsibility on the part of the medical staff, the assessment of the risks and advantages in relation to the illness that is being diagnosed, the mother's free and informed consent, the extent to which the tests are reliable in an area as delicate as this, and the choice of the most appropriate procedure.

b. General programmes of antenatal tests

It is very important here to distinguish between the various procedures that are being used. Blood tests, urine analysis and ultrasound are now carried out almost as a matter of routine in pregnancy care, and can be beneficial for both mother and child. Procedures of this type present no problems from a moral point of view.

There are other programmes, however, that incorporate other kinds of test that should never be carried out indiscriminately on pregnant women. They should be confined to women with particular problems, such as those aged over 35 who have given birth to children that were affected with congenital abnormalities, or have relatives with genetic and other problems. Procedures in this group vary considerably according to the doctors involved. They are currently likely to include taking samples of foetal blood, foetoscopy, chorionic biopsy and (most frequently) amniocentesis. General programmes of this type have no medical justification; they camouflage a hidden wish to eliminate mentally handicapped children, and can easily become discriminatory when used on ethnic groups, for example black people, threatened with a particular illness.

For systematic programmes of antenatal tests to be acceptable, they have to meet certain conditions. These are a clear definition of the kinds of risk involved, high quality laboratories, low admissible limits of positive and negative margin of error, follow-up and assessment of the procedures used to discover the effects on the foetus and the mother, information and counselling, confidentiality, an absence of discrimination, and a fair distribution of the resources available. They should not be used simply to find out the child's gender with a view to eliminating children of the wrong sex, to detect anomalies of little importance, or to facilitate birth control.

c. Carrying out the tests

There are still a few matters I want to refer to in addition to the conditions I listed in the last paragraph. These tests must always be carried out with the full and informed consent of the parties concerned, and the offer of a test must never be linked to an undertaking to have an abortion if a serious defect is detected in the embryo/foetus. Some people believe that there is no point to antenatal tests if abortion is ruled out. Such a position is unacceptable.

d. Tests with positive results

If, as usually happens, the test is negative, the parents experience a great feeling of relief. If the tests point to a serious congenital defect, we are faced with a much more difficult problem.

Far too often, some doctors see abortion as the only solution, whereas in reality there are still many more avenues left to explore. Other procedures might include the family accepting the handicapped child even after the gloomiest prognosis, or having therapy after the birth or even *in utero*. The link between genetic abnormality and abortion is quite unnecessary, and on no account should it be considered normal. Unfortunately, in our society, and not only among health professionals, the idea is spreading that there is a logical connection between the two. There are also plenty of people who wonder whether it is legitimate to allow the birth of a child whose quality of life is going to be poor. The lives of some handicapped children can bring great suffering, and normal mental development can be limited. However, a life which can appear frustrating and miserable to one person may be viewed quite differently by the individual living that life. In any case,

from a Christian point of view, even the most diminished existence has a value in itself. By allowing the selective abortion of
handicapped babies, our society is helping to reinforce a climate
that is hostile to all diminished beings who are not properly
formed.

It is true that handicapped people impose economic and social
charges on society as a whole, but the reality is never as difficult
to bear as is first feared. We must never fall into the trap of
assessing people in purely economic terms; this is particularly
true of the most needy. Social solidarity needs to operate more
effectively, and thereby take some of the weight off the family's
shoulders.

The Church's doctrine is summarized in *Donum Vitae* thus:

*If prenatal diagnosis respects the life and integrity of the
embryo and the human foetus and is directed towards its
safeguarding or healing as an individual, then the answer is
affirmative.*

For prenatal diagnosis makes it possible to know the condition of the embryo and of the foetus when still in the mother's
womb. It permits, or makes it possible to anticipate earlier and
more effectively, certain therapeutic, medical or surgical procedures.

Such diagnosis is permissible, with the consent of the parents after they have been adequately informed, if the methods
employed safeguard the life and integrity of the embryo and
the mother, without subjecting them to disproportionate results. But this diagnosis is gravely opposed to the moral law
when it is done with the thought of possibly inducing an
abortion depending upon the results: a diagnosis which shows
the existence of a malformation or a hereditary illness must
not be the equivalent of a death-sentence. Thus a woman
would be committing a gravely illicit act if she were to request
such a diagnosis with the deliberate intention of having an
abortion should the results confirm the existence of a malformation or abnormality. The spouse or relatives or anyone else
would similarly be acting in a manner contrary to the moral
law if they were to counsel or impose such a diagnostic procedure on the expectant mother with the same intention of possibly proceeding to an abortion. So too the specialist would be

guilty of illicit collaboration if, in conducting the diagnosis and in communicating its results, he were deliberately to contribute to establishing or favouring a link between prenatal diagnosis and abortion.

In conclusion, any directive or programme of the civil and health authorities or of scientific organizations which in any way were to favour a link between prenatal diagnosis and abortion, or which were to go as far as directly to induce expectant mothers to submit to prenatal diagnosis planned for the purpose of eliminating foetuses which are affected by malformations or which are carriers of hereditary illness, is to be condemned as a violation of the unborn child's right to life and as an abuse of the prior rights and duties of the spouses.[2]

NOTES

1. Great Britain Catholic Bishops' Joint Committee on Bioethical Issues, *Antenatal Tests: What You Should Know. Answers to Questions Which Face Every Pregnant Mother* (1990); D.C. Wetz and J.C. Fletcher, 'Fetal Knowledge? Prenatal Diagnosis and Sex Selection?', in *HCR* 19 (1989) no. 3, 21-27; M.T. Mennuti, 'Prenatal Diagnosis. Advances Bring New Challenges', in *NEJM* 320 (1989) 661-663; M. d'A. Crawford, 'Prenatal Diagnosis of Common Genetic Disorders', in *BMJ* 297 (1988) 502-506; E. Sherman and G.J. Annas, 'Routine Prenatal Genetic Screening', in *NEJM* 317 (1987) 1407-1408; D.J. Roy, 'First-Trimester Fetal Diagnosis: Prudential Ethics', in *CMAJ* 135 (1986) 737-739; B.M. Dickens, 'Prenatal Diagnosis and Female Abortion: A Case Study in Medical Law and Ethics', in *JME* 12 (1986) 143-144, 150; Comité Consultatif National D'éthique Pour Les Sciences De La Vie Et De La Santé, *Avis sur les problèmes posés par le diagnostic prénatal et périnatal*, 13 May 1985; Ch. J. Dougherty, 'Prenatal Diagnosis: A Reappraisal', in *LQ* 51 (1984) 128-138; M. Robertson, 'Towards a Medical Eugenics', in *BMJ* 288 (1984) 429-430; A.V. Campbell, 'Ethical Issues in Prenatal Diagnosis', in *BMJ* 288 (1984) 1633-1634; John Paul II, 'Allocution au Congrès Médical International du Mouvement pour la vie', in *DC* 80 (1983) 189-191; J. Mahoney, 'A Theologian's Reflections on Pre-Natal Screening', in *CMQ* 30 (1979) 121-126.
2. *Donum Vitae*, I, 2.

Chapter 8

Eugenics[1]

Eugenics is normally presented as an attempt to improve the human race. Francis Galton (1822-1911), who is credited as the first person to use the word, defined eugenics in 1904 as the study of socially controllable factors which can elevate or diminish the racial qualities of future generations both physically and mentally. From the end of the nineteenth century, when we began to talk of eugenics as a science, to the present time, each era has interpreted the word differently in the light of the preoccupations, scientific information and ideologies of the day.

8.1 Positive and negative eugenics

Eugenics follows the classical distinction of positive and negative, and the latter model has so far held sway.

Negative eugenics seeks to eliminate physical and mental characteristics that are not considered desirable for the human race. Measures adopted to achieve this objective are divided into two types: the first is the avoidance of conception; the second is the elimination of handicapped people early on, either before they are born or shortly afterwards.

In order to influence the processes of human reproduction, eugenics starts by identifying carriers of transmittable abnormalities, a task which can sometimes pose considerable problems. Once this identification has been carried out, an attempt is made to avoid conception in one of two ways. The first involves carriers behaving responsibly, avoiding marriage completely or certain kinds of marriage, or avoiding reproduction through appropriate contraceptive methods. The second approach does not demand free responsibility, but rather proceeds by imposing a way of life. It does so by prohibiting marriage, making sterilization compulsory, or locking the carriers up in institutions where relations with members of the opposite sex are extremely difficult.

The second measure adopted by eugenics consists of eliminating carriers of serious anomalies through abortion or ending their lives at an early stage after birth. The physical elimination of imperfect individuals after they are born is not now tolerated by even the most zealous eugenicists, such is the degree of opposition from society and legislation.

Positive eugenics seeks to improve humanity's genetic endowment. Until the development of new techniques of assisted reproduction such as artificial insemination, *in vitro* fertilization and embryo transplantation, natural reproduction as a method was almost out of the question. Today, new frontiers are being opened up thanks to selection of gametes and embryos, but the impact of these innovations is quite limited because of normal sexual behaviour and human reproduction. When the recombination of DNA (deoxyribonucleic acid) becomes possible at an early stage in human reproduction, new technical possibilities will become available, although widespread application will be unlikely for many reasons. Thought is being given to therapies for other procedures which may not completely cure genetic deficiencies, but rather compensate for them in other ways.

8.2 Historical development

Eugenics as a science-based discipline made its first appearance towards the end of the nineteenth century, although there had been many activities with eugenic objectives prior to that. People have dreamt since time immemorial of the ideal of the perfect human being, of a human race with no handicapped members, and over time this ideal found its way into a number of ideas which were of little value, but which none-the-less found support in a wide variety of ideologies.

Eugenics after birth was once practised in Sparta, where children considered to be weak or deformed were abandoned in a pass on Mount Taygetos. Strictly speaking, abortion was not eugenic, and it was practised for quite different reasons. There was very little scientific and technical knowledge around, and it was therefore not possible to diagnose hereditary defects. It was only when it was thought that the child was the fruit of incest or some other kind of unacceptable sexual relationship that abortion took on a eugenic complexion, in the way we understand it today. The custom that was most effective from a eugenic point of view was the regulation of marriages between closely related people. The reasons for this were religious, moral or social and, with hindsight, we can detect an element of some understanding of genetics.

For decades, eugenics was thought to have a great future in countries like the United States, Britain and Japan; this was based on the belief that control over reproduction would lead to the disappearance or reduction of inherited genetic defects. In consequence, radical measures such as sterilization and castration were imposed on defenceless individuals in the name of science; it was, however, a science based on quite false assumptions. At one stage, the United States introduced rigid rules on immigration, and prohibited entry to anyone from the south and east of Europe. Some countries used to demand a health certificate that was issued to couples before they got married. It had a specific purpose: sometimes it was simply used to detect certain contagious illnesses, and there was no form of prohibition attached to it; sometimes it meant that the holder could not marry, and failure to obey this instruction could result in punishment. Eugenic tendencies were to be found in a Nazi law of 14 July 1933 which had the avowed aim of preventing the birth of children with hereditary diseases; under this legislation, anyone with a hereditary illness could be sterilized. This law was effectively the starting point for a broad eugenic programme which dealt with the destruction of unvalued life.

Eugenic movements fell back substantially after World War II, largely as a reaction to the horrors committed by the Nazi regime, but also thanks to scientific advances. Increased sensitivity to the rights of the individual and improved legal protection also made compulsory sterilization unthinkable. Moreover, the development of antenatal tests made it possible to diagnose hereditary abnormalities and non-hereditary embryo malformations caused by X-rays, rubella and various teratogens, thereby widening the scope for eugenic abortion. However, this type of abortion was not carried out as a way of preserving the genetic stock; the purpose was to deal with the family and social problems that flowed from having children with serious abnormalities. The development and

general availability of contraceptive devices and genetic counselling helped to avert pregnancies which had previously been quite
unavoidable. The other route that was open to eugenics was
provided by the new techniques of assisted reproduction which
made it possible to select gametes and embryos *in vitro*. Their
impact on eugenics was small because of the prevailing patterns of
sexual behaviour.

8.3 Moral questions

Concerns on behalf of future generations – like trying to
ensure the best living conditions for them and avoiding obstacles
to their general well-being – are quite legitimate in themselves.
They are even obligatory for public authorities, scientists and
private individuals. These concerns, when they are reduced to
simple terms like 'promoting good and eliminating bad', were
recognized as valid and worthy of encouragement by Pius XII in
1953.[2]

There are moral reservations about both the assumptions underlying eugenics and its procedures and policies. Here are some
issues that help to discredit ideas with a eugenic component:

– racism;
– the wish to discriminate – for example, against immigrant
workers;
– imposing measures on people, rather than seeking their free
and informed consent;
– no respect for the beginning of human life;
– the violation of sexual and marriage rights, even going so
far as to claim that no one has a right to have children.

Apart from the scientific and technical difficulties associated
with positive eugenics, the main problem we come across concerns the model or desirable characteristics of future generations,
the criteria for this selection, and the individuals who will do the
selecting.

NOTES

1. M. Robertson, 'Towards a Medical Eugenics?', in *BMJ* 288 (1984) 429-430; H. Wattiaux, 'Eugénisme et morale catholique', in *NRT* 113(1981) 801-817; K.M. Ludmerer, 'Eugenics I, History', in *EB* I, 457-461; M. Lappe, 'Ethical Issues', Ibid., 462-468; D.M. Fieldman, 'Jewish Religious Laws', Ibid., 468-470; W.W. Bassett, 'Eugenics and Religious Law. Christian Religious Laws', Ibid., 471-472; L.S. Dawidowicz, 'The Failure of Himmler's Positive Eugenics', in *HCR* 7 (1977) no. 5, 43-44.
2. Pius XII, 'Allocution of 7 September 1953', in *AAS* 45 (1953) 605.

Chapter 9

Abortion

It is all too common for the strong to attempt to impose their will on the weak. To make matters worse, these two groups are never equal in number. In our society, an unborn life must surely be one of the weakest and most threatened of all lives, and cries out for special support.

In this discussion of abortion, I will deal with the classical questions of the status of the embryo/foetus and the moral and legal dimensions, and as far as the moral position is concerned, I will devote a separate section to co-operation. This will be preceded by some considerations that will serve to focus the matter correctly within our society.

9.1 Background

Like all human problems, abortion is one that must be described in meticulous detail if a solution is ever to be found. I have therefore decided it would be useful to make a few extra preliminary remarks before I get down to dealing with the issues that normally come under the heading of abortion.

I have a feeling that there is something quite fundamental to this lively social debate that has been obscured. Abortion is emphatically undesirable in a human society that has a developed moral sense. It is nothing for our society to feel proud of – nor is it a sign of progress – yet preventing it should be a shared task that rises above the debates on the morality of abortion and its decriminalization. There are a lot of complex motives standing in the way of a preventive policy based on consensual programmes. However, in a pluralistic society it is possible and desirable that there should be substantial agreement on views if the number of abortions that take place is to be reduced.

Abortion is not even a pleasant experience for the woman, even if it is she who has requested it in the first place. The fact that it appears to have a liberating dimension does not prevent the woman being afflicted by a degree of solitude, and beset with anxieties and pressures. In principle, we should encourage all attempts to help the woman resolve the problems that encourage her to believe that abortion is a liberation.

Given the complex world we live in, it is self-evident that the prevention of abortion is the great moral challenge of our time. To look upon it as merely a matter of personal responsibility for the people involved is quite wrong; to leave it like that falls a long way short of addressing the problem properly. A vast social framework has been constructed, and within it the termination of a human life in its early stages seems to be logical and tragically coherent. Insistence on the macrosocial aspect of abortion can encourage the individual to think of him/herself as the mere plaything of alien forces, like a defenceless victim of powerful circumstances which release him/her from all personal responsibility, or which dismiss personal responsibility to the sidelines. Recognition of the impact produced by interpersonal factors must not deny each person his/her intellectual freedom, given that each individual is not obliged to repeat moves that are already fixed.

Talking about the complexity of the social framework that is the breeding ground for abortion can encourage a certain feeling of impotence, particularly when one is trying to think of the best 'therapy' to adopt. What can a person or a group – even a country – do to throw off the mentality, the attitudes and the social and economic conditioning that are so favourable to abortion? It would be sad if legitimate awareness of the complexity of the situation derived from a form of paralysis that is effectively an end to action in favour of unborn life. The outlook is unquestionably bleak, but I must here explain why I am still optimistic.

First of all, I must acknowledge that the background is not encouraging. The strong emotions that many people bring to this subject make it even more difficult to treat it with the seriousness and calm that it demands. As a result, the outlook is none too hopeful, and positions are taken up with such fanaticism that any intellectual debate is more or less pointless. What is more, the verbal aggression, the accusations and the diatribes that the various groups hurl at one another contribute to a most unedifying spectacle. Ideological and political interests seem to carry more weight than serious thought, and the manipulation and distortion of data make serious discussion even more remote.

Much time is spent concentrating on three points – the moral status of the embryo and the foetus, the ethical focus of abortion, and moral judgement of legislation in this area – but I wonder if this betokens a sign of clear thinking, however important the three issues may be. I acknowledge that these matters need to be studied with due seriousness; however, I also think that we can provide more effective support to an unborn human life on a long-term basis if we give more consideration to the numerous concepts that contribute to making abortion more acceptable, even normal, in our society.

Another activity that could prevent abortion would be to look at pregnant women who see it as a way out of their problems. Such '11th hour' actions are frequently necessary, but it would be much better to prevent these situations in the first place, either by preventing unwanted pregnancies or by eliminating the unsatisfactory circumstances that women so easily find themselves in. This '11th hour' approach can be made in two ways: offering the women opportunities for kindly, supportive discussion (acknowledging that abortion is often associated with loneliness) and providing social welfare systems to remedy other problems.

There is another factor that favours the prevention of abortion, but it is difficult to identify. It consists of the various aspects of economic, cultural and social family policy which are designed to give the child a welcome, instead of encouraging fears and anxieties at the thought of another child.[1] There is a danger that some groups will insist on adopting some of these measures only because they are associated with the prevention of abortion; in fact, they are more important for the value that they bring to a wholesome family life, irrespective of anything they do for human life prior to the birth. Such health measures include facilities for pregnant women at the workplace and improved adoption systems, although the latter must always have the main criterion in mind – that of the interests of the child who is to be adopted.

The most difficult, but perhaps most decisive, way of correcting the increase in the number of abortions takes the form of what we might call a broad educational campaign, although not one restricted to young people. A campaign of this kind would seek to eliminate, or modify, those parts of our social mentality and other widespread attitudes that discourage the welcoming of a new human life. By the same token, the campaign would aim to create an entirely new mentality and set of attitudes.

Education generally is opposed by an unco-operative type of freedom that claims 'rights over one's own body'; it should therefore call for a form of freedom that incorporates solidarity. Despite advances that have been made on behalf of handicapped people, there is still a broad social climate that is very hostile to anyone with major physical or mental problems. Legitimate pleasure at personal well-being, and ambiguous praise for the so-called good things of life, can sometimes produce people who think of nothing but their own interests, and who cannot tolerate the most minor personal restrictions, even when they affect a neighbour's basic needs. The effect is that the weakest people, in this case the embryo and the foetus, are victims in our society. It is a society that is unable to harmonize well-being, self-realization and pleasure with respect for other people's basic rights even though they place restrictions on us. We are faced with the danger of confusing legal and moral legitimacy, and of slipping from what is technically possible into what is morally possible.[2] Lastly, I want to say that sex education must include responsibility for fertility. These are a few notes for a broad, unhurried education programme in support of unborn life.

A moral 'crusade' that aims to underline the inhuman and unchristian side of abortion has to be part of preventive action on a world scale. We have to be realistic, and acknowledge that we cannot have high expectations for campaigns of this type in our society. Such ideas must of course be encouraged, but sadly there are not many people listening. Numerous conditioning factors of human behaviour stand in the way of this moral message being heard more widely. Be that as it may, all efforts to convince people of the immorality of abortion must remain part of moves for worldwide prevention, the basic tenet of this section.

Discussion on the law as it relates to abortion tends to be passionate. There is a link between the number of abortions and what the law says, but it is difficult to quantify; this is partly because the situation is already fairly obscure, and as a result there is little clear evidence to go on. Those who favour permissive legislation give the impression that they have fulfilled their 'duty' by defending such a position. It seems to me that insistence on the freedom to have abortions is only part of the story, and does little more than attract attention. Such insistence should put the same amount of energy into defending the duty of solidarity, whereby the woman will not find herself in circumstances that 'encourage' her to get rid of the embryo or foetus. Insistence on the freedom to have abortions often implies a degree of cynicism and hypocrisy, not to mention a lack of solidarity. On the other hand, too much confidence is sometimes placed in the law as an ally against abortion. The effectiveness of penal sanctions is markedly reduced in a society that is broadly tolerant about terminating pregnancies, and where new techniques are appearing that enable abortions to be carried out at an early stage. Wide-ranging debate on abortion and the law is therefore wholly legitimate, but this must not monopolize our attention as it tends to distract us from a number of other issues.

Current differences should not stand in the way of the various groups working together, and taking part in activities aimed at drastically reducing the number of abortions. In this way, it would give the best human and Christian witness to the unborn life; the unborn life is the weakest, poorest and most silent life that has no voice of its own and, because of its extreme fragility, it relies on the solidarity of others.[3]

9.2 What is the 'status' of life before birth?[4]

If we could find a common, shared reply to this question, its repercussions on a moral assessment of abortion and associated legislative problems would be enormous.

However, the differences in opinion originate in the way the question is formulated, and are an indication of how complex the issue really is. We use a range of words and phrases like the status of life before birth, the beginning of human life, humanized life, humanization, the person, specifically human life, biologically human life, animation and infusion of the soul. However, I have chosen the formulation 'the status of (human) life before birth', and I obviously mean its anthropological status, and not just the legal status.

It is still not easy to find a reply to the question 'What is the status of life before birth?' because it is bound up with many issues like biology, ethics, philosophy, cultural ideas and psychological experiences. There is also the problem of which criteria we need to adopt.

I am going to confine myself to the most important of the many solutions available. It is the teaching of the Catholic Church, and of many other groupings outside the Church, that the decisive moment is fertilization. Some people acknowledge the undeniable importance of fertilization, but give weight to a combination of conception and individuation. There are others who locate the principle of a truly human condition at the beginning of the formation of the cerebral cortex.

a. Fertilization

Fertilization of the ovum by a human spermatozoon is the start of a life that biologically belongs to the human species. This union will not be the beginning of a life that will eventually give us an elephant or a rat. Furthermore, we are talking about a human life that is biologically separate from that of the mother, and consists of a 50 per cent complement received by the father and another 50 per cent received from the mother. Biologically speaking, there is no question that the zygote is not simply part of the mother's body, just like any other cell, organ or tissue. It is sometimes thought that the embryo, and even the foetus, belong to the mother, but from a biological standpoint such language is manipulative and imprecise. Any form of rational discussion with people who do not accept this scientific evidence will be difficult, not to say impossible.

For all practical purposes, this life that is biologically separate from that of the mother is unrepeatable and unique. Apart from monozygotic twins, it is almost a miracle for the same genetic complement to be repeated in two individuals. From its earliest forms and stages, this new life possesses internal mechanisms which, in favourable circumstances, will enable the individual to be a fully developed human being. The process of development and growth are not, however, ordained by the mother but by the embryo itself. From the very beginning, this minute being possesses the basic programme to enable him/her to be a future individual, within the context of the environment in which s/he lives.

The Congregation for the Doctrine of the Faith has this to say on the subject:

> From the moment that the ovum is fertilized, a life is begun which is neither that of the father nor of the mother; it is rather the life of a new human being with his own growth. It would never be made human if it were not human already... Modern genetic science ... has demonstrated that from the first instant there is established the programme of what this living being will be: a man, this individual man with his characteristic aspects already well determined. Right from fertilization the adventure of a human life begins, and each of its capacities requires time – a rather lengthy time – to find its place and to be in a position to act. The least that can be said is that present science, in its most involved state, does not give any substantial support to those who defend abortion.[5]

b. Implantation

Some writers lay great stress on implantation, and their reason for so doing is to be able to argue for termination of the process that was initiated at fertilization. Round about the sixth or seventh day after fertilization, the fertilized ovum implants in the uterus, and a week later the process of conception stops.

The reasons for giving so much weight to implantation are these. Until the very end of the process, individuation is not irreversibly defined, and there is still a possibility that it could be two or more children, or just one. We cannot talk of individuals until we have moved past this period of ambiguity and uncertainty about number. Häring has said that the argument that the fertilized ovum cannot yet be a person or an individual with all the rights of the human species seems convincing as long as we stay with our traditional concept of the person.[6]

On the other hand, it is widely (though not universally) accepted by the scientific community that a large number of zygotes are expelled spontaneously by nature before implantation takes place, and that there is very little natural elimination subsequent to that. On this basis, some writers deny the inviolability of the fertilized ovum before implantation. If nature seems too wasteful, why should we not be able to terminate at this early stage? Is it possible that this large number of lives cut off so prematurely by nature are human beings with eternal fates and vocations?

This approach presents a number of problems. We do not know until after implantation the exact number of individuals that have been conceived, but this does not mean that the conception that started with fertilization is without human life. Nature's prodigality in eliminating a lot of abnormal beings does not allow us to increase that number of lost beings by artificial means. Implantation of the ovum, a delicate and important moment in the genesis of any human life, nevertheless adds nothing to the internal process of development of a human being which has already begun.

c. Development of the cerebral cortex

Conscious, rational life is specific to the human species, and the potential of this superior life is linked to the development and functioning of the brain. These days, it is generally accepted by scientists and the law that clinical death takes place when the brain irreversibly ceases to function. A brain that is observed no longer to be functioning is dead; in these circumstances, we say that the person is clinically dead. On the basis of this accepted definition of the end of life, some people see a parallel with the principle of human life itself. They say that, until the first indicators of basic brain life appear, we cannot speak of a human being. However, life which has started with fertilization, although worthy of respect, is not completely inviolable until the end of the second month when we begin to see the first signs of the future brain. They also refer, although less emphatically, to the process of the evolution of the species. As we do not speak of the human species until a particular stage in the configuration of the brain, why not apply the same hypothesis to ontogenesis or the genesis of individuals?

Everybody acknowledges the importance of the brain to a human life, but does denying human status to a being that has no cerebral structure – but will clearly have one if we wait a short period of time – justify a lower assessment of that life? Any similarity with anencephalic patients misses the point. In both cases, there is a material similarity in that the brain is silent, but there is a fundamental difference just the same. An anencephalic person is irreversibly lost, whereas there is every hope for the future in the developing foetus.

d. Relationship criteria

Many people believe that the biology and development of the embryo and foetus cannot solve this problem. Human life cannot be reduced to biology. They therefore use other criteria whereby the person is a member of society and has a range of relationships. These relationships consist of being accepted by parents, of being acknowledged by society, of being wanted children, of being destined to live (despite laboratory experiments), and being pro-created intentionally.

Of the many theories that have been produced on this subject, one that comes from a group of celebrated French scholars deserves special attention. This draws a distinction between human life and humanized life, and the step between the two phases is marked by the relationship of recognition. Human life needs to be protected from the earliest moments, and until the step of recognition is made, its inviolability is not complete. 'We think,' write the French thinkers referred to above, 'that a distinction can be drawn between human life and humanized life. If it is really true to say that the individual is only humanized in his/her relationship with people, and for and by other people – his/her very being is received from others – the relationship of recognition, as we have outlined it, reveals, rather than installs, the fully human character that is developing. To put it in another way, just as a human being does not exist without a body, so it cannot be humanized without this relationship with other people.'

One of the positive aspects of this position is that it underlines a human being's social dimension. Important questions now arise. Is recognition so important for society and parents that life is not fully human without it? What is introduced by the recognition that the embryo or foetus do not already possess in themselves as far as intrinsic dignity is concerned? Why limit this interpretation, as its authors do, to the first stages of unborn life? Why not apply it equally to life after birth?

e. Some conclusions

When we speak of abortion, we do not always draw a clear distinction between the scientific facts revealed by empirical sciences and the interpretations and assessments that are made of them.

The Catholic Church's position affirming the inviolability of all human life from the moment of fertilization is the most coherent, in that it envisages a continuous development with no qualitative leaps. And this view is in accord with scientific evidence.

As for attributing personhood to all phases of human life prior to birth, the situation is immensely uncertain and will remain so for some time.

9.3 A moral assessment of abortion[7]

In our society, people often attempt to avoid discussing the morality of abortion by claiming – as they frequently do on other subjects – that it is exclusively a matter for one's personal conscience. However, recognizing the value of our consciences does not mean we can avoid determining what we mean by 'individual'. A Christian has the experience and wisdom of humanity, but also has the model of Jesus of Nazareth, and the secular and current experience of Christian communities seen in the light of the Church's magisterium.

a. The Bible's teaching

Neither the Old nor the New Testament provides us with a moral standard on abortion that enables us to decide with any certainty on the complex situations that life throws up. The Greek Septuagint Old Testament offers an approximate distinction between abortion and murder: 'When people who are fighting injure a pregnant woman so that there is a miscarriage, and yet no further harm follows, the one responsible shall be fined what the woman's husband demands, paying as much as the judges determine. If any harm follows, then you shall give life for life.'[8] The sense of the text is as follows: if the woman (and not the foetus) dies, the guilty one shall pay with his life in accordance with the law of the *lex talionis*; if she does not die, the guilty man shall be punished with a fine.

The New Testament refers to the Baptist before his birth as if he was already born:

When Elizabeth heard Mary's greeting, the child leapt in her womb. And Elizabeth was filled with the Holy Spirit and exclaimed with a loud cry, 'Blessed are you among women, and blessed is the fruit of your womb. And why has this happened to me, that the mother of my Lord comes to me? For as soon as I heard the sound of your greeting, the child in my womb leapt for joy.'[9]

This extract is mainly interesting for its support for the Church's interest in the value of life in the womb.

The New Testament's abundant teaching on the Commandment to love your neighbour, together with Christ's attitude towards the poor and defenceless, produce a framework that can be applied worldwide; it also contains substantial meaning for a life as fragile and threatened as that of the embryo or foetus.

All things considered, the Bible contains a large corpus of teaching that comes down clearly in favour of human life. However, it cannot be understood as a clear, decisive norm, rather as a framework of inspiration and reference, and it is on this basis that the Church has continued to reflect ever more deeply, and taken many other circumstances into account. The Spanish bishops present a brief summary of this teaching as follows:

God is the only lord of life and death. Except in extreme cases of legitimate defence, man may not make an attempt on human life. The Old Testament expresses this very idea in various ways: life, whether it is one's own or another's, is a gift from God which man must respect and care for, and may not dispose of. God, the living, created 'humankind in our image, according to our likeness' (Gen 1:26) and wants humankind to live, and 'God is not of the dead, but of the living' (Mk 12:27) also wants humankind to live. To achieve this, he protects people's lives by prohibiting murder (Gen 9:5-6, Ex 20:13). In the New Testament, he continues with the high esteem for human life that he has referred to in the Old Testament, by demonstrating his preference for marginalized and less important lives and saving them for the true life. By so doing, he unequivocally revealed the value of every individual's life, irrespective of its qualities and social usefulness. The right to life is inherent to life itself as an intangible value in itself which must be respected and safeguarded.[10]

b. The Church's secular experience[11]

It is fair to say that the Church has not changed its position on the morality of abortion down through the centuries. There has been, it is true, a range of views and slight differences of opinion, but these have not invalidated the Church's main thesis.

During the time of the Roman Empire, when abortion was endemic, the early Christians affirmed a new attitude that consisted of respect for unborn life. There were, however, disagreements about the type of moral disorder that abortion implied – violation of love for one's neighbour, lack of maternal love, a lack of reverence for the work of God the creator, a sign of sexual disorder, magic, idolatrous practices, and the like.

The distinction between a formed and unformed, or animated or unanimated, foetus has served to justify a range of views on the morality of abortion. These views constitute a common stand of opposition to abortion as something that is not part of the Christian conscience. The death of an unformed or unanimated foetus is completely unacceptable, although it is less serious than the elimination of a foetus that has been formed or in which the soul has been infused. This distinction found its way into the arena of canonical penalties and irregularities relating to the exercise of the priestly ministry.

An instance of the Church's position on abortion is to be found in penal legislation. Punishment varied from church to church, but generally speaking it was severe and rigorous, although it was rarely as harsh as the penalties meted out for deliberate murder.

It is also believed that the liturgy collaborated with the Church's traditions with regard to the unborn life. The feasts of Christ's conception, or the Annunciation, (nine months before Christmas) and the Immaculate Conception of Mary (nine months before the celebration of her birth) have both been celebrated in the East since the seventh century. Apart from their immediate and relatively limited significance, they may well have helped in some way to give a holy character to all human life after conception.

Theologians are divided as to the moment of animation or the infusion of the spiritual soul. Some say it occurs at the moment of conception, while others opt for a later stage. Either view supports the moral outlawing of abortion whether it occurs before or after animation.

c. Current doctrine

In its current teaching on abortion, the Church distinguishes between the objective plane and the subjective plane, as it does with all doctrines. When the Church proclaims a doctrine, it does not set itself up as the judge of a given individual. Without ever approving of abortion, the Church never ceases to be sensitive to those cases where the circumstances are exceptional and involve particular conflict. This shows the Church's pastoral skill in being able to approach these situations in the same spirit as Christ.

On an objective plane, the Church expresses its doctrine by means of formulas that have become clearer with the passing of time. Abortion that has been brought about directly is never legitimate, whereas indirect forms can sometimes be so. The category of indirect abortions includes the removal of a cancerous uterus during pregnancy, and the termination of an ectopic pregnancy when it becomes dangerous for the mother. By contrast, direct abortions are those carried out for the purposes of birth control, because of family or social difficulties, in the event of rape, and for other therapeutic reasons.

The Church arrives at these formulations from two carefully considered points of view. In the first place, it is based on the principle that an innocent human being may never be deprived of life by a direct action. Speaking of induced abortion, the

Congregation for the Doctrine of the Faith states that, 'Divine
law and natural reason, therefore, exclude all right to the direct
killing of an innocent man.'[12] On the other hand, the existence of
an innocent human life is admitted from the moment of conception, or fertilization. The uncertainty surrounding whether the
concept of 'a person' can be applied from the very beginning
does not prevent us from demanding absolute respect for it. The
condition of innocent human being for the embryo and foetus is
a basic assumption: 'Respect for human life is called for from
the time the process of generation begins. From the time that the
ovum is fertilized, a life is begun which is neither that of the
father nor of the mother; it is rather the life of a new human
being with his own growth. It would never be made human if it
were not human already.'[13]

The Catholic Church's position on abortion attempts to be
unconditional and coherent; it is there to defend life. It must also
be emphasized how clearly such a basic, fundamental question is
dealt with. Catholic teaching lays down objective criteria for the
protection of life, and believes that fertilization is the decisive
moment for moral assessment. For that reason, the embryo and
the foetus's growth into life are removed from all considerations
of conflict of values, tastes and customs. It also appears more
coherent because of the continuity which underpins the whole
process of human life. Furthermore, it is free of the difficulties
which beset other opinions. These include views which give a
moral value to the implantation of the ovum and the forming of
the cerebral cortex, and views which allocate a moral importance to a human being's social dimension. With its position on
abortion, the Catholic doctrine also believes it is providing support for other lives in danger of being considered less valuable,
such as the lives of old people and others with terminal illnesses.
This clear, unambiguous argumentation is a barrier preventing
us from becoming increasingly aggressive towards those who
are regularly discriminated against in our society. Lastly, nobody has the right to terminate the process started at fertilization,
and the State and all other institutions and authorities similarly
have no entitlement to have a say in the life of a human being at
this initial stage.

It is proving very difficult to have Catholic doctrine accepted
in today's world.[14]

9.4 Co-operation in abortion

The question whether certain actions mean co-operation in abortion or not, and whether they are justified for a sincere conscience, needs to be answered whether abortion is legalized or not. Even in a society with permissive laws, there are more and more situations and actions which clear-thinking health professionals and others are beginning to question. These uncertainties tend to centre on the steps taken in the period leading up to a legal abortion, rather than on the actual carrying out of an abortion or of subsequent interventions.

Can a Catholic carry out clinical examinations or put forward medical opinions which are going to leave the door open to a legal abortion, for example by certifying a serious genetic defect? Can one occupy the post of director, administrator or head of department in a centre or clinic where abortions are being performed? What can we say of a judge who acts for wards of court and whose intervention is going to allow a minor to have an abortion? Does it make sense for religious communities to be on the premises of health centres where abortions are carried out? These questions identify only some of the many problems faced by certain individuals.

a. General considerations

The subject of co-operation relies on two closely linked points of reference. For one thing, it is inseparable from the conception one has of a Christian's mission and presence in the world; for another, it cannot be isolated from the concrete configuration of the world in which each one of us has to live.

Our world is a lot more complicated than it was in centuries gone by. We are much more interdependent, ethical pluralism is more established, the idea of scandal resulting from co-operation is understood quite differently, and good and evil often seem to be so closely intertwined that it is difficult to tell them apart. Once upon a time, evil was looked upon more objectively, whereas today it is personal affairs that are more accentuated. These circumstances, and others which I could mention, go towards explaining the context of co-operation.

Co-operation also influences how we determine a Christian's mission and presence in society. God has called us to be his collaborators, and instruments in the construction of his kingdom far from the complicity of the forces of evil. In reality, good and evil are intimately mixed together, and it is not easy to work out how to separate them. If we withdraw to the sidelines so as to avoid being accomplices in evil, we are compromising our collaboration in God's projects. If we opt for a more compromising life in this world, we can then give the impression of colluding with the powers of evil.

Will Christians have to stand aloof from the world, from economic, social and cultural activities, just to stay absolutely pure, like a chosen group sheltering from the contagion of the masses? If so, how can we then be witnesses of divine charity in the world, and collaborate in the establishment of a friendly community that is open to all? Matthew said, 'In gathering the weeds you would uproot the wheat along with them. Let both of them grow together until the harvest',[15] and St Paul has written, 'I wrote to you in my letter not to associate with sexually immoral persons – not at all meaning the immoral of this world, or the greedy and robbers, or idolaters, since you would then need to go out of the world'.[16]

Many Christians emphasize other aspects of the Church's sensitivity to such issues and interpret life differently. So, for instance, they decide to spend time in compromising situations and run the risk of contaminating themselves. Häring has written that it is easy for anyone who has retired from the world and is concentrating on his/her own salvation to take an impeccably rigorous line and say that no material co-operation is legitimate. For those who live in the world, Häring points out, this is a very delicate matter as they work for the establishment of the Kingdom of God and the salvation of those who are in danger.[17]

Before I finish with these general considerations, I would like to add a brief word on some people's wish for a good understanding of this particular issue, and their desire that all situations should be defined morally and with absolute clarity. It is understandable for people to want to be clear on matters of this type; it can be very frustrating not to know where one stands. However, while we must never dismiss efforts to reach clear convictions, sometimes all we can do, even when it comes to important questions, is to make do with half-measures. Sometimes, we have to accept the fact that we are just human beings with limited insight and humble convictions.

b. Concrete situations

– Participation in carrying out an abortion. It is here that co-operation with abortion can be at its most intensive, while at the same time attracting the fiercest moral reservations.

– Participation in stages prior to abortion. This situation can arise particularly in countries that have legislation in favour of abortion. There is no shortage of laws insisting that health professionals have to be involved in the performance of certain functions. Such professional activities are frequently legitimate in themselves, but the law considers them necessary for abortion to be legal. They are closely linked to abortion, however, because of the way the law links them together, not because of the action in itself. They include analyses and diagnoses which are in themselves independent of abortion; they are designed, for instance, to see whether the foetus is normal, or to decide whether continuing with the pregnancy could endanger the mother's life. Guidance on such a complex situation as this appears in a general principle set out in a document produced by the CEI (Conferenza Episcopale Italiana), the Italian bishops' conference. It states that, 'Early treatment is legitimate and appropriate as long as abortion is not the specific and necessary aim.'[18]

– Treatment following abortion. This type of treatment does not present moral objections, even for people with a strict moral conscience. To quote again from the Italian bishops, 'Treatment following abortion ... is legitimate and appropriate ... and is an example of affection and love in the midst of the difficulties, which the termination often aggravates instead of eliminating'.[19]

9.5 Abortion under the law

In this section, I am going to deal with four issues:

– certain legislative questions;
– the legal situation in Great Britain and Europe;

- the ethics of legislation;
- objection of conscience.

a. Legislative models[20]

Although there is no such thing as two identical laws, it is just about possible to suggest three types or models. They are:

1. laws that permit abortion with a maximum time limit;
2. laws that allow abortion only for medical reasons;
3. laws that prohibit abortion.

1. Laws in the first category all have one thing in common: that is, that abortion is possible up to a certain stage in the pregnancy, and is essentially at the woman's request. The woman can have an abortion, if she wants one, up to a certain point in the pregnancy; this varies from 10 to 12 weeks or even three months, according to the legislation. There is no need for another person (e.g. a doctor, psychologist or social worker) to certify that there are good reasons for proceeding with the intervention. These laws also contain a large amount of relatively unimportant detail. Beyond the final point at which the woman has unimpeded access to abortion, these laws often additionally allow limited access for various other reasons including danger to the woman's life and eugenic abortion.

2. Under the second group of laws, abortion is not simply a matter of the woman asking for it. Abortions may only be performed legally if there are particular circumstances. These are known as indications, and are confirmed by persons other than the woman; these people are usually doctors. There are four indications used to justify abortion. They are medical (a serious threat to the pregnant woman's physical or mental health which cannot be dealt with in any other way), eugenic (the certainty, probability or suspicion that the foetus is suffering from a serious physical or mental defect), social (factors that have an impact on the woman or her family like economic problems, housing and other children) and humanitarian or 'ethical' (when the pregnancy is the result of rape or incest or results from sexual relations with a minor or someone who is mentally handicapped). Not all legislation in this group includes all four indications.

Legislation that technically falls into this second category is sometimes interpreted so broadly by society that there is little practical difference from laws in the first group.

3. Restrictive legislation includes laws which completely prohibit induced abortions, or only allow them in very limited circumstances (e.g. saving the mother's life or following rape).

[*b. Editor's note: Abortion legislation in Britain*

It is not possible here to summarize the many and varied examples of abortion law in European countries or North America. As an important example one may offer the UK Abortion Act of 1967, which permitted medical termination of pregnancy for the first time in British law. Conditions are that two registered medical practitioners are of the opinion, formed in good faith, that there is risk to the life of the woman, or of injury to the physical or mental health of the woman, or any existing children of her family, greater than if the pregnancy were terminated; or that there is a substantial risk that if the child were born it would suffer from such physical or mental abnormalities as to be seriously handicapped. After prolonged campaigning by the anti-abortion lobby, a gestational time limit of 24 weeks was imposed by Parliament in a clause of the Human Fertilization and Embryology Act 1990 on abortions for therapeutic and social reasons. However, this limit explicitly does not apply to abortions in case of handicap to the child, nor to cases where grave permanent injury to the physical or mental health of the pregnant woman is virtually certain, or where there is risk to her life. Moreover, in these latter circumstances (of injury or death for the woman), the requirement of the 1967 Act for the agreement of two registered medical practitioners no longer applies. A doctor can act on his own judgement.

The vast majority of 180,000 or so abortions performed each year in Britain are for therapeutic reasons. Mason and McCall-Smith are of the opinion that the scope of the Act approximates to abortion on demand and probably exceeds that envisaged by its originators. They doubt whether it is now possible to perform an illegal abortion in Great Britain provided the regulations are observed (*Law and Medical Ethics*, 105-6).]

c. *The ethics of legislation*[21]

For legislation to be ethically acceptable, it is not enough for it to go through the legally correct process of drafting and approval. Observation of procedures only provides juridical legitimacy; only justification from the point of view of the common good can invest it with moral value. It is not easy to reach agreement on what the demands of the common good are under a given law. The origins of these differences are legion. They include the many, varied ideas that human beings and societies have on the subject, different scales of values, and an analysis that does not coincide with reality – for example, an analysis of the predictable negative and positive consequences of the various possible alternatives.

From the standpoint of political ethics, different options have to respond honestly to the following question: What are the favourable and the unfavourable consequences for individuals and society in the short, medium and long term?[22]

Supporters of decriminalizing abortion put forward numerous arguments in support of their contentions, and I will set out a few here. For one thing, they say, this legislative model is the only one that is capable of eliminating clandestine abortions and the damage subsequently suffered usually by the woman: this typically includes danger to her life and fertility, and economic exploitation. In this way, the door is also closed on discrimination brought about by repressive legislation of the type that militates against working-class people. The rich can always travel abroad to have their abortions, whereas the poor cannot. Permissive legislation does not force abortion on people; it simply legalizes it by creating a framework that respects freedom of conscience and the peaceful co-habitation of differing personal opinions. The woman's autonomy is safe, something that cannot be said of the alternative legislative model.

The Church is opposed to the decriminalization of abortion. It is the Church's view that the outlawing of abortion is necessary if life before birth is to be effectively protected. If this protection did not exist, millions of human beings would be lost. Here, we are talking of the weakest human beings, those who have no way of speaking up for themselves and have no means of defending themselves. Permissive laws are the most discriminatory because they deny human beings their most basic right – the right to life. Prohibiting abortion closes the door on possible threats to the lives of others like the elderly and mentally and physically handicapped. If we are going to leave that door open, who is to say that tomorrow human wickedness will not take more aggressive steps against the lives of beings who have already been born? The task of laws is to protect the rights of human beings, especially the most basic rights, and even more particularly the rights of the most defenceless individuals.

d. Objection of conscience[23]

Some health professionals ask themselves to what extent their convictions of conscience are protected when abortion is decriminalized. They wonder how they are expected to respond to activities related to abortion, especially if they were employed in public health centres. These situations could arise in a surgical team, among doctors who are obliged to have given opinions for the abortion to be legal, among nursing staff and judges who are responsible for wards of court, and among employees of a hospital run by a Catholic foundation. Is objection of conscience a right even when there is a risk to the mother's life unless she has an abortion? And if abortions are available on Social Security or the National Health Service, can one object to one's contributions being used for this purpose?

The issue of objection of conscience arises when a law permits conduct that is opposed to an individual's convictions of conscience, and when the individual realizes that s/he may be asked to carry out an action that is legal, but in his/her view immoral. This is the point at which there may or may not be objection of conscience. The greatest dignity of a human being is rooted in fidelity to the dictates of his/her own conscience. It follows that true objection of conscience contains a lofty moral message which is an expression of human freedom in the face of human powers and laws.

If objection of conscience is not legally recognized, those who have objections find themselves in a very awkward situation, and can even find themselves subjected to various forms of discipline. Fortunately, respect for objection of conscience is on the increase in certain democratic countries, and this is sometimes even protected in law. Such legal recognition is to be welcomed. It reveals maturity in a society where fidelity to one's conscience is an important element of personal dignity and the common good. At the same time, it is also a case of public authorities showing an element of humility. Legal protection for objection of conscience must not be looked upon as a gratuitous, generous concession, or some sort of privilege or dispensation; nor should it be seen as a strategic or tactical move or a piece of political opportunism.

Regulating objection of conscience can be done in many ways. It can be guaranteed by general provisions, for example by recognizing freedom of conscience, or by introducing an express condition that contains a conscience clause covering every activity such as abortion, contraception, techniques of assisted reproduction, euthanasia and military service.

In the case of abortion, a vital element is the possible need for a prior declaration of the objector's condition. Under French law, there is no need for a prior statement to be handed to the health authorities; it is sufficient for the woman to ask for an abortion. Other legislation, such as that in force in Italy and Norway, requires prior communication to be made to the health authorities. Defenders of the first model believe that it gives better protection for the health worker's freedom and provides a better guarantee for the objector against reprisals, discrimination and threats. Those who support the second type claim that, if there are a lot of objectors, some women would not be able to do as they wish because they would fall foul of arguments that were held to be legal.

Legal recognition of objection of conscience eliminates a lot of problems for objectors, but they do not disappear altogether. Difficulties can arise in the law itself; this may be because the objection does not incorporate certain situations such as the need for intervention to save the pregnant woman's life. In other cases, objectors are subjected to unfair discrimination both at work and outside. As the Italian bishops' conference has pointed out, the dangers of discrimination which conscientious objectors encounter require a much more lively and effective spirit of solidarity both among medical and para-medical staff and in the Christian and civil communities.[24]

NOTES

1. Bishops of Ireland, 'Yes to Life' (from the pastoral letter *Human Life is Sacred*), in *Doctrine and Life*, May/June 1992, 326-335; 'The Sacredness of Human Life, Statement issued after meeting of 9-11 March 1992', in *Doctrine and Life*, May/June 1992, 345-346; Archbishops of Great Britain, 'Abortion and the Right to Life', in *Doctrine and Life*, May/June 1992, 336-344.

2. On the incidence of the use of technology in abortion, cf D. Callahan, 'How Technology Is Reframing the Abortion Debate', in *HCR* 16 (1986) no. 1, 33-42.

3. In search of common ground, see C.S. Campbell and others, 'Abortion: Searching for Common Ground', in *HCR* 19 (1989) no. 4, 23-37.

4. W.N. Clikenbeard, 'On the Trail of the Holy Humanhood', in *JME* 15 (1989) 90-91; Ch. Bernard and others, 'Le statut de l'embryon humain dans l'Antiquité gréco-romaine', in *LTP* 45 (1989) 179-195; J. Croteau, 'Le foetus humain, une personne? Essai philosophique', in *LTP* 45 (1989) 209-227; C.A. Bedate and R.C. Cefalo, 'The Zygote: to Be or not to Be a Person', in *JMPh* 14 (1989) 641-645; C. Strong and G. Anderson, 'The Moral Status of the Near-Term Fetus', in *JME* 15 (1989) 25-27; J.F. Malherbe, 'L'embryon est-il une personne humaine?', in *LV* 34 (1985) no. 172, 19-31; C.A. Tauer, 'The Tradition of Probabilism and the Moral Status of the Early Embryo', in *TS* 54 (1984) 3-33; P.A. Smith, 'The Beginning of the Personhood: A Thomistic Perspective', in *LTP* 39 (1983) 195-214.

5. Sacred Congregation for the Doctrine of Faith, *Declaration on Procured Abortion* (1974), text in A. Flannery (ed.), *Vatican Council II: more Post-Conciliar Documents*, Dominican Publications, Dublin 1984, 441-453.

6. B. Häring, 'New Dimensions of Responsible Parenthood', in *TS* 37 (1976) 127.

7. J.T. Noonan, *The Morality of Abortion. Legal and Historical Perspectives*, Harward University Press, Cambridge, Massachusetts, 1972; D. Callahan, *Abortion: Law, Choice and Morality*, MacMillan, New York 1970; F.J. Elizari, *El aborto ya es legal, ¿qué hacer ahora?*, PS, Madrid 1985; R.A. McCormick, 'Notes on Moral Theology: 1983', in *TS* 45 (1984) 119-122; A. Hortal, 'Abortion: a necessary and difficult dialogue', in *ST* 71 (1983) 19-29; M. Wreen, 'Abortion: the Extreme Liberal Position', in *JMPh* 12 (1987) 241-265; G.M. Atkinson, 'Is Abortion a Religious Issue?', in *HCR* 9 (1979) no. 1, 4 and 28; R.J. Lilford and N. Johnson, 'Surgical Abortion at Twenty Weeks: Is Morality Determined Solely by the Outcome?', in *JME* 15 (1989) 82-85.

8. Ex 21:22-23; cf J. Alonso, 'El aborto desde la Biblia', in *VN* 1367 (1983) 60-62; W.S. Kurz, 'Genesis and Abortion: An Exegetical Text of a Biblical Warrant *Ethics*', in *TS* 47 (1986) 668-670.

9. Lk 1:41-44.

10. Episcopal Commission for the Doctrine of Faith, 'Notes on Abortion', in *Ecclesia* 1712 (1974) 13. See S. Congregation for the Doctrine of Faith, *op.cit.*, no. 5.

11. See the study cited by J.T. Noonan, 1-59.

12. Sacred Congregation for the Doctrine of Faith, no. 14.

13. Ibid., no. 12.

14. J.M. Gustafson, 'A Protestant Ethical Approach', in J.T. Noonan, *op.cit.*, 101-122. For non-Catholic arguments see J. Durand, 'L'avortement thérapeutique dans le protestantisme', in *ScEc* 19 (1967) 445-464; *Abortion. An Ethical Discussion*, Church Information Service, London 1965; 'Les Luthériens des États-Unis et l'interruption de la grossesse', in *Idoc* 2 (1969) 11-16.

15. Mt 13:29f.

16. 1 Cor 5:10.

17. B. Häring, *The Law of Christ*, II, Herder, 1968, 470.

18. Standing Committee of the Italian Bishops' Conference, *Pastoral Instruction* (8 December 1978) no. 44.

19. Ibid.

20. *La législation de l'avortement dans le monde*, OMS, Geneva 1971; F.J. Elizari, *El aborto ya es legal, ¿qué hacer ahora?*, PS, Madrid 1985.

21. D. Callahan, *Abortion: Law, Choice and Morality*, MacMillan, New York 1970; W.E. May, 'Abortion, Catholic Teaching and Policy', in *LQ* 52 (1958) 38-44; P. Hannon, *Church, State, Morality and Law*, Gill & MacMillan 1992; 'The Conscience of the Voter and the Law-maker', in *Doctrine and Life*, May/June 1992, 224-252; W. Robinson, 'European Dimension of the Abortion Debate', in *Doctrine and Life*, May/June 1992, 267-281; S. Lee, 'Abortion Law: the Tragic Choices', in *Doctrine and Life*, May/June 1992, 282-297; G. Whyte, 'Abortion and the Law (Irish)', in *Doctrine and Life*, May/June 1992, 253-272.

22. See The Declaration of Belgian Bishops' Conference on 'The depenalization of abortion', in *DC* 86 (1989) 760-761.

23. F.J. Elizari, 'La objeción de conciencia en materia de aborto', in *Moralia* 5 (1983) 489-500, and in *RF* 207 (1983) 687-692.

24. Standing Committee of the Italian Bishops' Conference, *op.cit.*, no. 45.

Chapter 10

Use and donation of embryos and foetuses[1]

10.1 History

The use of embryos for reasons other than human reproduction is now very common, particularly since *in vitro* fertilization became widespread. In addition to this technique, there are new scientific and technological developments which make it possible to study, and carry out experiments on, embryos and foetuses *in vitro*. There are also various applications with embryos and foetuses following spontaneous and induced abortions.

Since the 1930s, foetal tissue has been used as the source of cell lines used in virus research and in the preparation of vaccines, particularly against poliomyelitis.

More recently, research has concentrated on transplanting foetal material into live patients for therapeutic purposes. Foetal material has three properties which appear to make it particularly interesting from the point of view of transplants. They are rapid growth, adaptability, and the fact there is very little or no immune response from the host. The three illnesses for which foetal grafting is currently part of the treatment are Parkinson's Disease, diabetes, and anaemia caused by radiation. All of this work is at an experimental stage.

It has also stimulated advances in diagnostic, preventive, therapeutic, pharmacological, scientific, industrial and clinical medicine. Sometimes, the aim of this work is beneficial for embryos and foetuses; sometimes the aim is increased knowledge and technical expertise which we will be able to take advantage of in the future. Occasionally, though, the embryos and foetuses are used as donors of tissue and organs for medical and other, less edifying, purposes. The fact that there are so many objectives has a profound influence on the moral position[1].

There is a huge range of situations for which embryos and

foetuses are used, and these situations are closely involved with moral questions. These situations include the question whether the people are alive or dead, laboratory embryos, embryos or foetuses *in vitro*, embryos and foetuses from a spontaneous or induced abortion, whether the embryos and foetuses are viable,[2] embryos created in a laboratory solely for the purposes of study and experiment, or surplus embryos of an *in vitro* fertilization intended for reproduction.

10.2 Live embryos and foetuses

Interventions on live embryos and foetuses have two objectives: the first is the health of the embryo or foetus; the second consists of other scientific, experimental and therapeutic objectives.

From the Church's standpoint, as is so often the case, research and experimentation are only admissible for the benefit of the embryo or foetus. When the objective is therapeutic, there are no moral problems as long as the following conditions are fulfilled:

– there is a possibility of making a clear and precise diagnosis;
– the illness, dysfunction or defect to be cured, prevented or diagnosed must be serious, and the prognosis a matter of urgent concern;
– intervention is essential as there is no other, more reasonable alternative available;
– there is a good chance of success (except when the risk to life is such that experimental treatment is considered legitimate);
– the doctors are suitably skilled;
– the parents have given their consent;
– the interventions must not be aiming to influence non-pathological hereditary characteristics or racial selection.[3]

Donum Vitae has pronounced thus on the subject: 'One must uphold as licit [those] procedures carried out on the human embryo which respect the life and integrity of the embryo and do not involve disproportionate risks for it but are directed towards its healing, the improvement of its condition of health, or its individual survival.'[4] On the assumption that the interventions have a therapeutic objective, even if they are experimental, if they are 'used for the benefit of the embryo itself in a final attempt to save its life, and in the absence of other reliable forms of therapy, recourse to drugs or procedures not yet fully tested can be licit.'[5]

Study and experiments whose objectives are not the health of the embryo and foetus may also be legitimate if certain conditions are met. These conditions may be difficult to achieve for the time being, but none-the-less they are as follows: there should be no risk to the embryo's life or integrity; earlier tests must have been carried out on animals; the parents must have given their informed consent; there must be no interference in non-pathological genetic inheritance; the doctors must be highly skilled, and the scientific aims must be serious, properly drawn up by their authors, and evaluated by independent, qualified and sensible bodies or individuals.

It follows that research, even if it is limited to simple observation, will not be legitimate if the methods employed or the effects brought about imply a risk to the embryo's life or physical integrity.[6] The creation of embryos in laboratories for research purposes or as donors of biological material is immoral.[7] It cannot be justified by any aim, however noble – whether it be scientific advance or their usefulness for other specified individuals or for society as a whole. Not even the informed consent of the parents makes it legitimate.

10.3 Dead embryos and foetuses resulting from spontaneous abortion

Even when the human embryo or foetus is dead, it possesses a value based on morality, and it therefore merits a form of dignified, respectful treatment which is different from that accorded to animals or to dead children or adults. The most striking difference about adults is that, while they are alive, they can give authority for their bodies to be used for scientific or therapeutic purposes for the benefit of others.

The conditions that have to be met are:

– clinical death;[8]
– an aim in accordance with respect for the embryo or foetus.

Objectives include an attempt to confirm a diagnosis *in utero*, a search for the cause of a spontaneous termination of pregnancy, a possible transplant to benefit other human beings, and scientific study and experimentation. Objectives associated with obtaining beauty products are particularly shocking to moral sensitivity;[9]
– the parents' consent.[10]

Even when these conditions are fulfilled, there are many who believe that the use of dead embryos and foetuses should be kept to a minimum.[11]

Respect for the dead embryo/foetus should have nothing to do with a position that grants greater moral value to it than to a dead child or adult.

10.4 Dead embryos and foetuses resulting from induced abortion

On the face of it, one might imagine that the cause of death should be irrelevant to the donation of a dead person's organs or tissue for medical purposes, as long as the aim of the medical intervention did not lead to the death in the first place. However, it is not as straightforward as that.

There are two main reasons why some people are opposed to the use of tissue or organs from dead embryos and foetuses resulting from induced abortion. They are the connection between the abortion and an intention to acquire embryos and foetuses, and the link between the use of this material and the fact that the abortion was carried out at all.[12] They think that abortions could be encouraged which would not otherwise have taken place. According to other reports, there are women who have announced they are prepared to have an abortion in order to give foetal tissue to specified recipients. There are even people who believe that these practices can succeed in encouraging pregnancies (with subsequent abortion and intention to transplant) which would otherwise not have come about.

A number of measures are proposed to avoid such links being established. They include not allowing women who abort to profit in any way from the abortion, preventing the doctors who carry out the abortion from deriving any advantage, and, therefore, insisting on complete independence between the doctors carrying out the abortion and those involved in the transplant. The decision to abort should be made independently of the possible use of tissues or organs, and taken prior to discussion on this. Nor should the timing and method of abortion be influenced by therapeutic needs. Even when these conditions are met, there will still be those who consider it unacceptable to use bodies that have been the victims of human irresponsibility. Lastly, some people point out the risk that induced abortions can be presented as spontaneous.

[*Editor's note*: For the use of foetal ovarian material in the treatment of infertility, see appendix to chapter 4, p. 87.]

NOTES

1. Recommendation 1100 of the Council of Europe, 'On the use of embryos and human fetuses', in *MM* 39 (1989) 404-411; Official English Text, Ibid., 397-404; Medical Centre Committee on Ethics (Stanford), 'The Ethical Use of Human Fetal Tissue in Medicine', in *NEJM* 320 (1989) 1093-1096; G.J. Annas and S. Elias, 'The Politics of Transplantation of Human Fetal Tissue', in *NEJM* 320 (1989) 1079-1082; J.A. Robertson, 'Rights, Symbolism, and Public Policy in Fetal Tissue Transplant', in *HCR* 18 (1988) no. 6, 5-12; K. Nolan, 'Genug Ist Genug: A Fetus Is Not a Kidney', in *HCR* 18 (1988) no. 6, 13-19; A. Fine, 'The Ethics of Fetal Tissue Transplants', in *HCR* 18 (1988) no. 3, 5-8; 'Report on the use of embryonic tissues for therapeutic, diagnostic and scientific purposes', National Ethical Commission for life and health matters, in *LH* 209 (1988) 222-223; M.B. Mahowald and others, 'The Ethical Options in Transplanting Fetal Tissue', in HCR 17 (1987) no. 1, 9-15; H.-M. Sass, 'Moral Dilemmas in Perinatal Medicine and the Quest for Large Scale Embryo Research: A Discussion of Recent Guidelines in the Federal Republic of Germany', in *JMPh* 12 (1987) 279-290; Recommendation 1100 of the Council of Europe, 'On the use of embryos and human fetuses', in *Il Regno* 32 (1987) 250-251; H. Caton, 'The Ethics of Human Embryo Experimentation', in *LQ* 54 (1987) 24-42; R.M.L. Winston, 'Why a Ban on Embryo Research Would Be a Tragedy', in *BMJ* 295 (1987) 1501-1502; A.P. Cole, 'The Issue of Human Embryo Research', in *CMQ* 38 (1987) 16-20; Bishops' Conferences of England and Wales and Scotland, *The Duty to defend the embryo*; T. Phipps, 'Embryo Experimentation. An Ethical Examination', in *CM* 38 (1987) 50-55; J. Brown, 'Research on Human Embryos. A justification', in *JME* 12 (1986) 201-205; C. Grobstein, 'The Moral Uses of "Spare" Embryos', in *HCR* 12 (1982) no. 3, 5-6.

2. Viability, as applied to the embryo, means the absence of biological characteristics likely to hinder development. The non-viability of embryos or foetuses has to be determined exclusively with objective biological criteria based on intrinsic defects. See *Recommendation 1100* of the Council of Europe, appendix 1-3.

3. See *Recommendation 1046* of the Council of Europe, appendix b), 1.2.4.5.

4. *Donum Vitae,* I, 3.

5. Ibid., I, 4.

6. Ibid.

7. Ibid., I, 5.

8. In this respect, it is necessary to differentiate between total death (clinical and cellular) and partial death (after clinical death, cells, tissues, and organs can survive). See *Recommendation 1100,* no. 15.

9. *Recommendation 1046* of the Council of Europe (1986), requests an investigation into 'the rumours circulating among the media into the sale of embryos and dead fetuses and the publication of the results', no. 14, a. 1.

10. The culmination of this condition can result in spontaneous abortion; the petition for its authorization could perhaps be deemed inopportune.

11. *Recommendation 1046,* appendix b, 6.

12. C. Gorman, 'A Balancing Act of Life and Death', in *Time* (1-2-1988) 49; E. Thorne, 'Trade in Human Tissue Needs Regulation', in *Wall Street Journal* (19-8-1987) 3.

Chapter 11

Handicapped newborns[1]

Scientific and technical advances in neonatal care mean that many
human beings now survive whereas, only a few decades ago, they
would have died in a matter of days, months or years. At one time,
doctors and families had no alternative but to accept the inevitable;
nowadays, barriers that were hitherto insurmountable have been
overcome, although there are still many that remain impracticable
or present major difficulties. Progress has provided a solution for
many problems, and has stimulated many others. In many cases,
individuals can benefit from treatment; in others, there is no point
in making any effort to save their lives – and in the middle there is
a grey area where decisions are far from clear. Prognosis is
frequently difficult, and it is not at all uncommon for there to be an
element of urgency. This explains why decisions are so complex.

There is now an additional problem – that of children with
severe and permanent physical or mental abnormalities which
may or may not involve a risk to their lives. These young people
occasionally have a problem which endangers their lives, and this
may or may not be curable with the right treatment. Sometimes
they are refused a form of treatment that is used on children with
no handicap at all; the explanation given is simply that these
children do have a handicap.

The situation is therefore very confused from both a medical and
a moral standpoint. Laws, courts and morals have attempted to
provide a solution to these problems; I will confine myself basically
to moral considerations and only a few excursions into other fields.

Ethical debates on kinds of treatment designed to keep seriously ill newborns alive began in the 1970s. They took place first
among health professionals, and later on among moralists, jurists
and families, and in the media and parliaments. Attention focused
on just two groups of sufferers: mentally handicapped children
who needed surgery to save their lives by correcting fatal physical

problems, and children with spina bifida. Whether the latter were operated on or not, either they would die soon or they would live on with severe disorders and, even if they were operated on in time, they would survive with physical and/or mental handicaps of some type.

There are two big questions to deal with, one to do with the background information, the other to do with procedure. The first concerns the indications and criteria used for taking decisions; the second relates to the people who are responsible for that decision. From a moral point of view, the first question is more important by far.

We need to know what the indications are, so let us start by enumerating the values involved in such cases. In the first place, there is the child's life (how long it has survived and in what conditions). The family and society also have interests, but of very different magnitudes. The arrival of the newborn may appear to be a very positive thing for the family, but there is also a negative side involving economic problems, deterioration of the couple's relationship and so on. In our society, great emphasis is laid on how much handicapped people cost; on the other hand, there is a danger of devaluing the concept of humanity and taking risks, especially on behalf of the weakest members of society. Some people with an interest in eugenics draw attention to the fact that there is a danger for the human species in an excessive number of handicapped people.

So much for the values and interests. Let us now move on to some indications:

– no handicapped person should be denied, just because of his/her handicap, the appropriate amount of reasonable means and resources that are considered right for children with no handicap. Anything else would amount to morally indefensible discrimination;

– nor should such treatment be withheld for institutional or administrative reasons;

– the family's inability to cope with the situation satisfactorily does not justify the refusal of interventions that are considered 'normal'. Society must demonstrate its solidarity in situations like this, and there must be no reduction in respect for life simply because of the family's economic or emotional difficulties;

– there can be different complications arising from mental handicap which justify the failure to use treatment that might be given to non-handicapped patients. In such a case, there would be no discrimination;

– if the treatment only serves to prolong life for a short period of time, reducing it or stopping it would not present any moral problems;

– if the treatment might extend life for a longer period of time, and this will involve repeated, difficult and problematic interventions with poor prospects of recovery, failure to use the treatment would not be irrational.

When a decision is being taken whether it is sensible to proceed with a given form of treatment, thought has to be given to the same issues that are looked at in other cases. These are the type of therapy, the degree of complexity and the risks, the cost, how easy the application is, and the likelihood of success – in fact, everything that concerns the patient's condition and resilience.

This area is varied and complicated, and decisions sometimes have to be taken very urgently. In these circumstances, there are no procedures or indications that can substitute for the good sense of those involved in deciding; nor can these procedures take the place of these people's responsibilities. By the same token, it is impossible to eliminate completely the uncertainties, doubts, conflicts and tensions involved. There is inevitably a margin for error.

As for those who have to take the decisions, a number of solutions have been proposed by courts and some writers. Some see the decision as the parents' exclusive responsibility; this is presumably on the grounds that they are best placed to see to the child's well-being, and above all it is they who have to accept the consequences if they decide to try and save his/her life. There is sometimes the danger that they place their interests above those of the child, or else a false sense of guilt encourages them to demand everything possible for their child.

Others give the parents the first and most decisive word, but not the only word as they may counterpose their interests to those of the child. There needs to be, therefore, a quick way of getting a court ruling. Then there are those who see the decision as purely medical and hand it over entirely to health professionals; it is difficult to go along with this view, even though the medical implications cannot be denied. There is also a need to build in issues relating to the origin, destiny and meaning of life and death.

Given the social and cultural values of the society in which we live, I think the decision basically has to be that of the parents, as long as they receive the relevant medical information and psychological counselling. Hospital ethics committees can be of tremendous help both to families and to doctors, as long as the decisions are not urgent. Recourse to the courts should be kept to a minimum, particularly when the family members are divided or when their opinion not to go for medical treatment is clearly opposed by medical opinion.

None of these decisions guarantees a correct moral position, whoever takes the decision. For that reason, I believe that, from a moral standpoint, the person who has to take the decision should consider all these alternatives. What is important is that the criteria should be the right ones and the situation correctly assessed, irrespective of who is taking the decision.

NOTES

1. T.A. Long, 'Infanticide for Handicapped Infants: Sometimes It's a Metaphysical Dispute', in *JME* 14 (1988) 79-81; D.D. Raphael, 'Handicapped Infants: Medical Ethics and the Law', in *JME* 14 (1988) 5-10; M.A. Gardell, 'Jane, Bioethics and the Supreme Court', in *JMPh* 11 (1986) 285-290; K.M. Mason and D.W. Meyers, 'Parental Choice and Selective Non-Treatment of Deformed Newborns: A View from Mid-Atlanta', in *JME* 12 (1986) 67-71; Pro-Life Commission of the US Bishops' Conference and Pro-Life Commission of American Jewish Congress, 'Principles in the treatment of handicapped newborns', in *MM* 35 (1985) 819-822; B.V. Johnstone, 'The Sanctity of Life, the Quality of Life and the New Baby Doe Law', in *LQ* 52 (1985) 258-270; W.G. Bartholome and J. Arras, 'Imperiled Newborns Raise Moral Doubts', in *HCR* 15 (1985) no. 1, 46-47; K. Kipnis and G.M. Williamson, 'Nontreatment Decisions for Severely Compromised Newborns', in *Ethics* 95 (1984) 90-111; Commission for the Study of Ethical Problems in Medicine and Biomedical Research, *Deciding to Forego Life-Sustaining Treatment*, Washington 1983, 197-299 and 467-492; C. Gillespie, 'Letting Die Severely Handicapped Children', in *JME* 9 (1983) 231; R.A. McCormick, 'Notes on Moral Theology: 1982', in *TS* 44 (1983) 71-122; 'Withholding Treatment in Infancy', in *BMJ* 282 (1981) 925-926; R.C. Coburn, 'Morality and the Defective Newborn', in *JMPh* 5 (1980) 340-357; J.K. Mason and R.A. McCall-Smith, *Law and Medical Ethics* (1991), ch. 7, 'Neonaticide and selective non-treatment of the new born', 150-159.

Chapter 12
Genetic engineering[1]

12.1 Ideas

The term genetic engineering is used in very different contexts. Used inappropriately, the term is applied to processes, ancient and modern, in the cultivation of plants and animals; to assisted reproduction; and sometimes, also, to prenatal diagnosis and genetic screening.

Used appropriately, it is understood to mean the amalgamation of techniques which permit intervention in genetic information, at the level of the molecular structures and mechanisms involved in the transmission of inheritance.

Genetic engineering presupposes a knowledge of the chemical and physical properties of DNA (deoxyribonucleic acid), and depends on the techniques used for intervention in this field. DNA is the repository of biological specificity and individuality. It is found in the nucleus of chromosomes, of which each non-germ cell has 23 pairs. It is a chain which takes the form of a helix with an additional double strand. It is the chemical equivalent of genes; and the gene is a fragment of DNA that contains all the information relative to a protein. A human being has some 100,000 genes.

12.2 Technology[2]

The advent of molecular biology and an increasingly accurate knowledge of the structure and function of genes has facilitated the design of various techniques which can be used to manipulate and alter the genetic inheritance of living cells.

Micro-techniques mean that fertilized eggs and foreign genes can be inserted into the nuclei of cells. In this way, the information contained in these genes can be incorporated into the individual who develops from the egg cell, thus ensuring that it will be passed on to descendants. This is a completely artificial technique with no parallel in nature.

On the other hand, cellular fusion can occur all by itself, and is much more common in germ cells than in somatic cells. It can also arise artificially as a result of the fusing of the cellular membranes of neighbouring cells, thus forming a hybrid – that is, a new cell with a hybrid chromosomal endowment. This technique has been used to produce monoclonal antibodies.

The most commonly used technique is the recombination of DNA. This entails the production of hybrid DNA molecules by means of inserting DNA fragments from other organisms into host bacterial cells.

This artificial procedure does have its corollary in nature. Without any artificial interference, bacteria spontaneously transfer DNA to one another through processes known as conjugation and transduction. In conjugation, bacteria fuse temporarily and one of them (donor) transfers part of its DNA to the other. The passing on of genetic material is carried out directly by one bacterium to another. In transduction, a virus acts as a mediator: the bacterium transfers part of its DNA to the infecting virus. This then incorporates it for subsequent transfer to another bacterium. This procedure, then, comprises bacterium-virus-bacterium.

For a better understanding of the formation of recombinant DNA, or the formation of a molecule of DNA with a foreign gene, let us take as an example the gene for human insulin. Core elements of a bacterium which colonizes the human intestine, *Escherichia coli*, are cultured in the laboratory. Plasmids (small circular strands of DNA in the cytoplasm) are extracted from the bacteria and through means of restriction enzymes, the plasmid is cut at a determined site. For the other component, DNA containing the gene for human insulin is extracted from the pancreas, and, using restriction enzymes, this gene is separated out and incorporated into the plasmid. The new hybrid enzyme, which now contains the gene for human insulin, is introduced into the *Escherichia coli* cells, which will now produce human insulin. Given that the plasmids have a replicative mechanism that is independent of the bacterial cell, within a very short space of time there will be a huge number of hybrid plasmids; and the rapidity with which bacteria reproduce ensures that a vast quantity of human insulin will also be rapidly produced.

The applications of recombinant DNA are manifold and can be used in all sorts of ways, as we shall see.

12.3 Pharmacological applications

The pharmaceutical industry has been among the first to take advantage of the advances made in genetic engineering. These results have been made possible thanks to the extremely high rate at which bacteria reproduce. In less than 15 hours, and in suitable conditions, one bacterium is capable of reproducing itself 1000 million times. In this way the preparation of a vast quantity of product from a rare source represents significant savings on costs – a saving made possible because the technology, once developed, will not lead to increased costs. Furthermore, this line of production has another advantage: quality, the high level of purity of the product, and consequently, its greater therapeutic efficacy.

Human insulin – Compared with the insulin derived from the pancreas of slaughtered pigs and cattle, which used to be used in the treatment of diabetes, that produced by genetically manipulated bacteria represents huge advantages in terms of quality, quantity and costs.

Human growth hormone – This hormone is only produced by the brain; as a result, the only source was human cadavers. It was thus both scarce and expensive. This hormone is much more biochemically complex than human insulin and is used in the treatment of dwarfism with pituitary deficiency, bone fractures, for regrowth of the skin after burns, and for ulcers, etc.

Human interferons – Interferon is a protein which regulates the body's immune response to viral infections and the abnormal proliferation of malignant cells. Derived from blood, its natural production requires extremely expensive procedures for a small quantity. Genetic engineering can substantially increase production whilst keeping costs low.

Production of vaccines and other substances – This includes factor VIII for blood coagulation in the treatment of haemophilia, etc.

12.4 Uses in ecology and agriculture

Nitrogen fixation – Nitrogen is found in the atmosphere: plants need this for their development, but none of them can convert it unaided. This is done by micro-organisms in the soil or by feeding plants nitrogen-enriched fertilizers. Biotechnology enables plants to extract the nitrogen they need from the atmosphere with the consequent saving in fertilizers.

Creation of crops – capable of growing in saline and acid soils.

Hydrogen production – by biophotolysis.

Ecology – A great deal of pollution comes from non-biodegradable materials and chemical effluents produced by many different industries. Given the rate at which these harmful products accumulate, nature is unable to eliminate them. The solution would lie in genetically transformed bacteria, capable of breaking down and destroying crude residues.

Frost-resistant strawberries – sprayed with a bacterium from which the genetic material, corresponding to the protein which favours the formation of frost in leaves, has been removed.

12.5 Uses in animals

Gene grafting has succeeded in correcting some hereditary diseases in animals. In 1982 this process allowed the normal red colour in the eyes of vinegar flies to be restored. In 1984 rats with hereditary dwarfism had this condition corrected with injections of the gene for rat growth. In 1985 an inherited defect in rats was corrected.

12.6 Ethics of genetic engineering in subhuman species

Genetic engineering carried out on subhuman species – plants and animals – does not raise objections, in principle, if done within reason and with a sense of responsibility. After all, technological possibility alone does not constitute a moral issue. And to speed up artificially the evolutionary process using this technology does not create profound ethical problems either. On the other hand, we must not forget, when we create new species, the interdependence of ecosystems and the holistic nature of the biosphere. Intervention necessitates that we are mindful of these facts without imposing absolute limitations on what can be done. It has already been pointed out that we run the risk of reducing and impoverishing the rich variety of species in order to pursue our utilitarian ends. This is a real danger, but we must also bear in mind that genetic engineering is capable of increasing the variety of species.

The many advantages which the various applications of genetic engineering offer mankind mean that we must always bear the aforementioned aspects in mind, and that the techniques themselves provide sufficient assurance – that is, that there will be no risks of a serious uncontrollable epidemic because of mistakes made during genetic manipulation, fears, which, for the moment, appear to be unfounded.

12.7 Human genetic engineering[3]

Genetic engineering can change radically if it is focused directly on the human body. To untangle the different strands, we must differentiate between gene therapy (directed to correcting a disease or defect) and genetic improvement or perfective genetic engineering (the aim of which is to enhance by creating physical or mental features which we consider to be desirable). In both categories, we need to distinguish between what is feasible in germ cells (eggs, sperm) or in early stage embryos, and what actually happens in other cells in the human body – known, respectively, as germ cell and somatic cell genetic engineering.

Taking the two criteria together, ends achieved (treatment or enhancement) and the object of the intervention, the cells (germ or somatic) there are four possible options: genetic germ cell treatment, somatic cell treatment, genetic germ cell enhancement and somatic cell enhancement.

a. Technical possibilities

This is an area which is entirely subject to technological advances, and so the outlook is very changeable. The proven or

anticipated benefits to mankind and pressing economic concerns
have acted in concert to stimulate this extremely promising field
of investigation, which, on the other hand, has to surmount
technical difficulties. I shall refer to those achievements already
made, even though these may be in the early stages in some
cases, or to hopes which can expect to be realized within the
near future.

The first application for recombinant therapy used retroviruses,
and was approved by reputable North American organizations
on 19 January 1989. With the aim of achieving a better understanding of new treatments for cancer, cells which fight this
disease were targeted. Experiments had already been conducted
for some time in which cancerous cells had been taken from a
patient, submitted to a particular treatment, and then reinserted
into the patient's body. This technique was successful in 50 out
of every 100 cases, but once reinserted, it was impossible to
continue monitoring the progress of these cells, and to discover
why some worked while others did not. In an attempt to study
their progress in the blood and in the tumour cells, these cells
were tagged with a vector (a virus that transfers genetic material
from one cell to another). In this way, it is hoped that new
treatments for cancer will be discovered.

Other uses are also likely within the next few years, particularly those diseases attributable to a single gene – mono-
genetic disorders, such as adenosine deaminase deficiency, the
illness which affects 'bubble children', and haemophilia, etc.
Among the objectives for treatment are certain types of cancer,
viral illnesses like AIDS, and some types of cardiovascular
disorders.

Somatic cell therapy eliminates many obstacles and opens up
many possibilities for perfective genetic engineering or somatic
enhancement from a technological point of view. But not all the
technological difficulties will be overcome and some ethical problems will inevitably result.

As for germ cell therapy (gametes or early stage embryos), it
is highly unlikely that this type of technology will be in clinical
use for several years yet. But once this step has been successfully taken, then perfective germ cell engineering will not be far
behind.

b. Moral values[4]

Let us begin with somatic gene therapy. This type of therapy creates permanent and intrinsic modifications in the body, unlike other treatments which require the repeated administration of an external substance, and so, in a certain way, is similar to organ transplantation which requires the integration of foreign DNA. Mindful of these features, there is no cause for moral reservations, so long as the intention is the good of the patient. It presupposes the existence of a serious illness for which there is no better alternative treatment. As with any other form of treatment, informed consent must be obtained from the patient concerned, or in the event of their not being physically capable of giving their consent, from a person who is responsible for them.

Germ cell therapy usually refers to early stage embryo manipulation, and it throws up rather more tricky issues than somatic cell therapy. There would be no good reason to oppose it by claiming a special sanctity for human gametes, or in thinking that we are on a slippery slope, and that once the boundary had been crossed, there would be no going back. We have to trust in the fact that human beings are capable of setting themselves limits and of acting responsibly. If intervention falls back on the embryo, the fundamental principle is to respect its dignity.

As to perfective or enhancing genetic engineering, if it is somatic, there are fewer medical and ethical problems to be faced. At the moment, such renowned scientists as W. French Anderson see in it a threat to 'important human values in two ways: first, it could be risky medically, and that the risk might outweigh the potential benefits, and might even cause harm; secondly, it could produce moral uncertainties – that's to say, it would require ethical decisions to be taken which our society is not prepared to take, and which could lead to greater inequalities and an increase in discriminatory practices.'[5]

There is a difference between treatment and enhancement. Although the introduction of a normal gene to correct a defective one will probably not create any greater problems than exist already, we do not as yet know if such a procedure in a normal person, for the purposes of enhancement, might not produce important alterations in the functioning of the affected cells. It is here that the risks could outweigh the advantages.

Apart from the potential medical dangers, certain aspects would need to be clarified: which genes would be considered desirable; on what criteria would such an opinion be based? Who would be nominated as suitable candidates; what criteria would be used to determine candidacy to avoid discrimination between those who receive a certain gene and those who are precluded from receiving it?

NOTES

1. M. Lappé, 'The Limits of Genetic Inquiry', in *HCR* 17 (1987) no. 4, 5-10; President's Commission for the Study of Ethical Problems in Medicine and Biomedical and Behavioral Research, *Splicing Life: A Report on the Social and Ethical Issues of Genetic Engineering and Human Beings*, U.S. Government Printing Office, Washington 1982; R.F. Chadwick, *Ethics, Reproduction and Genetic Control*, Croom Helm, London 1987; J. Glover, *What sort of People Should There Be?*, Penguin, London 1984; E.K. Nichols, *Human Gene Therapy*, Harvard U.P., Cambridge, Mass and London 1988; T.E. Kelly, *Clinical Genetics and Genetic Councelling*, Year Book Medical Publishers, London 2nd edn 1986; European Parlament, Committee on Legal Affairs and Citizen's Rights, *Ethical and Legal Problems of Genetic Engineering and Human Artificial Insemination*, Luxembourg 1990.
2. C. Alonso Bedate, 'Biologia molecular y transferencia del ADN', in *LH* 214 (1989) 255-270; L. Hood, 'Biotechnology and Medicine of the Future', in *JAMA* 259 (1988) 1837-1844.
3. W.F. Anderson and others, *Human Gene Therapy. Preclinical Data Document*, Government Printing Office, Washington 1987; Id., 'Genetics and Human Malleability', in *HCR* 20 (1990) no. 1, 21-24.
4. W.F. Anderson, 'Human genetherapy: why define limits', in *LH* 214 (1989) 298-302; B.V. Johnstone, 'Genetic technology: historical-moral perspective', in *Moralia* 11 (1989) 297-314; F. Abel, 'Genetic engineering and bioethics', in *LH* 214 (1989) 250-254; 'Resolution of the European Parliament on the ethical problems and judicial issues of genetic engineering', in *LH* 214 (1989) 336-339; C.K. Boone, *Bad Axioms in Genetic Engineering*, in *HCR* 18 (1988) no. 4, 9-13; K. Nolan and S. Swenson, 'New Tools, New Dilemmas: Genetic Frontiers', in *HCR* 18 (1988) 5, 40-46; World Council of Churches, *Manipulating Life. Ethical Issues in Genetic Engineering*, Geneva 1982.
5. W. French Anderson, *op.cit.*, 299.

Chapter 13

Mapping and sequencing of the human genome[1]

The mapping and sequencing of all the genetic information of a human being is a unique piece of biological cartography, and is without question the most ambitious project ever dreamt up by biologists. By identifying human genes and establishing the sequencing of their nucleotides, a stimulus will be provided for several major advances for the well-being of humanity; they will make it possible for medicine to diagnose, and possibly treat, genetic illnesses or, at least, prevent them.

It appears that the first person to propose such a vast programme was R. Dulbecco in 1986. The scientific community mobilized rapidly around the suggestion, although the idea attracted comments from some and powerful reservations from others. At the present moment, opinions that are favourable to the project are clearly in the ascendant, although they lack the messianic fervour that characterized the early days.

There seem to be three geographical areas that are covered in the 'human genome' project – the United States, Europe and Japan. The huge financial cost (it is thought to be in the region of $3000,000), the technical complexity and the need for highly skilled staff have meant that the project was too much for the resources of a single country. HUGO (the Human Genome Organisation) was set up in Montreux, Switzerland at a meeting held on 6-7 September 1988 and is responsible for international co-ordination of the research. The objectives are to establish the location and sequencing of all the genes in the human body, and to do so by the end of the first decade of the twenty-first century. The results will fill an encyclopaedia of 1000 volumes, each volume being of 1000 pages, and each page containing 1000 words. This information will tell us the position of around 100,000 human genes and the sequencing of the three billion nucleotides that make up the genes and govern the production of proteins.

The project has attracted a wide range of objections. They include the assertion that it lacks significant scientific interest, the claim that money has been siphoned off from more interesting biological activities, the alleged inadequacy of science in general for advances of this sort (on the grounds that the work of relatively small groups is more effective), and the absence of the right type of technology to put the project into practice. There have also been some ethical issues raised.

Benefits to be derived from the project include the identifying of the genes that cause genetic illnesses and of the majority of genes involved in the development of the human body, the development of new technology related to recombinant DNA, and the opportunity to study the complex physiological changes that occur in cell differentiation.

Discussion around the project now centres equally on its scientific interest and the ethical repercussions. It is thought that the flow of information will be so colossal that it will be difficult to retain control of it. Furthermore, in view of the genetic variety of human beings, there is some doubt that the information obtained from a handful of individuals will provide us with adequate information.

From an ethical point of view, it has been observed that there is a danger in reducing human beings to a mere sequencing of four codes, and there have been questions about whether the project could be used to alter genetic inheritance or patent human genes. Moreover, there are fears that it is a small number of countries practising a form of scientific and technological colonization of all the other countries, and of the danger that the whole thing is dominated by economic interests.

The danger of neo-colonialism in science was raised by Pope John Paul II in his address of 10 November 1979 to the Pontifical Academy of Sciences. He said on that occasion that basic science is a universal good which all peoples must have the opportunity to cultivate, free from any form of international pressure or intellectual colonialism. He said he did not really believe that, in the competitive field of biotechnology, the less developed countries were going to be able to match the impressive momentum achieved by more powerful countries like the United States, Japan, Germany, Great Britain, Switzerland and France. On the other hand, he wondered whether less developed countries really had to throw in the towel and allow themselves to be colonized scientifically, technically and commercially. He speculated that they should try not to lose their own momentum, even if it meant making an economic effort that was out of proportion to their resources.[2]

Apart from the problem of fair distribution of resources, there has been plenty of debate around the real potential for predictive and preventive medicine to be derived from the human genome project, and around the consequences for the project. Those who defend the project argue from the premise that all illnesses have genetic components, however small – that is to say we all have a genetic predisposition to have particular illnesses in the course of our lives. The mapping and sequencing of the human genome would allow us to identify the genes that are responsible for our susceptibility to certain illnesses. DNA probes would make it possible to diagnose which illnesses one was likely to have later on in life. This diagnosis would suggest preventive action in the form of hygiene, diet and medication, and it is thought there could thereby be great savings for social security. Cardiovascular diseases and cancer would be the areas to be treated first by this medicine.

Such an optimistic view is not shared by others, who harbour ethical and social fears. There are those who maintain that predictive and preventive medicine is nothing but sheer utopianism. Is it possible, they ask, at a distance of, say, 20 years, to predict the likelihood of somebody catching an illness and then to prescribe the right medicine? Nobody denies that it is possible to identify a defective gene, but how do we know which people will get ill? Apart from the genes, we need to know the environmental factors necessary for the illness to establish itself; we still do not know exactly which those factors are that have to converge (at the same time as the genetic cause) for the illness to erupt. Forecasting each person's medical future may be little more than sheer fantasy.

For predictive medicine to be useful, it will have to produce effective prescriptive indications at a preventive stage. However, such prediction involves prescriptions relating to hygiene, diet and medication for the whole of one's life, and the person concerned would thereby be turned into a patient for the rest of his/her days. Would social security save money that way, or would costs simply mount up elsewhere? Is it not utopian to expect people to impose a lifestyle on themselves for 20 years, when the results of campaigns against tobacco (when we know exactly what the danger is) are so ineffective? Preventive medicine, not just predictive medicine, would be a mistake.

This kind of medicine could be used to carry out diagnoses of people's susceptibility to disease in certain industrial environments, and thereby produce categories of workers who would be excluded from certain jobs – so-called 'work lepers'. These discoveries could also be used to classify people according to various characteristics – suitability for intellectual and other kinds of work, or a predisposition to mental illness. This information could shape exclusive attitudes and deny these people access to particular forms of education simply because certain genes had been detected. We would then be in a position to control and guide people because of their genes. In short, we would have a society based on genetic classification. We would be generating a new form of eugenics.

None-the-less, despite its ambiguities and uncertainties, the project is attracting enormous support. Let us hope that the dangers listed above will be avoided by the skills and good sense of responsibility of the people involved. It is also to be hoped that there will be compensations for the dangers in the shape of benefits for humanity, and that there will be no manipulation of people, particularly those who are already most discriminated against. A word in favour of the project as a whole appears in recommendations adopted by delegates attending the 1988 Rome Bioethics Summit.[3] There are no intrinsic limits to the acquisition of knowledge about the human genome, and there should be no attempt to dilute encouragement being given to this field of research. For the project to achieve success, though, there will be have to be concerted efforts at both national and international levels. The publication and use of reports on the structure of the genome and other genetic information must respect the rights and interests of the individuals and groups from whom the information has been obtained. This will be a way of ensuring self-determination, confidentiality, and non-discrimination. The use of genetic therapy of somatic cells for specific genetic illnesses has to be assessed by using the same criteria as for other experimental treatments, such as effectiveness, safety, consent and confidentiality. As for interventions on germ cells, there are at present no medical indications or ethical justifications for intentional genetic manipulation. As for the training programmes around the human genome, we will have to rely on the assistance of ethics committees in education, on careful deliberation and on the development of sound policies. It is essential to explore and debate the following points that have been raised on the subject of the human genome project:

- the prediction of risks;
- screening;
- future diagnostic methods;
- the setting up of DNA banks for the study of family pedigree based on the genetic history of peoples and human illness;
- applicability and adequacy of patents and copyright.

NOTES

1. R. Smith, 'The Race for the Human Genome', in *BMJ* 297 (1988) 577; L. Hood, 'Biotechnology and medicine of the Future', in *JAMA* 259 (1988) 1837-1844; 'Mapping the Human Genome', in *Lancet*, 16 May (1987) 1121-1122; A.M. Capron, 'The Rome Bioethics Summit', in *HCR* 18 (1988) no. 4, Spec. Suppl. 11-13.
2. *AAS* 71 (1979) 1462.
3. A.M. Capron, *op.cit.*

PART III

The final phase of life

Chapter 14
Death

In the past, the final phase of a human being's life was very uncomplicated from a moral point of view. In our present day society, thanks to technical developments, advances in medicine and certain aspects of our culture, the last stage of life is now the subject of much moral reflection, and also presents some of the most difficult decisions in the practice of medicine.

From an ethical standpoint, there appear to be three important questions:

- the desire for a dignified, humane death, something that is increasingly accepted by certain sectors of our society;
- euthanasia;
- the use or rejection of extraordinary, disproportionate or unreasonable means to prolong life.

These three central themes are preceded by two more issues: what it is like to die these days within the socio-cultural framework of our society, and the notion of clinical death.

14.1 Dying nowadays[1]

Although it is often said that death is a great leveller, and in a very real sense that is true, the world offers us a wide range of images about death and the process leading up to it. Even within a given geographical area, death has a wide range of different qualities that vary from one historical period to the next. These days, death takes place in a variety of different settings according to what part of the world we happen to be in. Here I am going to confine myself to a consideration of what we call developed western society, and briefly indicate some of the characteristics of this society in the process leading up to death. Quite a large number of the changes that have come about in connection with death, apart from its medical sense, have thrown up a number of human problems and also pose certain moral questions.

Cause of death has changed enormously since the beginning of the twentieth century. In the early years of the century, there were numerous infectious or contagious diseases such as influenza, pneumonia and tuberculosis; today, death is more frequently caused by cardiovascular disease, cancer and road accidents, and chronic and degenerative illnesses are also on the increase.

Death also comes later these days, and it finds people at a stage in their lives when they are needy and very dependent. Thanks to technical progress and better health care, death also comes more slowly. To put it in another way, the process of dying is getting longer. People are also beginning to die in different places: we die at home much less often than we used to, and tend to finish our days in institutions or clinics, far from the familiar settings in which we have spent our lives.

Nowadays, the road leading to death is much more controlled by technology, and this is particularly so of time spent in intensive care units. The climate surrounding the final stages of life is also much more dehumanized than before, and it is also becoming less and less common for a priest to be in attendance. People's attitudes have become more conscious and well formulated; they say that dying is a more human affair, and that they are entitled to more independence in the decisions they take around that time.[2]

These days, society appears to be keen to conceal death from the person who is dying. This trend is extremely common in Europe, but has no parallel in North America where little is hidden from the patient. The personal feelings of health professionals have a strong influence on which way it goes. These attitudes of our society during the period leading up to death have had a lot to do with changes in moral attitudes to dying.

14.2 Clinical death[3]

In clinical death, we have a concept of death that enables us to pin-point as precisely as possible the moment it takes place, and this raises a large number of social and personal questions. Perhaps the most pertinent issue from a medical standpoint concerns transplants, although that is by no means the whole story.

The death of a human being is a complex reality which we can look at from a variety of angles – religious, philosophical, medical, legal, economic and socio-cultural. Let us take a closer look at clinical death. For a long time, the popular view and the professional medical position of clinical death were the same: a person died when s/he stopped breathing and his/her heart stopped beating. These signs were easily detectable, and their validity was not in doubt.

Scientific and technical advances then demonstrated how difficult it was to say that a person's clinical death was the same thing as the respiratory and circulatory functions coming to a halt. For one thing, thanks to resuscitation techniques, it is now possible to restore heartbeat when the heart has spontaneously stopped beating. For another, technology even enables us to stop the heart deliberately in order to carry out an operation – and then get it to function normally afterwards.

All this has forced us to give serious thought to the scientific validity of traditional indicators. Medical experts have gradually come round to identifying clinical death with the irreversible cessation of cerebral activity. An important step in this direction was taken by P. Mollaret and M. Goulon in 1959[4], but the most decisive impetus was provided by a report produced by the Harvard Medical School in 1968.[5] Since then, contributions from scientists all over the world have clarified the criteria and tests used to certify irreversible cessation of cerebral activity. However, although there is substantial agreement on many points, there is still significant dissent, for example in respect of anencephalic newborns, foetuses and small children.

Identifying a person's clinical death on the basis that the brain has irreversibly stopped functioning does not necessarily mean that there has to be somebody observing the brain with the help of special equipment. In most cases, death is a slow process. The various organs and systems that support life begin to fail and stop working at different times; it is exceptional for death to be instantaneous and sudden, or almost instantaneous. Brain death, on the other hand, normally comes about as a result of successive organic failures. Otherwise, any doctor is qualified to certify brain death and the person's death without needing to pronounce on the functioning of the brain.

There are three models of legislation in existence:

– laws that set out two alternative definitions of clinical death, the classical and modern, and leave it to the doctor to choose;
– laws that establish the classical definition as the main one, and leave the modern definition for special cases (e.g. when the respiratory and circulatory functions are being artificially maintained);
– laws that accept brain death to the exclusion of all other definitions.

Of these three, the third is the most common.[6]

14.3 A dignified death[7]

Support for the idea of a dignified death represents not only a moral victory, but increased concern for a dignified and humane life. In our culture, this new attitude is slowly gaining ground, although the rate of progress varies from one part of the world to the next. However, in many parts of the world where people can scarcely think beyond the basic need for survival, the matter remains somewhat academic by comparison with what obtains in developed countries.

There used to be popular images of what might be considered a desirable death (at home with the family, in the company of friends and neighbours and comforted by the last rites) or an undesirable death (a violent death, suicide or condemned to death). Just the same, there was no clear or systematic idea. The notion of a dignified death is something that has sprung up in our culture.

A variety of terms is used in an attempt to express the idea, and they will be examined in depth later on. They include dignified, humane, happy and natural death, the right to die, the right to die with dignity or with serenity, and the right to be conscious up to the very last moment.

Even if we acknowledge each person's right to determine exactly what a dignified death is, there is a substantial ethical issue surrounding what is really meant by the phrase. In many respects, there is much agreement despite the pluralistic nature of our society, but on some issues there is serious disagreement.

The ethical imperative of looking upon a death in the context of personal dignity can be translated into numerous concrete, basic issues and minutiae. A combination of love for humanity, skill and imagination can give reasonable shape to a request for a dignified death in line with the needs and wishes of those involved. Later on, I will be looking at the main components of a humane death.

a. Solidarity

Although this is an all-embracing demand, it is important to emphasize that it is very difficult to conceive of the process of dying as dignified if there are not other people present playing a supportive role. Their presence will take different forms according to circumstances. I do not think it is an exaggeration to say that solidarity is a priority component of a humane death, perhaps even more important than freedom. Human beings are social beings. We need others in order to be ourselves in life, and this condition is no less decisive in our final moments. Solitude, lack of interest, and forgetting on the part of others prevent a person from being able to live his/her death as befits a human being. Dying alone without the company and support of society at such decisive moments is cruel, and is not in keeping with humanity's social nature or dignity. The Conference of German bishops commented that, 'Nobody can live his/her life alone, nobody can face his/her death in solitude. "Alone" means without the fundamental support of others. For many people, death is preceded by a decisive, and sometimes brutal, break with the world surrounding them, and is also accompanied by a growing solitude. [...] For that reason, everybody at the last stage of his/her life needs intensive help to be able to die a death that is worthy of a human being.'[8]

b. Relief from pain

The elimination of pain, or at least relief from it, is essential if death is to be approached more humanely. In an extended state-

ment from which I am about to quote, the Congregation for the
Doctrine of the Faith's *Declaration on Euthanasia* raises a number
of issues related to pain. These include the misery it causes so
often to people's well-being, and above all the legitimate recourse
to various procedures and medications to reduce pain and even
eliminate it.

Physical suffering is certainly an unavoidable element of
the human condition; on the biological level, it constitutes a
warning of which no one denies the usefulness; but, since it
affects the human psychological make-up, it often exceeds its
own biological usefulness and so can become so severe as to
cause the desire to remove it at any cost.

According to Christian teaching, however, suffering, especially suffering during the last moments of life, has a special
place in God's saving plan; it is in fact a sharing in Christ's
Passion and a union with the redeeming sacrifice which he
offered in obedience to the Father's will. Therefore one must
not be surprised if some Christians prefer to moderate their use
of painkillers, in order to accept voluntarily at least a part of
their sufferings and thus associate themselves in a conscious
way with the sufferings of Christ crucified (Mt 27:34). Nevertheless it would be imprudent to impose a heroic way of acting
as a general rule. On the contrary, human and Christian pru-
dence suggest for the majority of sick people the use of medicines capable of alleviating or suppressing pain, even though
these may cause as a secondary effect semiconsciousness and
reduced lucidity. As for those who are not in a state to express
themselves, one can reasonably presume that they wish to take
these painkillers, and have them administered according to the
doctor's advice.

But the intensive use of painkillers is not without difficulties, because the phenomenon of habituation generally makes
it necessary to increase their dosage in order to maintain their
efficacy. At this point it is fitting to recall a declaration by Pius
XII, which retains its full force; in answer to a group of
doctors who had put the question: 'Is the suppression of pain
and consciousness by the use of narcotics... permitted by religion and morality to the doctor and the patient (even at the
approach of death and if one foresees that the use of narcotics

will shorten life)?', the Pope said: 'If no other means exist, and if, in the given circumstances, this does not prevent the carrying out of other religious and moral duties: Yes.' In this case, of course, death is in no way intended or sought, even if the risk of it is reasonably taken; the intention is simply to relieve effectively, using for this purpose painkillers available to medicine. However, painkillers that cause unconsciousness need special consideration. For a person not only has to be able to satisfy his or her moral duties and family obligations; he or she also has to prepare himself or herself with full consciousness for meeting Christ. Thus Pius XII warns: 'It is not right to deprive the dying person of consciousness without a serious reason.'[9]

c. Psychological help

Psychological counselling is always useful, but it is rarely more urgently required than when death is at hand. It is hardly surprising that there should be an element of anxiety about the process of dying, and it sometimes makes other worries even more difficult to cope with. The period leading up to death includes not only depression, but a reaction on the part of the patient to chronic illness, the inexorable loss of faculties and independence, chronic pain and the prospect of an imminent death. The dying person should be in a position to entrust all these personal matters to skilled professionals. If there is to be relief from suffering, attention should also be paid to the patient's accommodation and living conditions; however, for various reasons it is difficult to ensure that decent conditions and company are available in today's health services.

d. Religious help

Spiritual counselling means that there must be facilities for the dying person not to have to deal with religious problems alone. This does not mean confession; it is quite simply a matter of respect for the sick person who should not be confused in the head when s/he goes into hospital.

e. Telling the patient the truth

Telling the sick person the whole story is an integral part of the respect due to his/her dignity. This matter is dealt with in chapter 18.

f. Other ways of caring

One's health frequently declines in the final stages of one's life, especially following a long illness. Problems include nausea, vomiting, loss of appetite, constipation, debilitation, breathlessness, itching, dry mouth, incontinence, insomnia, bed sores, and problems caused by probes. These matters have to be sorted out if the patient is to have reasonable peace of mind.

This can in part be achieved by material comforts such as a properly adapted bed, a reasonably large room with pleasant, tasteful decorations, and a rhythm of life modified to fit in with what the patient is capable of doing. Opportunities for the patient to spend some time on his/her own can also help to ensure that his/her final days are spent in conditions of human dignity.[10]

g. Freedom

One of the most popular ideas associated with a dignified death is the need to give the person enough freedom to deal with decisions that affect him/her personally. This reclaiming of personal autonomy is particularly relevant to two decisions that the patient may have to make. They are the right to reject a prolongation of life through extraordinary, disproportionate or futile means, and the freedom to ask for euthanasia. I will deal with these two issues in the remainder of this chapter.

14.4 Rejecting extraordinary means[11]

a. Limits to the prolonging of life

Christian morality and any reasonable code of ethics would defend the need to protect human life, and to care for someone's health – but not at any price. Among all the formulas used to define the limits of this duty, the Christian tradition places great emphasis on the distinction between ordinary and extraordinary means. According to this doctrine, the obligation to protect life extends as a general rule only to ordinary means and not to extraordinary means.

The Spanish Dominican Domingo Báñez is said to have coined the phrase in the sixteenth century to express this aspect of morality. The distinction, widely used by moralists, has been endorsed by Pius XII,[12] and is used in bishops'[13] conferences and by non-religious organizations.[14]

The distinction has recently been heavily criticized, to the extent that it is now losing ground to other formulations. It is significant that the Holy See's document on euthanasia does not go out of its way to defend the idea:

In the past, moralists replied that one is never obliged to use 'extraordinary' means. This reply, which as a principle still holds good, is perhaps less clear today, by reason of the imprecision of the term and the rapid progress made in the treatment of sickness. Thus some people prefer to speak of 'proportionate' and 'disproportionate' means.[15]

The main criticism is that the distinction is so unclear as to be unusable. Paul Ramsey describes the distinction as incurably circular unless we fill it with concrete and descriptive meaning.[16] There is also a danger that the use of these words can encourage discrimination or inequality by placing too much emphasis on the financial side.

For all its limitations, though, the ordinary/extraordinary distinction has been useful in the teaching of moral issues. It achieved this by encouraging reasonable attitudes to the prolongation of life and caring for the sick. It was completely different from idolatrous and reverential vitalism, and steered well clear of obscure guilt feelings that are aroused if 'not everything is being done'.

For these reasons, there are those who prefer to draw distinctions between reasonable and unreasonable, useful and futile, and proportionate and disproportionate. We must not fall into the trap of assuming that new terminology will solve all problems. The

problem is immensely complex, and it is even more difficult to
pin down because of variable factors such as rapid scientific and
technological advances, personal wishes, socio-cultural questions,
and the patient's current health.

b. Criteria for taking decisions

Irrespective of the words used to describe the distinction, it is
important to use clear guidelines if we want to come to sensible,
reasonable solutions. The Vatican's statement on euthanasia gives
useful indications in this respect:

> In any case, it will be possible to make a correct judgment as to
> the means by studying the type of treatment to be used, its
> degree of complexity or risk, its cost and the possibilities of
> using it, and comparing these elements with the result that can
> be expected, taking into account the state of the sick person
> and his or her physical and moral resources.
>   In order to facilitate the application of these general princi-
> ples, the following clarifications can be added:
> – If there are no other sufficient remedies, it is permitted,
> with the patient's consent, to have recourse to the means
> provided by the most advanced medical techniques, even if
> these means are still at the experimental stage and are not
> without a certain risk. By accepting them, the patient can even
> show generosity in the service of humanity.
> – It is also permitted, with the patient's consent, to interrupt
> these means, where the results fall short of expectations. But
> for such a decision to be made, account will have to be taken
> of the reasonable wishes of the patient and the patient's fam-
> ily, as also of the advice of the doctors who are specially
> competent in the matter. The latter may in particular judge that
> the investment in instruments and personnel is disproportion-
> ate to the results foreseen; they may also judge that the tech-
> niques applied impose on the patient strain or suffering out of
> proportion with the benefits which he or she may gain from
> such techniques.
> – It is also permissible to make do with the normal means that
> medicine can offer. Therefore one cannot impose on anyone the

obligation to have recourse to a technique which is already in use but which carries a risk or is burdensome. Such a refusal is not the equivalent of suicide; on the contrary, it should be considered as an acceptance of the human condition, or a wish to avoid the application of a medical procedure disproportionate to the results that can be expected, or a desire not to impose excessive expense on the family or the community.

– When inevitable death is imminent in spite of the means used, it is permitted in conscience to take the decision to refuse forms of treatment that would only secure a precarious and burdensome prolongation of life, so long as the normal care due to the sick person in similar cases is not interrupted. In such circumstances the doctor has no reason to reproach himself with failing to help the person in danger.[17]

Let us now move on from general indications to two concrete situations – artificial feeding and resuscitation.

c. Artificial feeding[18]

Of all the 'treatments' used to maintain life, one that has aroused most debate in recent times is that of artificial nutrition and hydration. The question whether it must be used and whether it is legitimate to withdraw it, or not use it in the first place, can occur in a wide range of situations. These can involve people who are close to death, permanently comatose patients, and patients whose health is in serious decline but whose lives are not in danger. For many decades now, Catholic scholars have said that it is legitimate to withhold intravenous feeding in particular circumstances, on the assumption that it was not a case of ordinary means.[19]

Within the Church, we find two points of view. G. Durand and J. Saint-Arnaud set them out thus:

There are those who believe that respect for human life demands that we continue feeding seriously ill people, even artificially, and that includes people in irreversible comas, because feeding and hydration are part of the minimum care that compassion demands. On the other hand, there are theologians and philosophers who maintain that recourse to artificial nutrition and hydration does not involve the same moral obligation as the natural process of ingesting solids and liquids. This is a medical technique that is more akin to treatment than to everyday care.[20]

By contrast, the Pontifical Academy of Sciences inserted a statement on feeding under the heading of health care rather than treatment.[21] D. Callahan describes the struggle between heart and mind on this issue; although he admits the legitimacy of not using artificial nutrition in some circumstances, he is fully aware of the profound significance of feeding. As it is 'the most fundamental of all human relationships', it would be most dangerous, he says, to play with such a basic moral emotion. Therefore, continuing with the feeding is 'a tolerable price to pay to preserve [...] one of the few moral emotions that could just as easily be called a necessary social instinct.[22] The same idea is used when arguing with those who defend euthanasia, and who would not consider artificial nutrition to be obligatory.[23]

[*Editor's note*: In Britain, controversy has centred upon what is now called 'persistent vegetative state' (PVS), in which a person's higher brain functions have ceased, although the brain stem is still alive and he continues to breathe unaided. Survival is possible for 30 years or more, provided water, food and antibiotics are administered. PVS is seen by the medical profession as a new phenomenon resulting from advances in medical technology which prevent natural death after the occurrence of acute brain damage.[24] In 1992-93 controversy focused around the tragic fate of Tony Bland, a young man who had been in this condition since the Hillsborough football disaster of 1989. His parents and the hospital authorities applied to the High Court for leave to discontinue the life support and let him die. The dominant medical and legal opinion was that tubal feeding should be seen as medical treatment. Others argued that it was elementary care and that the intention to bring about certain death through the withdrawal of food and water would amount to murder. The courts eventually ruled that the feeding should be seen as medical treatment and its withdrawal was lawful. Acute differences appeared among Catholic commentators on the morality of this decision, although the bishops opposed it on the grounds that it amounted to involuntary euthanasia.[25]]

d. Resuscitation[26]

This word has come to mean many things, but I should like to concentrate on the procedures that have been developed in the last few decades in the field of restoring heartbeat after cardiac arrest. If the heart does not resume beating after a few minutes, the brain suffers total and irreversible damage. Cardiac arrest occurs at some moment in anybody's dying process, whatever the cause of death may be; hence, the decision to resuscitate or not is of the highest importance.

The history of resuscitation is closely linked to the development of medical equipment, and to advances in anaesthetics, surgery and medical research in general.

Decisions in this field are highly complex. On the one hand, they have to be taken very quickly, as any delay in resuscitation limits the chances of success. If the heart does not start beating again within a few minutes, the brain suffers irreversible damage. On the other hand, consideration has to be given to how successful resuscitation is likely to be, given that it is not just a question of prolonging life, but is also connected to the circumstances surrounding the patient's hospitalization. It may be, for instance, that the patient is in one of those hospitals where there are clearly established procedures about when resuscitation should not be attempted. It can be no easy matter determining the categories of patient or situation to be excluded from resuscitation, but there do not appear to be any grounds for believing that any application of this sort should in principle be rejected. As long as there is no naive belief that these policies can cope with all circumstances, they can be a most useful aid to health professionals, providing they have been drawn up by a multi-disciplinary team.

The ideal of the patient's autonomy presents some difficulties, given the sick person's health and the urgency with which the intervention must take place. The same goes for the involvement of the family.

Finally, there are other situations that throw up questions similar to those presented by resuscitation and artificial feeding. These situations include whether or not to continue with mechanical ventilation, dialysis after chronic renal failure, and antibiotic treatment when it only serves to maintain the patient artificially in a vegetative state.[27]

14.5 Living wills[28]

People believe they have the right freely to take the decisions that are most directly related to the process of dying. This is another example of the importance given to the idea of freedom in western society. It is also a new expression of the principle of autonomy, and it is being increasingly canvassed in the fields of bioethics and medical practice. However, the demand for dignity during the period leading up to death becomes less and less easy to understand without respect for freedom.

These days, people are demanding greater personal freedom in respect of the decisions most directly connected with the final phase of life, and particularly the right to ask for euthanasia and reject the prolongation of life by disproportionate means. I will now confine myself to ways in which our society expresses the right to reject treatment prolonging life when it appears futile. Of all the formulas used, I will only deal with the living will (sometimes known as the 'advance directive').

When somebody on the point of dying is still conscious, and is capable of saying that s/he does not want his/her life prolonged by extraordinary means, that in itself should be a sufficient indication for family members and doctors.

The most difficult situations arise when, as so often happens, the person is unconscious and incapable of expressing his/her wishes. There are two solutions to this type of problem:

– the living will, whereby the patient him/herself gives instructions about the decisions to be taken if s/he is close to death and can no longer express his/her wishes;
– designating a representative as the person authorized to take decisions on behalf of the patient at such a time.

The living will is a document in which someone in complete control of his/her faculties requests that certain wishes relating to his/her health care should be carried out. The wish most frequently expressed in these documents concerns not prolonging life by disproportionate means.

The phrase 'living will' seems to have been coined by a Chicago lawyer, Louis Kutner, in 1967. The first draft of a living will appeared in 1969 and was submitted to the Euthanasia Educational Council. In the next 20 years or so, it is estimated that over 20 million people have signed declarations of this type in the United States.

There are many models of a living will, and the differences reflect the individuals and groups that have drawn them up. They may be classified under three headings. The first are living wills of a religious inspiration, for example those produced by the American Association of Catholic Hospitals, Protestant hospitals and even bishops' conferences (the North American conference several years ago, and the Spanish conference more recently in 1989). The religious component means that they contain specific provisions relating to issues such as the meaning of life and death.

Other living wills originate in professional groups such as the American Public Health Association. These documents contain highly technical medical details, and sometimes even list forms of health care and treatment which must be started or stopped, as well as types of pain or other conditions which must be avoided in the last few days.

Lastly, there are groups which we might call 'educational', such as the Society for the Right to Die with Dignity. Living wills drawn up by these organizations adopt a rather general approach, and in this way are similar to models in the first group, except that they sometimes also allow for euthanasia.

[*Editor's note*: The editor has been unable to trace examples of living wills or advance directives issued by English-language Bishops' Conferences comparable with that issued in Spain. However, there have been some prepared by Catholic medical ethics centres, e.g., J. De Blois, M. McGrath and K.D. O'Rourke, 'An Advance Directive for Future Health care Decision: A Christian Perspective', in *Health Progress*, July-August 1991, 27-31 (may be obtained from Center for Health Care Ethics, 1402 S. Grand Bulvd, St Louis, MO 63104).]

'Living wills' contain the personal details of both the person writing the declaration (some people add the names and signatures of witnesses) and those to whom it is addressed (e.g. family, doctors and priests); the text of the will consists of whatever wishes the patient may have. A living will produced by Spanish bishops, for instance, contains five provisions:

- the appropriate treatment to be used to relieve pain;
- rejection of disproportionate or extraordinary treatment;
- rejection of active euthanasia;
- no painful or unreasonable prolongation of the process of dying;
- a request for help in dying in a humane and Christian manner.

There are several issues surrounding the value of a living will. For the person making out the living will, it is a humane act performed after mature reflection, and it is assumed to have been carried out freely, consciously and responsibly. The people to whom the living will is addressed are asked to acknowledge and respect the document in the same way as if it were a normal will. In some countries, the living will has legal status.

As for the term of the document, or the period of time during which it is in force, it begins to apply when the patient is no longer capable of expressing his/her wishes and is in a critical situation from which s/he will not recover.

It is common for living wills to make reference to the meaning of life and death. The Spanish bishops' document speaks of life as a gift and a blessing of God, without being a supreme and absolute value. Death is seen as an inevitable reality, the end of life on earth and gateway to eternal life.

There is no consensus on the meaning and usefulness of a living will. Some people look upon it as unnecessary from a practical point of view, because its terms are so vague. The reason for this is that medical practice is becoming increasingly obsessed with therapeutic treatments, and there are those who believe that a living will actually could stand in the way of what it sets out to do – to defend the patient's freedom.

Others see it as being morally and socially useful. Personally, I think we should give it a positive welcome. Basically, it is no more than a modern version of the traditional moral doctrine on ordinary and extraordinary means. It attempts to introduce an element of common sense and rationality into decisions concerning one's final moments – a time one is spending far from obsessive concentration on life on earth. Amidst this effort to achieve rationality, the patient is granted a few words of his/her own. They signify a serene acceptance of the limitations of the body, of science and of technology – and opposition to Promethean and Faustian attitudes, or to an unreasonable attachment to life. This can be very helpful for families and health professionals. We have to acknowledge that it is instructive as an indicator of values and directions for moral action. As the meanings and values set out in living wills are slowly incorporated into our social mentality and professional practice, it may be that interest in them will start to decline. For the moment, I think it is a good idea for these values to become better known; they symbolize a moral approach that is worth promoting in decisions related to the last days of a person's life.

14.6 Euthanasia

a. A confused debate

Public debate on euthanasia frequently falters for lack of clarity. To an extent, this is inevitable. There are several factors that contribute to this uncertainty, but I want to focus on the way in which ambiguous language is used both to express and feed this confusion. Let us take a fresh look at what the word actually means, otherwise we will never be able to introduce any semblance of order into public debate on the subject.

The etymological origin of the word 'euthanasia' is 'good death' and, although it has acquired various other meanings over the years,[29] it might be useful to see how the word is normally used today.[30]

It would be a lot clearer, in fact, if certain interventions and situations were not called euthanasia at all, even when the word is preceded by adjectives like 'indirect', 'passive' and 'negative'. An indication of the prevailing ambiguity is that people who use the word loosely find that they then have to explain what they mean in order to be understood properly. As there are other, less ambiguous expressions in the language, it would be a good idea if we started using them, thereby avoiding much confusion.

Necessary treatment designed to eliminate, alleviate or prevent pain may well have the secondary effect of accelerating death, but it should never be called euthanasia.

A refusal to accept, or to continue with, disproportionate or futile means with a view to prolonging life should not be described as euthanasia either, even when it is qualified as 'indirect', 'passive' or 'negative'. The same goes for treating illnesses or secondary pain in a patient who has irreversibly lost consciousness.

With these sensible exclusions, we can avoid overloading the word 'euthanasia'. Even if we add adjectives like 'indirect', 'passive' and 'negative', the situation remains somewhat unclear, as we can see from the confusion that many people, not least health professionals, labour under.

The most illuminating definition of euthanasia that I have come across is the one put forward by the Congregation for the Doctrine of the Faith's *Declaration on Euthanasia*. This describes it as 'an action or an omission which of itself or by intention causes death in order that all suffering may in this way be eliminated.' Euthanasia is all about intentions and the methods used.[31] I therefore think it is correct to look upon euthanasia as an act of commission as much as one of omission. The word should be used to describe not only positive actions, but also decisions not to carry out normal, proportionate health care which could save a life. I also think it is relevant to point out that there can be an element of euthanasia in an action arising out of the intention of the person concerned or the methods used. Just the same, I find the addition of the phrase 'in order that all suffering may in this way be eliminated' more debatable. This is very often the case, but it must have been possible to use a more general expression.

Things would be a lot clearer if we omitted the word 'euthanasia' altogether in the circumstances referred to above, and also dispensed with paired terms such as 'direct/indirect', 'passive/active' and 'positive/negative'. Much more relevant words are 'voluntary' and 'non-voluntary' (or 'involuntary') according to whether the dying person has asked for the intervention or not.

b. *The morality of euthanasia*[32]

According to Catholic doctrine as it is normally taught, euthanasia is not morally acceptable; this is true even if it is considered objectively, either from Christian standpoints or from more specifically humane points of view. There are, however, some who believe that outright condemnation of euthanasia is not completely correct from a humane point of view.[33]

A document produced by Spanish bishops on euthanasia provides a detailed position on the Christian basis for condemning
euthanasia:

Neither the New Testament nor the Old Testament tackled
euthanasia directly and explicitly. The Bible, however, contains a fundamental affirmation: God is the Lord of life and
death. It is God who has called men and women into existence
and given them life as a gift, and as a blessing which they must
look after and cherish, and never dispense with. Within the
biblical tradition, there is a line of progress which increasingly
underlines the value and sacrosanct nature of all human life.
'Thou shalt not kill' thereby acquires much more relevance, to
the extent that the principle of the inviolability of human life is
now extended to everyone. Jesus gives special impetus to the
demand for respect for all human life. As the Church examines
the principle further, it teaches explicitly that the inviolability
of all human life extends to any phase of human life.[34]

There is something morally objectionable about non-voluntary euthanasia, whereby a quality as basic as life itself is taken
away without the wishes of the person concerned being taken into
account. If the aim of such a practice were eugenic or racist, or
encouraged by public authorities or other influential bodies, the
moral outrage would be colossal.[35]

We should not try and place the morality of euthanasia within
a narrow, individual, moral framework. As Pope John Paul II has
pointed out, the issue contains a genuine cultural option:

The task which is imposed on the Christian community in a
similar socio-cultural context is more than mere condemnation
of euthanasia or a simple attempt to prevent its dissemination
and subsequent legalization. The fundamental problem above
all is this: How can we help men of our time to become aware
of the inhuman character of some aspects of the dominant
culture and to rediscover the most precious values guaranteed
by it?

The Pope understands very well how, in places where certain
socio-cultural values are well established, 'bringing one's own or

somebody else's life gently to a close may well appear to be a logical, humane solution.'[36] We can none-the-less pick out a number of factors that favour a growing trend in support of euthanasia. To quote again from the Spanish bishops' statement on euthanasia, these factors include 'the process of secularization, the crisis of religious values in the west, and the prioritizing of the freedom of the individual which ultimately affirms that a terminal patient has the right to dispose of his/her life as s/he wishes. It is equally undeniable that the legalization of abortion has an impact in the area of euthanasia. When the law allows a life in gestation to be disposed of, it is on its way to accepting that other human lives can also be disposed of.'[37]

c. Euthanasia under the law

Before we look at the question of euthanasia under the law, this might be a good moment to recall how ambiguous the word 'euthanasia' is when we are talking about legislation and de-criminalization.

Sometimes – and this makes the confusion even greater – laws are held to be decriminalizing simply because they attach legal status to living wills, or to the appointment of a representative with the power to turn down the opportunity to prolong life by means of disproportionate procedures.

There are laws which decriminalize 'mercy killing' by attaching to it relatively mild penalties. It is in fact nothing short of murder. We feel the same about legislation whereby judges are given the right to reduce penalties for certain murders that have been committed for 'honourable' reasons. We can only properly talk of decriminalization when we acknowledge that we are taking someone's life in particularly painful or wretched circumstances.

At one time, there were campaigns and proposals around the idea of the social and legal acceptance of euthanasia, including non-voluntary euthanasia. These fleeting attempts took place in the first quarter of the twentieth century, but the Nazis' use of euthanasia for eugenic reasons meant that moves to legalize voluntary euthanasia lost their impetus after World War II. Since then, however, proposals for legalization have reappeared in certain countries, although no legislation has yet been passed.[38]

[*Editor's note*: Attempts to legalize euthanasia include the Voluntary Euthanasia Bills put before the British Parliament in 1936 and 1969, and a successful referendum in the Swiss Canton of Zurich in 1977. But the most important by far is the recent legislation in the Dutch Parliament (1993), designed to regularize an already existing practice. According to an intensive survey among doctors sponsored in 1991 by the Dutch Government, an average of 2,300 requests for euthanasia are granted annually, although more than four times that number, 9,000 are refused – largely by general practitioners. Nevertheless, euthanasia was – and still remains – illegal and liable to conviction in the courts. But the courts would allow a defence of medical necessity. Contrary to some reports, the new law, which came into force early in 1994, did not legalize the practice, but guaranteed doctors immunity from prosecution provided they follow a 28-point checklist of conditions. These include evidence that the patients are terminally ill, that they are in unbearable pain and that they have, in front of witnesses, repeatedly asked to die. The doctor must also have consulted relatives and at least one other medical professional. Finally, it must be reported to the public prosecutor, who has to decide on a case-by-case basis whether to prosecute. If the active ending of life was not carried out at the express request of the patient, the prosecutor will in principle start proceedings.[39]]

The innumerable reasons adduced by groups and movements supporting the decriminalization of euthanasia are varied in content and importance. The reason most frequently put forward is the person's autonomy. Laws and societies that prohibit euthanasia are accused of hypocrisy and inhumanity on the grounds that they do not grant someone who is suffering greatly the right to ask for his/her sufferings to be brought to an end. Another criticism of these laws is their alleged illogicality and cynicism. If suicide is not penalized, and the patient is granted the right to reject treatment, is there such a great difference between a fatal injection and refusal to have certain treatment?

On the subject of the efforts to decriminalize euthanasia, I would like to add one small point. If all this support for a person's right to ask to die were accompanied by comparable interest in demanding and providing the best care for the terminally ill, would this euthanasia campaign not lose much of its interest and meaning? On the one hand, we have requests for the freedom to ask to die; on the other, however, we hear nothing about effective assistance to ensure that the person spends the last days of his/her life in as humane a manner as possible; this is quite absurd and almost beggars belief.

The arguments in favour of keeping euthanasia outside the law are many and powerful. A survey that was unofficial, but one which none-the-less faithfully reflected informed opinion within the Anglican Church in Great Britain, came out opposed to legalizing voluntary euthanasia as it believed that such an idea presented more disadvantages than advantages:

> If all the care of the dying were up to the standards of the best, there would be few cases where there was even a prima facie argument for euthanasia; better alternative means of alleviating distress would almost always be available if modern techniques and human understanding and care of the patient were universally practised.
>
> ... to justify a change in the law in this country to permit euthanasia, it would be necessary to show that such a change would remove greater evils than it would cause. We do not believe that such justification can be given; for
>
> a. such cases are very few, and would be fewer still if medical, and in particular hospital, practices were sounder;
>
> b. a change in the law would reduce the incentive to improve these practices;
>
> c. the legalization of euthanasia would place some terminal, and even some non-terminal, patients under pressure to allow themselves to be put away – a pressure which they should be spared;
>
> d. it would also, in practice, be likely to result in recourse to euthanasia in many cases in which it was far from morally justified, and performed for unsound reasons;
>
> e. in the rare cases (if such there are) in which it can be justified morally, it is better for medical men to do all that is necessary to ensure peaceful dying, and to rely on the flexibilities in the administration of the law which even now exist, than to legalize euthanasia (which would have to be subject to rigid formalities and safeguards) for general use;
>
> f. although there may be some patients whose relationship

with their doctor would not suffer, we believe that for the great
majority of patients their confidence in doctors would be gravely
weakened.[40]

In fact, patients who ask for euthanasia are really asking for
better care, a more humane support system and fewer technical
tricks. It is important to be able to make sense of what the patient
is really saying on such occasions. Many requests for euthanasia
do not so much express the patient's wishes as criticize the
shortcomings of medicine and society, the lack of solidarity, and
the incapacity for sacrifice by the suffering human being.

NOTES

1. E. Mansell Pattison, *The Experience of Dying*, Prentice Hall, Englewood
    Cliffs, 1977; J. Basurko, 'La cultura dominante ante el problema de la
    muerte', in *IV* 62 (1976) 103-122; L.H. Lofrand, *Toward a Sociology of
    Death and Dying*, Sage Publ., Beverly Hills 1976; VV.AA., *Les hommes
    devant la mort*, Cerf, Paris 1975; Ph. Ariès, 'Death in reverse', in *STeol* 11
    (1972) 19-28; Thomas Nagel, 'Death', in Nagel, *Mortal Questions*, CUP,
    Cambridge, 1979, 1-10.
2. M.W. Linn and others, 'Impact of Nursing Home Staff on Training about
    Death and Dying', in *JAMA* 250 (1983) 2332-2335.
3. Ethics Committee, Hospital of St John of God, Barcelona, 'Criteria for brain
    death', in *LH* 212 (1989) 148-151; J.M. Stanley, 'More Fiddling with the
    Definition of Death?', in *JME* 13 (1987) 21-22; S.J. Younger, 'Framing the
    Line of Brain Death', in *HCR* 17 (1987) no. 4, 43-44; S.G. Potts, 'Headaches
    in Britain over Brain Death Criteria', in *HCR* 17 (1987) no. 2, 2-3; S.F.
    Spicker, 'Philosophical Aspects of Brain Death', in *JMPh* 9 (1984) 373-375;
    D. Shrader, 'On Dying More than One Death', in *HCR* 16 (1986) no. 1, 12-
    17; D.N. Walton, *Brain Death. Ethical Considerations*, Purdue Univ., West
    Lafayette 1980; J. Korein, *Brain Death*, N.Y. Academy of Sciences, New
    York 1978; A.M. Capron, 'Legal Aspects of Pronouncing Death', in *EB* I,
    296-301; H.M. Sass, 'Brain Life and Brain Death: A Proposal for a Norma-
    tive Agreement', in *JMPh* 14 (1989) 45-59; R. Gillon, 'Death', in *JME* 16
    (1990) 3-4; B.A. Rix, 'Danish Ethics Council Rejects Brain Death as the
    Criterion of Death', in *JME* 16 (1990) 5-7, and reactions against it, 8-13.
4. P. Mollaret and M. Goulon, 'Le coma dépassé', in *RN* 101 (1959) 3-15.
5. 'A Definition of Irreversible Coma.' Report of the Ad Hoc Committee of the
    Harvard Medical School to Examine the Definition of Brain Death, in *JAMA*
    205 (1968) 85-88. Pius XII, in an allocution of 24-11-1957, in *AAS* 49
    (1957) 1027-1033, recognizes that it is up to the skill of the doctor to define
    with accuracy what is meant by death and the moment it occurs; it is not the
    responsibility of the Church.

6. A.M. Capron, 'Determining Death: Do We Need a Statute?', in *HCR* 3 (1973) no. 1, 6-7.
7. P. Caucanas-Pisier, 'Associations for the Right to Die in Dignity', in *Concilium* 21 (1985) 50-63; A. Autiero, 'Experiencing one's own death', in *CC* 134 (1983) I, 348-356; D. Callahan, 'On Defining "Natural Death"', in *HCR* 7 (1977), no. 3, 32-37; D.M. High, 'Is "Natural Death" an Illusion?', in *HCR* 8 (1978) no. 4, 37-47; J.H. Blits, 'Natural Death and Moral Individuality', in *JMPh* 5 (1980) 236-245.
8. German Bishops' Conference, *Human Death with Dignity and Christian Death* (1978).
9. Sacred Congregation for the Doctrine of Faith, *Declaration on Euthanasia* (5 May 1980), reprinted in *The Pope Speaks* (Winter 1980), 284-296 and in S.E. Lammers and A. Verhey, *On Moral Medicine*, 441-444.
10. On care at the end of life see R. Bayer and others, 'The Care of the Terminally Ill: Morality and Economics,' in *NEJM* 309 (1983) 1490-1494; 'Soins in phase terminale', in *Laennec* 35 (1986) 1711-1713; E. Kübler-Ross, *On Death and Dying,* New York 1969.
11. Pius XII, in *AAS* 49 (1957) 1030; Sacred Congregation for the Doctrine of Faith, *Declaration on Euthanasia* (1980) 30; D.A. Cronin, *The Moral Law in Regard to the Ordinary and Extraordinary Means of Conserving Life*, P.U. Gregoriana, Rome 1958; R. O'Neil, 'In Defense of the "Ordinary/Extraordinary" Distinction', in *LQ* 45 (1978) 37-40; J.J. McCartney, 'The Development of the Doctrine of Ordinary and Extraordinary Means of Preserving Life in Catholic Moral Theology. Before the Karen Quinlan Case', in *LQ* 47 (1980) 215-224; Ch. Meyers, 'Intended Goals and Appropriate Treatment: An Alternative to the Ordinary/Extraordinary Distinction', in *JME* 10 (1984) 128-130; J.V. Hickey, '"Ordinary" and "Extraordinary" Vary with the Care', in *HCR* 13 (1983) no. 5, 43-44; J.B. Balsam, 'To Sustain Life or to Allow to Die?', in *Ang* 66 (1989) 264-281; J.P. Mullooly, 'Ordinary/Extraordinary Means of Euthanasia', in *LQ* 54 (1987) 50-57.
12. Pius XII, in *AAS* 49 (1957) 1030.
13. For example, the North American Bishops in *The Ethical and Religious Directives for Catholic Health Care Facilities*, 1971.
14. The House of Delegates of the American Medical Association, in 1973.
15. *Declaration on Euthanasia,* 30.
16. P. Ramsey, 'Euthanasia and Dying Well', in *LQ* 44 (1977) 43.
17. *Declaration on Euthanasia,* 30.
18. G. Grisez, 'Should Nutrition and Hydration Be Provided to Permanently Comatose and Other Mentally Disabled Persons?', in *LQ* 57 (1990) no. 2, 30-43; D.J. Horan, 'Hydration, Nutrition and Euthanasia: Legal Reflections on the Role of Church Teaching', in *CMQ* 40 (1989) 57-69; R. Steinbrook and B. Lo, 'Artificial Feeding. Solid Ground, Not a Slippery Slope', in *NEJM* 318 (1988) 286-290; R.D. MacKay, 'Terminating Life-Sustaining Treatment. Recent US Developments', in *JME* 14 (1988) 135-139; J.R. Connery, 'The Ethics of Withholding/Withdrawing Nutrition and Hydration', in *LQ* 54 (1987) 17-26; S.T. Helsper and J.J. McCarthy, 'Foregoing Artificial Nutrition and Hydration. Some Recent Legal and Moral Implications for Catholic Health Care Facilities', in *LQ* 54 (1987) 39-46; E. McMillan, 'The Catholic Moral Tradition on Providing Food and Fluids', in *LQ* 54

(1987) 55-66; E.F. Diamond, 'Nutrition, Hydration and Cost Containment', in *LQ* 53 (1986) 24-35; G.J. Annas and others, 'Do Feeding Tubes Have more Rights than Patients?', in *HCR* 16 (1986) no. 1, 26-32; G.J. Annas, 'Elizabeth Bouvia: Whose Space Is This Anyway?', in *HCR* 16 (1986) no. 2, 24-25; R.A. McCormick, 'Notes on Moral Theology: 1983', in *TS* 45 (1984) 80-138, D. Callahan, 'On Feeding the Dying', in *HCR* 13 (1983) no. 5, 22; VV.AA., 'No feeding Tubes for me', in *HCR* 17 (1987) no. 3, Spec. Supp., 23-26; A.M. Capron and E.J. Cassell, 'Care of the Dying Withholding Nutrition', in *HCR* 14 (1984) no. 5, 32-37.

19. G. Kelly, *Medico-Moral Problems*, Catholic Hospital Association, St Louis 1958, 130; C.J. McFadden, *Medical Ethics*, F.A. Davis, Philadelphia 1967, 246-247; G. Healy, *Medical Ethics*, Loyola, Chicago 1956, 80.

20. G. Durand and J. Saint-Arnaud, *op.cit.*, 301.

21. Pontifical Academy of Sciences, 'Le prolongement artificiel de la vie et la détermination du moment de la mort', in *DC* 82 (1985) 1169.

22. D. Callahan, *op.cit.*, 22.

23. D.J. Horan, *op.cit.*

24. 'Discussion paper on treatment of patients in persistent vegetative state', Medical Discussion Committee of the BMA, September 1992, 4.

25. See, for instance, Kevin Kelly, 'Rest for Tony Bland', *The Tablet* 13 March 1993; The Linacre Centre for Health Care Ethics, 'Submission to the select Committee of the House of Lords on Medical Ethics', in Luke Gormally (ed.), *Euthanasia, Clinical Practice and the Law*, Linacre Centre 1994.

26. G.J. Annas, 'CPR (Cardiopulmonary Resuscitation): The Beat Goes On', in *HCR* 12 (1982) no. 4, 24-25; K. Nolan, 'In Death's Shadow: The Meanings of Withholding Resuscitation', in *HCR* 17 (1987) no. 5, 9-14; S.J. Younger, 'Do-not-Resuscitate Orders: No Longer Secret, But Still a Problem', in *HCR* 17 (1987) no. 1, 24-33; M. Gillick, 'The Ethics of Cardiopulmonary Resuscitation: Another Look', in *ESM* 7 (1980) 161-169; J.M. Stanley, 'The Appleton Consensus: Suggested International Guidelines for Decisions to Forego Medical Treatment', in *JME* 15 (1989) 129-136.

27. L.J. Schneiderman and R.G. Spragg, 'Ethical Decisions in Discontinuing Mechanical Ventilation', in *NEJM* 318 (1988) 984-988.

28. R. Gillon, 'Living Wills, Powers of Attorney and Medical Practice', in *JME* 14 (1988) 59-60; L.L. Heintz, 'Legislative Hazard: Keeping Patients Living, against Their Wills', in *JME* 14 (1988) 82-86; C.L., 'Do Nurses and Doctors Put off Signing Living Wills?', in *HCR* 16 (1986) no. 3, 3; 'A Christian Living Will', in *HCR* 17 (1987) no. 5, 47; J.B., 'Livings Wills: When Do They Mean What They Mean?', in *HCR* 13 (1983) no. 4, 2; S.J. Eisendrath and H.R. Jonsen, 'The Living Will. Help or Hindrance?', in *JAMA* 249 (1983) 2054-2058; T. Harrington, 'Living-Will Legislation Opposed: Massachusetts', in *Origins* 9 (1980) 650-651; M. Lappe, 'Dying While Living: A Critique of Allowing-To-Die Legislation', in *JME* 4 (1978) 195-199; 'Christian Alternative to the Living Will', in *HCR* 5 (1975) no. 1, 3 and 55. *The Living Will: Consent to Treatment at the End of Life*, joint report by Age Concern and King's College Centre for Medical Law and Ethics, Edward Arnold, London and New York 1988; J. Finnis, 'Living Will Legislation' in Gormally (ed.), *Euthanasia, Clinical Practice and the Law*, Linacre Centre, London 1994; British Medical Association, *Statement on Advanced Directives*, May 1992.

29. M. Vidal, *Bioética*, Tecnos, Madrid 1989, 62-73.
30. Sacred Congregation for the Doctrine of Faith, *Declaration on Euthanasia*, 29.
31. *Declaration on Euthanasia*, 29.
32. W.B. Smith, 'Judeo-Christian Teaching on Euthanasia: Definition, Distinctions and Decisions', in *LQ* 54 (1987) 27-42; H. Trowell, *The Unfinished Debate on Euthanasia*, SCM 1973; P. Foot, 'Euthanasia', in *Virtues and Vices*, Oxford, Blackwell 1978; R.G. Twycross, 'Euthanasia', in Duncan, Dunstan and Welbourn (eds.), *Dictionary of Medical Ethics*, DLT 1981; T. Wood, 'Euthanasia', in Macquarrie and Childress, *A New Dictionary of Christian Ethics*, SCM Press 1986; L.S.Cahill, 'A "Natural law" Reconsideration of Euthanasia', in Lammers & Verhey, *op.cit.*, 445; D. Maguire, *Death by Choice*, NY 1975 and 'A Catholic View of Mercy Killing', in M. Kohl (ed.), *Beneficient Euthanasia*, Buffalo, NY 1975; *On Dying Well: An Anglican Contribution to the Debate on Euthanasia*, London: Church Information Office, 1975; L. Gormally (ed.), *Euthanasia, Clinical Practice and the Law*, Linacre Centre, 1994; British Medical Association, *Euthanasia*, 1988.
33. I. Giunchedi, 'L'eutanasia e l'arbitrio della ragione', in *RTeol* 25 (1984) 508-520.
34. Spanish Bishops' Conference's Committee on Faith, 'Notes on Euthanasia', in *Ecclesia* 2265-2266 (1986) 53.
35. For information on other issues raised, see A. Holderegger, 'A Right to a Freely Chosen Death', in *Concilium* 179 (1985) 90-100; F.J. Elizari, 'Is human life an absolute value? Towards a reworking of the value of "human life"', in *Moralia* 1 (1979) 21-39.
36. John Paul II, 'L'euthanasie, problème de culture et de foi', in *DC* 81 (1984) 1019.
37. Spanish Bishops' Conference's committee on Faith, 'Notes on Euthanasia', in *Ecclesia* 2265-2266 (1986) 52.
38. 'Final Report of the Netherlands State Commission on Euthanasia: An English Summary', in *Bioethics* 1 (1987) 163-174; R.M. Bratton, 'The Right to Die: A Constitutional One?', in *The Jurist* 41 (1981) 155-175; 'Initiative du Canton de Zurich', in *MH* 37 (1979) 205-208; 'Euthanasia and Doctors. A Rejection of the BMA's Report', in *JME* 15 (1989) 124-128.
39. Information from various reports in the *Guardian*, 3 November 1992, 10 February 1993, 11 January 1994; press release from the Netherlands Ministry of Justice, February 1993. See also J. Keown, 'Some Reflections on Euthanasia in the Netherlands' and 'Further Reflections on Euthanasia in the Netherlands in the Light of the Remmelink Report and the van Der Maas Survey', in L. Gormally (ed.), *Euthanasia, Clinical Practice and the Law*, Linacre Centre, London 1994; *Medical Practice with the Regard to Euthanasia and Related Medical Decisions in the Netherlands*, The Remmelink Report (upon which the 1993 legislation was based) was published in *The Lancet* 14 September 1991, 669-674.
40. *On Dying Well*, CIO, London 1975, 61-62.

Chapter 15

Hunger strikes[1]

15.1 History

Hunger strikes are not a product of the twentieth century. We have ample evidence of them taking place at many times in the past, not least the Middle Ages and the eighteenth century during the struggle for independence in the United States. They have become much more frequent in the twentieth century, and this is of no little significance. The best-known hunger strikes include those by Gandhi (17 of them during the period 1918-1948), and by members of the IRA in 1981 as a result of which 12 members of that organization died. Recourse to this extreme practice is not unknown in the Third World; examples include Kerala, India (1983), but most occur in Latin America: Bolivia (1977-78), Santiago de Chile (1978), and Miguel de Escoto, the Nicaraguan Minister of Foreign Affairs (1985).

For the most part, these protests centre on demands which concern public authorities; it is much less common for private sector organizations to be involved. These demands are very wide-ranging and vary greatly in moral importance.

The political, legal, social and moral dimensions of hunger strikes have much more impact when the strikers put their lives at risk, and when the health professional becomes involved.

In the next few pages, I am going to concentrate on the moral issue of force-feeding hunger strikers. It is clearly not possible to deal with this problem without acknowledging the highly complex nature of hunger strikes; there are many features that may not be superficially present at any given moment, but are none-the-less there at all times.

15.2 A definition of hunger strikes

Let us define a hunger strike in its strictest sense as total abstention from food for the successful prosecution of certain demands, and a preparedness to die if the demands are not met. There is much more to hunger striking from a phenomenological point of view, but these are the main issues; the others are secondary and of little relevance to this section.

Abstention from food and drink must be complete, apart from substances that are artificially placed in the striker's body. There is always a link in hunger strikes between abstention from food and death, as the striker is determined to sacrifice his/her life if his/her demands are not met. This deliberate attitude presents us with a dilemma: the person's moral right over his/her own life on the one hand, and society's attitude to this on the other. It is a matter of verifiable fact that the connection between abstaining from food and dying is more complex; the reason is that this connection depends upon unequal relationships between the striker and others' legal and moral responsibilities. The striker is primarily responsible for this link when he/she refuses to give up. However, there are other people who are also involved; these are people who refuse to accept the demands, public authorities which may outlaw forced feeding, and doctors who, for one reason or another, will not perform it. Then there are movements, groups and individuals which strengthen the striker's resolve by giving advice and putting pressure on him/her. Finally, in an ill-defined way, there is society and its attitudes.

On the other hand, we must acknowledge that the striker's primary intention is not to die. What he/she really wants is that his/her demands should be met. It follows that hunger striking does not necessarily have any connection with death. For this reason, some people have placed death resulting from a hunger strike in the moral category of indirect effect.

The reasons for the hunger strike and the context in which it takes place are vitally important for a moral consideration of the phenomenon. As for the reasons, it is usually a matter of the striker claiming basic human rights, since the strike has nothing to do with objectives related to health, safety or aesthetics. Sometimes, the demands appear to have little moral weight, and the aims are out of proportion to such a radical means.

Another characteristic of hunger strikes is publicity; this is fundamental if society is to ally itself with the striker by giving him/her support. If society abandons, repudiates or shows hostility towards the striker, his/her gesture loses all meaning and effectively counts for nothing.

15.3 The Church's official position

The Church's official position on this question is by no means clear. The Irish bishops gave no authority for the IRA prisoners' hunger strike, although it is doubtful whether their statement referred to the strike *per se*, but rather to the circumstances surrounding it. The Irish bishops' position was that contempt for human life, the incitement of revenge, the exploiting of hunger strikes to promote a campaign of murdering and intimidating innocent people, and the initiating of children in the ways of violence was utterly evil.[2]

In 1983, fishermen in Kerala, India, took part in a hunger strike, and nuns and priests subsequently joined forces with them. The bishops of Kerala responded in tones which seem to indicate outright condemnation. In no circumstances, they said, may hunger strikes be permitted if they can result in death; nor may the use of violence or taking part in demonstrations or protests which involve these practices.[3]

As for certain other hunger strikes that have taken place, bishops have indicated their solidarity with the objectives that were being pursued, while remaining silent about the problem of whether the hunger strike had any moral legitimacy.

15.4 Moral positions

Hunger strikes now bring us to a very broad general issue. This is a human being's ethical power over his/her own life, and the attitude which society should adopt towards a person who voluntarily puts his/her life in great danger. Many values are involved in such an antagonistic situation, and some of them, particularly personal autonomy and human life, are very important indeed.

1. *Putting life first*. In a moral conflict such as this, there are people who reject the notion that a human being has the ethical

freedom to sacrifice his/her life by hunger striking. Such a position has been, and continues to be, common among Christians who base their view on God's absolute sovereignty over human life.

Those who defend this position also support the legitimacy, even the obligatory nature, of forced feeding, although they usually draw distinctions between different phases of consciousness and actually losing consciousness. As long as the hunger striker is conscious, and is in a fit state to express his/her wishes, the doctor is not morally obliged to intervene because, although the striker's action is objectively immoral, each person is free to behave badly. Accordingly, forced feeding would be a violation of freedom and an attack on personal dignity. There are plenty of people, however, who believe that forced feeding is legitimate, even when the person is conscious. When, however, the striker has lost consciousness, the doctor does have the right or duty to intervene. None-the-less, to justify such a move, the doctor would have to base his/her actions on certain assumptions; one of these assumptions is seeing the strike as the result of frustration and misery rather than a lucid, free decision. The doctor might even feel that, even if the decision were taken clearly and freely, it could be assumed that there had been a change in the striker's will while faced with such a threatening situation.

The World Medical Association (WMA) is quite clear on forced feeding while the hunger striker is conscious, but is silent on the correct attitude to adopt when s/he has lost consciousness. Where a prisoner refuses nourishment, the WMA says, and is considered by the doctor to be capable of forming an unimpaired and rational judgement concerning the consequences of such a voluntary refusal of nourishment, he or she shall not be fed artificially. The decision concerning the capacity of the prisoner to form such a judgement should be confirmed by at least one other independent doctor. The WMA also states that the consequences of refusing nourishment should be explained by the doctor to the prisoner.[4]

This distinction drawn between the attitude to be adopted when the hunger striker is conscious and the attitude to be adopted when he/she is unconscious is bizarre and unsatisfactory. If the striker is not fed in the early stages so as not to oppose his/her will, how can forced feeding be justified later on when s/he is unconscious and has somehow managed to survive that long? Of course, there is a difference, and this way we are at least spared the 'spectacle' of someone resisting violence. This difference would presumably take the form of avoiding something that would be shocking to the most hardened sensitivity. It would make a lot more sense, in the view of many people, to say that forced feeding is morally acceptable whether the striker is conscious or unconscious.

2. *Putting autonomy first.* There are others, however, who would put freedom of the individual first in this situation. In our society, where personal autonomy is accorded cult status, it is by no means unusual to hear opinions that support a person's fundamental right over his/her own life. Taking that to its logical conclusion, voluntary euthanasia and hunger strikes become moral options. This moral current is not uncommon in what we might call secular morality.

Many who place such emphasis on personal autonomy add an important rider. The will, they say, must be involved in moral decisions, but it is not a sure and sufficient indicator of moral quality. In making such a decision, the will has to submit to responsibility and common sense. The basic problem, therefore, is whether it is possible to suggest objective criteria with which to determine responsibility in such decisions.

That being said, it is very common for secular morality to accept that a hunger strike can reach its logical conclusion. In such a case, doctors would have no reason to feel obliged to carry out forced feeding.

3. There is a third group that comes to conclusions that are similar to those of the second option. They get there by different routes, not from recourse to personal autonomy but from the indirectly voluntary. They argue that hunger strikes leading to death may be a moral possibility, since death is not sought directly, but it is the indirect result of an act whose primary and direct objective is the recognition of certain rights. If the remaining conditions set out in the principle of double effect are fulfilled, there are no reasons for moral rejection. In such circumstances, doctors would again not be obliged to carry out forced feeding.

NOTES

1. F.J. Elizari, 'Moralidad de la huelda de hambre', in *FC* 8 (15-4-1990) 20-23;
    Équipe of Theologians of the Justice and Peace Commission of the French
    Speaking Belgian Bishops' Conference, 'Comprendre la grève de la faim.
    Note de la faim. Note de travail', in *Supp* 158 (1986) 135-156; N. Selleck
    and others, 'When Patients Harm Themselves', in *HCR* 14 (1984) no. 2, 22-
    23; C.L., 'In Jail for Refusing to Testify: Is Forced Feeding Justified?', in
    HCR 14 (1984) no. 1, 2; E. McDonagh, 'To die for a Cause: martyrdom from
    an Irish perspective', in *Concilium* 183 (1983) 355-365; G.J. Annas, 'Prison
    Hunger Strikes: Why the Motive Matters', in *HCR* 12 (1982) no. 6, 21-22;
    R.A. McCormick, 'Notes on Moral Theology: 1981', in *TS* 43 (1982) 106-
    112; Justice and Peace Commission (Ireland), 'Hunger Strikers of Maze
    Prison', in *Origins* 11 (1981) 91-92; Irish Bishops' Conference and Justice
    and Peace Commission of Ireland, *The Hunger Strikers at the Maze Prison,*
    (1981); D. Dooley-Clarke, 'Medical Ethics and Political Protest', in *HCR* 11
    (1981) no. 6, 5-8; Bishops' Conference of North Ireland, *Appeal to the
    Hunger Strikers*; Ch. Mellon, 'Irlande du Nord: Bilan d'une grève', in
    Project 160 (1981) 1249-1256; H. McCabe, 'Thoughts on Hunger Strikes',
    in *New Blackfriars*, July/August 1981, 303-310.
2. Irish Bishops' Conference *op.cit.*, 711.
3. *Oriens*, December (1984) 9.
4. *Declaration of World Medical Association,* 1977.

Chapter 16

The elderly and the chronically sick[1]

16.1 The elderly and their increasing numbers in society

If the twentieth century has been dubbed the century of demographic growth, it may be that the twenty-first century will be called the century of ageing. Getting old is, of course, quite normal and is something which people come to expect, but it is nowadays very different from what it was in the past. The number of elderly people in western countries is very high both as an absolute and as a proportion of children, young people and adults. The situation in Third World countries is very different. It has been said that these demographic distributions are at least as important as the technological revolution and the biological revolution that await us.

Analysis of the population by age is influenced by trends that are associated with fertility and mortality – and occasionally migration, when there is enough of it to have an impact. In our society, the proportional increase in the number of elderly people has been more sharply accentuated by the dramatic drop in the birth-rate. However, there are also more old people living longer than average at the top of the pyramid; they are doing so thanks to medical advances, better social welfare and improvements in hygiene and diet. It is worth noting that there is a disproportionately high number of women in this group of old people.

This massive demographic shift impacts on every single person, both within the family and within society as a whole. The changes will affect the economic structure, the organization of social life, the way in which we view life and life cycles, and how relations are conducted between individuals and the various generations .

The increase in the number of old people is having a major economic effect on the rest of society; this has to be accepted in a spirit of solidarity. It is also bringing about a degree of social readjustment in many parts of the world. At the same time, there are repercussions in the field of medicine, because the elderly are more frequently victims of chronic illnesses and therefore are in most need of health care.

16.2 Medicine faces a new challenge

For centuries, medicine was not really capable of curing certain diseases. All it could do was to give a measure of comfort and relief. Today, the dominant medical ideology is to provide a cure, and thereby contribute to the prolongation of life. However, given the increase in the number of elderly people beset by chronic and non-chronic illnesses, the objective of medicine can no longer be solely that of curing. Acknowledging this is not tantamount to admitting that medicine has failed or that the objectives should be dropped. As far as the elderly are concerned, medicine can, and should, have new aims that are not so much to do with the number of years people live but with the quality of their lives. It means medicine will have to do a rapid re-think. We are in danger of reacting to the new situation too slowly, although it must be said that an element of fresh awareness can be detected on the part of politicians, doctors and people working in other social agencies. This can be seen in a large number of new initiatives.

If we look carefully at the conditions in which old people live, it is clear that we need to determine precisely what the new aims are. One of the first aims concerns the doctors who will have to look after these people. Health care is essential for this section of society. However, given the specific nature of the kind of care that is needed, I wonder if what the doctors who look after the elderly need is not medical knowledge after all. Perhaps what they really need are personal qualities of courtesy and patience, the ability to listen and exchange views, and a psychological awareness to enable them to perform a relatively unsatisfying job which does not end up with a cure. The direction that health care now needs to take should not be dictated by modern styles of medicine but by the elderly patients' actual needs.

There are many ways of dealing with this situation. One involves health professionals who have been trained in traditional ways, and who can be accompanied by other health workers who have specialized in working with elderly people. Another involves other kinds of health professionals being given not only scientific and technical knowledge but an understanding of human relations and attitudes that are appropriate to care of the elderly. For this kind of work, great skill and a true vocational calling are necessary. Of course, it is easier to teach the right sort of knowledge to people who already have a vocation to look after the elderly than it is to give vocational skills to someone who has this knowledge and nothing else. Just the same, it is obvious that we cannot delay these changes any longer; the well-being of the elderly demands it.

Another matter which society, like medicine, must sort out is the quality of life that the elderly should enjoy. It is no longer simply a matter of them living longer. Our culture should never be a paean to life at any price, or idolize existence for its own sake. Excessive concentration on living is immoral. Medicine has to accept both its own limitations and the limits of technology and the human body. Medicine has to adapt to the needs of old age, but each old person must also approach the situation realistically, according to his/her individual circumstances. We all need training in how to grow old in a humane, reasonable and sensible way. Assuming that an old person is not to suffer any form of discrimination nor to be denied appropriate health care, it follows that we must not forget the duty and obligation to use scarce health resources reasonably. It is certainly difficult to work out a just and comprehensible policy in this respect, but that does not mean that what we think of on the spur of the moment will do. We all need to sit down and think the issue through, so that we understand the issues as clearly as possible. Of course, while doing so, we must bear in mind the importance of solidarity between the generations.

Caring for older people is going to be problematic if we do not agree on a new culture for the elderly, and define it as a stage of life within a given society. The significance and position of the elderly can no longer be a purely individual matter; it must be a collective task. It will be difficult to develop this culture for the elderly if we reject the notion that death is normal and a natural point in life's cycle.

16.3 Caring for the elderly is the responsibility of the family and of society

The elderly are entitled to be looked after properly, although, as I have been trying to demonstrate, society needs to decide for itself what this looking after actually means. Let us now turn the spotlight on those who are responsible for this kind of work.

There is no single form of care that suits every time and place; for instance, the person's family and the way his/her life is organized can have a decisive influence. The number of parents living with their children has declined considerably in our society. One reason for this is that there are now fewer parents who rely financially on their children, and this in turn is partly due to social security and national insurance benefits such as pensions, sickness insurance policies, and other state subsidies and private schemes. There are also a lot of single-parent families, and family relationships have generally become more complex as a result of divorces, separations and remarriages. Families are now smaller and have fewer children, and it is often the case that, in families where the grown-up children are married, both spouses are out at work and this cuts down the amount of time that can be devoted to their parents. Traditionally, the wife used to take most responsibility for the ageing parents, but this is much more difficult to arrange these days for many reasons, not least the fact that she is often at work and out of the house. The family's job of taking responsibility for the old folk in those days was based on two assumptions: firstly, it was taken for granted that families could look after the elderly members with very little outside help; and secondly, it was assumed they had the moral, psychological and spiritual strength to see it through.

As far as financial assistance goes, it would appear that the family's obligation to provide monetary help has moved on considerably since the old days when there was no network of social services paid for out of general taxation. Nowadays, the idea of taking on the financial burden of caring for the chronically sick and the elderly quite often seems beyond public institutions, and we cannot expect families to deal with the problem on their own. This is the point at which there needs to be a degree of solidarity to ensure that the elderly receive the right kind of help. People in need have a moral right to be looked after, and the particular obligation that families share is related to the bonds that are created between people by biological links and living together. Love and a feeling of gratitude for what one's parents have done must not disappear, no matter what social and cultural changes may take place.

All in all, the response depends a lot on the type of relationship between parents and children when the latter are still young. Looking after elderly relatives should not be too much of a burden for the children, and seriously endanger their health, thereby making the situation even worse. Some people believe that society should not take over the entire economic burden in case the children wash their hands of it completely, and stop doing what they should be doing for their parents in the first place.

There is another kind of need that only the family, the children, the brothers and sisters and the spouse can meet. The elderly need their nearest and dearest around them at this point of their lives more than any other. The people who have been part of our personal lives cannot easily be replaced, and such gestures can sometimes be more important than the best medical care. For some elderly people, it is absolutely essential that members of the family are round about them at this time; to a lesser extent, this is also true of friends and the settings in which happy times have been spent together.

It is not part of any plan that society should play an exclusively economic role to enable the family to provide this dual service. The life of an elderly dependant or a chronically sick person can go on for years. To make matters worse, given the way that western society looks at these things, this situation can seem, at least unconsciously, to be a threat to the freedom of relatives and the realization of their expectations and legitimate plans. Prolonging such situations imposes various limitations, creates stress and causes suffering, and in our society the virtues that encourage us to show courage in the face of adversity sadly count for little. It is difficult to put up with the sacrifice and the failure to fulfil oneself, particularly when one has not chosen this situation in the first place, and nobody knows how long it will go on for. That is why society must help these families by arranging for neighbours to provide simple services and for groups of volunteers to give them a break from the non-stop pressure. Families in such circumstances may also need professional psychological support so that members do not have mental breakdowns; this should help them to look after the elderly relatives even better.

16.4 Chronic illness

Although chronic illness is not at all the same thing as being old, the fact that the population is ageing means that chronic illness is on the increase. A chronic illness is one that lasts for a very considerable amount of time, and which continues to have a debilitating effect for a long time thereafter. Some doctors define it by laying down periods of time: for example, chronic illness has been defined as one that interferes with daily activities for more than three months a year, or involves the patient being in hospital for 30 or more days every year, or it is thought during diagnosis that either of these could well come to pass. In short, chronic illness is marked by duration, the severity of the condition, and progressive debilitation.

The growing number of chronic illnesses means we have to rethink many of our ideas, and they pose a major dilemma for health care. Chronic illness is on the increase everywhere: it affects individuals, families, social relations, and health and welfare services. It also presents many challenges to medicine and bioethics. The task of medicine cannot simply be limited to preventive and therapeutic objectives, and we need a new vision based on an understanding of what it all means to human beings and society.

Other subjects dealt with elsewhere in this book such as euthanasia and medical experiments also refer to the elderly and the chronically ill. They are all of the highest importance in the current period.

NOTES

1. N.S. Jecker, 'Towards a Theory of Age-Group Justice', in *JMPh* 14 (1989) 655-676; Reply by Daniels, Ibid., 677-680; L.B. McCullough, 'Long-Term Care: Policy, Ethics and Advocacy', in *HCR* 19 (1989) no. 5, 45-46; M.B. Kapp, 'Medical Empowerment of the Elderly', in *HCR* 19 (1989) no. 4, 5-7; R. Barnet, 'Plato on Medicine's Role in Society: the Care of the Elderly', in *LQ* 56 (1989) 63-71; M.J. Yaffe, 'Implications of Caring for an Aging Parent', in *CMAJ* 138 (1988) 231-235; B. Jennings and others, 'Ethical Challenges of "Chronic Illness"', in *HCR* 18 (1988) no. 1, Spec. Supp.; 'Justice between Generations and Health Care for the Elderly', in *JMPh* 13 (1988) no. 1, Monograph; European Parliament, 'The EC's initiatives in improving the condition of the elderly', in *MM* 37 (1987) 500-507; UN (General Assembly Session on Ageing), 'Final Declaration', in *MM* 35 (1985) 424-450; D. Callahan, 'What Do Children Owe Elderly Parents', in *HCR* 15 (1985) no. 2, 32-37; J.W. Rowe, 'Health Care of the Elderly', in *NEJ* 312 (1985) 827-835; 'The Elderly Persons', in *MH* 187 (1990), Monograph.

PART IV

The doctor-patient relationship

Chapter 17
Patients' rights[1]

At one time, the relationship between doctor and patient was simply looked upon as one that existed between two people. These days, by contrast, the ramifications of health care are enormous and include huge numbers of individuals (carers, family, health workers, insurance officials, judges, members of ethics committees, the patient's lawyer and other patients) and a wide range of other issues and interests.

The relationship is characterized by both societal and medical factors and, given that it is based on health/ill health, it has features which are quite unlike those to be found in other relationships. The personal traits of the people who intervene medically add further complexity to the relationship, as each one of them brings along his/her own conscious and unconscious world.

When the doctor touches the patient's body, it is a gesture that is some way from being purely professional, and it arouses a variety of reactions. It is part of the doctor's training that s/he carries around an image of what a good doctor is like, and also an image of what a patient should be like.

The patient enters a strange land with images of what the doctor will be like, with expectations of what will happen, and with his/her personal history. However, the relationship is characterized by inequality at several levels, such as knowledge and power. There are also other important details like the fact that the doctor is dressed and the patient is naked, and the doctor is standing up and the patient lying down.

A comprehensive study of the doctor-patient relationship will raise many questions, as we have just seen. The Spanish philosopher Pedro Laín Entralgo has said that the components of the relationship are its basis and its diagnostic, curative, social and ethical elements.[2] I myself propose to ignore the historical development of the relationship; instead, I will concentrate on the most common ethical issues, and add a few more. These will include the doctor's professional responsibility, strikes in the health service and ethics committees.

17.1 Historical notes

The issue of health has only slowly become one of our rights, and it has only become established in the western world in the last few decades. In many parts of the world, such ideas are virtually unknown to large portions of the population. Indeed, the phrase 'patients' rights' falls far short of describing the wide range of health needs that will be faced in the future, but I am going to use it just the same. The real situation as regards rights is far from secure, and falls a long way short of the fine ideals that we might occasionally like to dream of.

For centuries, the very idea of patients' rights in a moral or legal sense was unthinkable. It was not possible to protest to the civil or legal authorities except in the most unusual circumstances. The basics of health care were Christian charity, public welfare for the poor, increased public health (through isolating and controlling, rather than curing, certain sick people), and occasionally a contractual relationship between doctor and patient. The notion of a personal right to health care still had some way to go.

Patients' rights, which are today set out in all manner of declarations, were inconceivable in the practice of medicine at the time. It was still dominated by a paternalistic attitude that had itself been modelled on the father-son or master-servant relationship. It was only in the affirmation that doctors made of their duties that there was a hazy, negative acknowledgement that the patient had certain needs. They were a far cry from rights.

Patients' rights have developed very slowly, some of the factors involved being of a general nature and some of them being more specific. The seventeenth and eighteenth centuries were an important period in this respect. This period has been called the 'period of natural rights', and it was during this time that these rights found their expression in civil and political rights. They were eventually felt to be too narrow, and in the late eighteenth century there developed a much broader vision that culminated during the nineteenth and twentieth centuries in a comprehensive range of economic, social and cultural rights.

In this social climate, in which people became increasingly aware of human rights, a small amount of space began to be accorded to what might be called health rights, although this phrase was not used at the time. These rights, such as they were, amounted to very little, but there was little awareness in those days, and medical and social resources were very scarce.

Patients' rights have gained ground in this general social context thanks to a number of factors, and particularly so in the United States. Here, much of the credit goes to the involvement of three movements: the civil rights movement, especially in relation to the black minority, and the feminist and consumers' movements. A high profile organization in the consumer lobby was the National Welfare Rights Organization which, in June 1970, produced a document that included 26 petitions. Amongst them was what might be termed the first all-embracing declaration of patients' rights from a consumer's point of view.

It is worth pointing out that the influence of health 'consumers' – in other words, patients – in this development was minimal. It was a general consumers' movement which did most to make people aware. The fact that patients' input was limited is understandable, since the standing of patients in a hospital is fairly low, and that makes it difficult for them to organize themselves into groups to defend their interests. After all, once a person has left hospital, the last thing s/he wants to do is to go back. Moreover, hospital in-patients are frequently quite ill, and are not really up to finding out their rights and claiming them.

A number of factors contributed to the emergence of a social awareness of patients' rights in the United States. Progressive health education stimulated growing expectations in this field, and these wishes then turned into demands. Moreover, the fact that health costs were rising in a predominantly private health sector did much to strengthen the impetus of these claims. An increase in the incidence of medical malpractice was another reason for examining rights much more closely, and scientific research and experiments by governments and private organizations meant it was vital to provide patients with some protection. Moreover, memories of the abuses carried out by the Nazis triggered calls for the setting up of legal frameworks designed to avoid any repetition. The ever-increasing powers in the hands of doctors had to be 'compensated for' by patients becoming more aware and involved.

17.2 What we mean by patients' rights

The phrase 'patients' rights' has a legal ring to it, but this does not tell the whole story as it also incorporates economic, social and moral issues.

In this book, it is important to emphasize the moral side of patients' rights. Here, we understand them as ethical matters, and as the expression of values related to the individual and such matters as his/her dignity, autonomy and equality. Ethical rights have no legal standing, but they are not without substance for all that. The current distinction between legal and moral matters demonstrates how the human conscience has ways of producing standards which are quite different from laws. An ethical right that has no legal basis may need strengthening if it is to be won; on the other hand, the absence of a legal basis does not nullify that right. When a human right is granted some legal formulation, it usually gains in clarity, but many would say that there is a danger that it will lose much of its validity if it is construed as nothing more than a piece of legislation. That is not to say that I am opposed to giving rights the backing of the law; all I am trying to do is explain what moral rights are and what they can do, and that not everyone thinks it is a good thing if society entrusts the protection of people's interests to the law.

As far as health rights are concerned, we have to draw a distinction between the ideal set out in declarations and what really happens when they are implemented. The fact that there is a distance between the two can be because the health policy is bad, society lacks solidarity, or there is a shortage of resources to meet all social needs.

The demand for rights in the field of medicine does not always meet with universal approval. Reservations come from all quarters. These include claims that there is no comparison with the world of work and the perspective is too individualistic, that there is the risk of raising excessive and unreal expectations, that there is a danger of prejudicing the doctor-patient relationship and an obscuring of the idea that the person primarily responsible for his/her health is the patient, an acknowledgement of the difficulty in determining what the rights actually say, and the possibility of practising bad medicine which will do the patient no good.

The possible dangers inherent in a demand for health rights neither invalidate these rights nor give grounds for distrusting them. Health rights are demanded by some of the more aware individuals in our society, but they also encourage people to destabilize established positions. Lastly, they help to demystify the idea of the doctor as the only person who can care for the patient's health, they provide better protection to disadvantaged people and groups, and they increase a person's dignity.

NOTES

1. G.J. Annas, 'Patients' Rights Movement', in *EB* III, 1201-1206; J. Feinberg, 'Rights Systematic Analysis', in *EB* IV, 1507-1511; R. Macklin, 'Rights in Bioethics', in *EB* IV, 1511-1516; R. Gillon, 'Rights', in *BMJ* 290 (1985) 1890-1891; R.L. Shelton, *Human Rights in Health*, Ass. Scientific Publisher, Amsterdam-London-New York 1974.
2. P. Laín Entralgo, 'History of the Relationship', in *EB* IV, 1655-1662.

Chapter 18

The truth[1]

18.1 The situation in the past

For centuries, the ethical medical tradition did not see the need to affirm the patient's right to know the truth about his/her health. On the contrary, patients were told nothing, and had to rely on the doctor's discretion. Such an attitude has to be understood in the context of the medical profession as it was practised a long time ago.

An exception to this general rule in Christian circles concerned the obligation to inform the patient when s/he was close to death.[2] This was justified by the need to make arrangements for a religious preparation for death, and to make decisions concerning the family and other matters.

That exception apart, the great ethical texts are silent on any duty to tell the patient. The American Medical Association's Code of 1847 even encourages an element of deception, the Geneva Convention of 1948 utters not a word.

18.2 The current situation

Things are changing gradually these days, although the degree of progress varies from one country to the next – and that includes Western countries. There is a trend to provide the patient with maximum information in those societies where relations are more egalitarian and less hierarchical, and where cultural and health standards are high; it also happens in areas of medicine which allow patients to claim their rights. However, less information tends to be passed on when the news to be communicated is not optimistic. In these cases, the information is usually given not to the patient but to the family, and it is left to them to decide whether to keep it to themselves or to tell the patient everything.

Health workers tend to keep well away from confronting the patient in these circumstances. In the United States, however, it appears to be the norm to inform patients, including terminal patients. Here, it seems to be widely accepted both in society and in medical practice; in Europe, the situation is very different.

Resistance to telling the patient in our society is based on a number of issues, for instance the patient's health, the problem of saying anything when the doctor is not sure, and difficulties the patient may have in understanding. Some health workers are convinced that making it an absolute duty to tell the patient could have a negative effect on medical practice, and end up forcing doctors to practise bad medicine. There is also a school of thought that says that information brings more disadvantages than advantages; it is claimed, for example, that there is frequently no real information to give because of doubts arising out of the diagnosis, prognosis or therapy. However, the idea of the all-knowing, all-powerful doctor is a myth that must be rooted out of the public's perception of medicine. None-the-less, it is argued that saying nothing sometimes allows the patient to gain confidence in the doctor, and this can be very important if the therapy is to be successful.

There are also problems on the patient's side. This may be because his/her intellectual ability is declining as a result of the illness, and because his/her emotional state is unsteady. It is not uncommon for the patient to be incapable of understanding certain information because it is too technical, although that should not stop him/her being given some idea of what is going on. Another obstacle to the correct information being given can be the patient's state of mind: the patient's memory may be selective, and s/he may unintentionally retain some information and offload the rest. Each person's perceptions are heavily conditioned by the priorities, needs, worries, beliefs and tensions that s/he brings to the situation.

For health workers to give the patient the right sort of information, they need to know the patient and his/her expectations and wishes. However, they can only know these things if they have opportunities and facilities to listen to what the patient has to say; such circumstances are few and far between.

Although the last few paragraphs show how difficult it can be to communicate satisfactorily, and that it is wrong to attempt the

impossible, that should not be used as an excuse for removing the
patient's right to know exactly where s/he stands. We must encourage the attitude that patients do indeed have this right. Human beings have autonomy that is worthy of respect, and a sick
person is no different. However, the ability to have true autonomy
is unjustly curtailed if the person concerned is denied the information s/he needs. There is also the view that, if the patient
comprehends what is happening, it helps to promote the relationship with the doctor.

The obligation to inform the patient should not be seen as
absolute. The patient's health, which should not be wholly determined by the doctors but also by the patient, will prompt the
major decisions that need to be made. Pius XII gave clear guidance on this when he said that there are cases when the doctor
cannot reveal the whole truth even if s/he is asked to, although
this does not mean that s/he should say anything that is specifically untrue. This is particularly the case, the Pope went on, when
it is known that the patient will not have the strength to cope with
the news. However, there are other occasions when the doctor has
a duty to speak out; it is then a duty that overrides all other
medical and humanitarian considerations. It is not legitimate to
lull the patient into a state of false security, as there is a danger of
thereby compromising his/her eternal salvation or the fulfilling
obligations of justice and charity.[3]

The American Hospital Association provides very detailed
information relating to the kind of health care obtaining in
the USA:

> The patient has the right to obtain from his physician complete
> current information concerning his diagnosis, treatment, and
> prognosis in terms the patient can be reasonably expected to
> understand. When it is not medically advisable to give such
> information to the patient, the information should be made
> available to an appropriate person in his behalf. He has the
> right to know, by name, the physician responsible for coordi-
> nating his care.
>
>   The patient has the right to receive from his physician
> information necessary to give informed consent prior to the
> start of any procedure and/or treatment. Except in emergen-
> cies, such information for informed consent should include but

not necessarily be limited to the specific procedure and/or treatment, the medically significant risks involved, and the probable duration of incapacitation. Where medically significant alternatives for care or treatment exist, or when the patient requests information concerning medical alternatives, the patient has the right to such information. The patient also has the right to know the name of the person responsible for the procedures and/or treatment.

A patient may be transferred to another facility only after he has received complete information and explanation concerning the needs for and the alternatives to such a transfer.

The patient has the right to obtain information as to any relationship of his hospital to other health care and educational institutions in so far as his case is concerned. The patient has the right to obtain information as to the existence of any professional relationships among individuals, by name, who are treating him.

The patient has the right to be advised if the hospital proposes to engage in or perform human experimentation affecting his care or treatment. The patient has the right to refuse to participate in such research projects.[4]

The above document clearly refers to matters that come up elsewhere in this book. An example is informed consent for treatment or research. I will here confine myself solely to the information that is given to the patient.

The question of whether or not to inform the patient cannot be looked at in isolation from the issue of prior counselling. Discussion frequently centres on the appropriateness or otherwise of giving the patient information, and insufficient attention is paid to the support that the patient will need.

18.3 Access to medical records

Another aspect of patient information is the patient's access to his/her medical reports.[5] We are here talking about information that does not relate to treatment currently being received, but to what has gone on previously. Let us first take a look at what medical reports are all about. More than anything else, they seem to have been designed to respond to the needs of health workers so that they can look after the patient better. What medical records have to say covers a wide range of issues including past and present conditions, treatment that has been received, various diagnoses, the results of laboratory tests, data referring to personal and family history, and sometimes information received from people other than the patient. The doctor, of course, can add his/her own personal comments. Medical records are summaries of information used by the doctor treating the patient, and when the treatment is over they become a tool for communicating between doctors and specialists to enable them to care for him/her later on.

It is widely acknowledged that medical records belong to the doctor or hospital, although in some countries, like the United States, this idea of ownership is frequently called into question.

As a general rule, the doctor must tell the patient about what his/her medical record says when requested to do so by the patient. That is not to say that there are not situations when, for the patient's state of health or because information has been supplied from other sources, certain items may legitimately be concealed. There are doctors, though, who take a less ambivalent line on informing patients by systematically handing the patient a copy of the record, except in unusual cases. The patient also has the right to have inaccurate information struck from the record and, given the increased use of information technology, to know what use is to be made of it. Confidentiality is clearly essential.

There are those who believe that giving the patient access to his/her medical record can reduce its value, since the doctor is likely to omit information and opinions which would otherwise have been inserted. The retention of such information, on the other hand, can help to make the treatment more effective.

NOTES

1. D.H. Novack and others, 'Physicians' Attitudes toward Using Deception to Resolve Difficult Ethical Problems', in *JAMA* 261 (1989) 2980-2985, 'Informing Patients about Clinical Disagreement', in *Lancet*, 12 August (1989) 367-368; B.P. Minogue and others, 'The Whole Truth and Nothing but the Truth?', in *HCR* 18 (1988) no. 5, 34-36; P. Skrabanek, 'Honesty with Placebos', in *Lancet*, 31 January (1987) 265-266; C. Dyer, 'Failure to Warn', in *BMJ* 294 (1987) 1089-1090; 'Patient's Access to Personal Health Information', in *BMJ* 292 (1986) 254-256; H. Sergeant, 'Should Psychiatric Patients Be Granted Access to Their Hospital Records?', in *Lancet*, 6 December (1986) 1322-1325; F.G. Reamer and S.J. Schaffer, 'A Duty to Warn an Uncertain Danger', in *HCR* 15 (1985) no. 1, 17-19; R. Gillon, 'Telling the Truth and Medical Ethics', in *BMJ* 291 (1985) 1556-1557; L. Goldie, 'The Ethics of Telling the Patient', in *JME* 8 (1982) 128-133; R.A. Wright, *Human values in Health Care: the Practice of Ethics*, McGraw-Hill 1987; R.F. Weir (ed.), *Ethical Issues in Death and Dying*, Columbia, New York UP 1977; J. Jackson, 'Telling the Truth', in *JME* 16 (1991) 185-186 (and debate in subsequent issues of *JME*); R. Higgs, 'On Telling Patients the Truth', in M. Lockwood (ed.), *Moral Dilemmas in Modern Medicine*, OUP, Oxford 1985.
2. A. Bernadou, 'La vérité au mourant et l'équipe soignante', in *MH* 81 (1976) 48-50; D. Lanzas, '¿Deben saber los enfermos que van a morir?', in *Palabra*, 141 (1977) 25; 'La mort et l'aide aux mourants: vérité et mensonge', in *Supp* 117 (1976) 165-170.
3. Cited by M. Zalba and J. Bozal, *El magistero eclesiástico y la medicina*, Razón y Fe, Madrid 1955, 154-155.
4. *Charter of the rights of the sick people*, American Medical Association, 6 February 1973.
5. D. Brahams, 'Access to Medical Reports', in *Lancet*, 18 February (1989) 395; D. McKie, 'Patients; Access to Medical Records: Manoeuvring in the Commons', in *Lancet*, 11 April (1987) 873; H. Sergeant, 'Should Psychiatric Patients be Granted Access to Their Hospital Records?', in *Lancet*, 6 December (1986) 1322-1325; 'Data Protection Act: Subject Access to Personal Health Information', in *Bulletin of the Royal College of Psychiatrists* 10 (1986) 185; D. Short, 'Some Consequences of Granting Patients Access to Consultant's Records', in *Lancet*, 7 June (1986) 1316-1318.

Chapter 19

Privacy and confidentiality[1]

19.1 Background

The issues of privacy and confidentiality are closely related. The word 'privacy' itself has many meanings:

- not to be subjected to intrusions or the unwelcome physical presence of others in a private place, and not to be subjected to irksome noise when the individual can be seen dealing with private affairs, nor obliged to observe things that offend his/her sensitivity;
- no divulging of confidential information, whether true or false;
- no violation of the person's autonomy in respect of personal decisions;
- respect for the individual's ideas, values and ways of doing things.

Of the above definitions, only the second one is of relevance to confidentiality.

19.2 Confidentiality and the society in which we live

For centuries, professional confidentiality has been one of the duties most energetically affirmed in the field of medical ethics; in some countries, it has even been given legal backing. Its popularity does not, however, mean that it always operates in the same way. Like everything in this world, it is set within its own social and cultural context, and can change at any time.

Let me quickly run through some of the things which characterize our society and medicine, and which help to give shape to confidentiality as we understand it in our Western culture.

These days we are much more sensitive to, and enthusiastic

about, personal autonomy and privacy than we used to be, and this attitude has found protection in statute law; at the same time, there has been a growth in the technological means to invade people's privacy. Moreover, certain news-gathering services adopt styles that have very little respect for privacy; they are carried along by a self-evident yearning to make money out of it, despite the fact that the self-same news media continue to make scarcely credible appeals for freedom of expression.

Like other fields of general social activity, medicine has developed in ways that have had an impact on confidentiality. Illness itself has come to mean something else. It often used to be associated with the world of the divine and the mysterious, and was swathed in feelings of shame and guilt. Today, thanks to scientific advances and the growing spread of knowledge about health, this mysterious halo has for the most part disappeared. We have moved from a form of medicine that was almost completely liberal to one in which social and public issues are heavily emphasized, and where management staff with no medical training are involved. Individual medicine has turned into team medicine, an important development given the growing specialization in knowledge and technology. Data processing, enormously useful for epidemiological studies and planning health policies, is a recent development. One way and another, health services have seen the introduction of several practices that do little to encourage confidentiality.

All these issues have an effect on the way we live, and also impact on the way we think about confidentiality.

19.3 The ethical value of confidentiality

In our culture, confidentiality, particularly professional confidentiality, is looked upon as an important, and widely accepted, ethical value. I say 'our culture' so that we can determine separately whether confidentiality is independent of any historical conditioning, and is essential to any culture.

The fact that confidentiality is clearly and widely accepted does not mean that there are not a number of minority positions that are either sceptical about its meaning, or downright critical of a practice which they consider to be out of date. It is claimed that confidentiality prejudices the individual by making him/her more vulnerable, whereas openness is a positive factor that makes for equality between everybody. Some of these minority positions also claim that there is something antisocial about confidentiality in that it stimulates behaviour opposed to solidarity and favours corporate attitudes of power.

These differing views in no way detract from the widespread acceptance of the moral value of confidentiality. It is not an end in itself; instead, it protects and facilitates realities of profound human importance. Confidentiality is linked to a person's dignity, autonomy, image and reputation. It is a fundamental issue because, between rational beings with an awareness of their own identities, it is very closely linked to the concept of individuality, of being different from everyone else. Confidentiality provides a defence for one's emotional life and feelings, and contributes to a feeling of greater tranquillity in this important area of life. Absence of confidentiality undermines one's capacity to choose and to act, and thereby alters the conditions for independent action. Confidentiality facilitates relationships that are important for a person's well-being and health, including loving, friendly and professional relationships. On occasions, for instance in the event of HIV infection, confidentiality can protect the individual from being socially stigmatized, discriminated against, marginalized and even subjected to violence.

By making so many positive things possible for the individual, confidentiality has a high social value, since society is intrinsically interested in protecting and fostering people's happiness. Without it, the doctor-patient relationship would be seriously jeopardized, and it would elsewhere have a negative impact on individual people's health and even on society.

19.4 A relative value

The principle of confidentiality is not an absolute On the contrary, it contains a number of intrinsic limitations. If the person concerned gives his/her permission either explicitly or implicitly to have certain information passed on, this exempts a professional worker from the moral obligation of confidentiality. The disclosure of confidential information may be justified by the needs of the common good, or to protect a third person's good which is intrinsically more important than the value of the confidence. It is also legitimate to break confidentiality for the patient's own benefit, although here we have to be careful to avoid being paternalistic, or interpreting events in a way that takes the medical questions into account but not the individual's overriding interests. There are times when the law insists that secrets must be revealed; an example would be notifying the appropriate authorities of a contagious disease and identifying the sufferer so that s/he can be treated, and infection avoided. In these circumstances, the strength of the law is based on a sound moral basis, but there may be cases in which conflict can arise between implementation of the law and personal convictions; such conflict can be extremely difficult to resolve. Ideally, the law respects true conscientious objection, but does not ignore the demands of the common good.

A new problem has developed in the context of the spread of computers and new information technology (IT) systems. Computerization of medical records and other medical data is on the increase, and has been made possible by technical advances in IT which allow huge amounts of information to be stored, quickly accessed and easily transmitted. These advances enable us to know more about illnesses and to work out causes that had never previously been suspected. They also permit us to have a better idea of the mortality rate in the population, they facilitate the introduction of better planning for sickness prevention, they encourage health services to move to meet people's needs, and they make it possible to draw up statistics as a basis for medical research and to provide economic forecasts in the health field generally. It is clear that these systems are extremely helpful for research, welfare and even penal matters.

At the same time, an even greater danger of violating a person's privacy seems to come from the vast amount of information that is accumulated about each one of us, and from the fact that many people have access to these files and data banks.

For the time being, we can derive great advantages from the computerizing of personal medical data, and we can do so without our privacy being threatened because all the data are transmitted in code. However, for privacy to be safeguarded properly, those who have responsibility for information which can be identified with individuals must have respect for people. In order to guarantee patients' rights as far as possible, we have to start off by acknowledging that everyone is entitled to know that information relating to him/her will be stored in a computer, and that s/he can refuse to allow this to happen. The individual must similarly have access to files that refer to him/her in order to make sure that they are accurate, and must have the right to demand that details are corrected or erased, as the case may be. Equally, the patient should be told what use is to be made of the information. Just the same, people who are aware of how useful these modern data systems are should not be obsessively concerned about their privacy, but rather encourage a sense of solidarity so that information that is generally useful can be shared.

NOTES

1. M. Pringle, 'Using Computer to Take Patient Histories', in *BMJ* 297 (1988) 697; C.S.C., 'The Pure Church and the Problem of Confidentiality', in *HCR* 18 (1988) no. 1, 2; *BMA* 'Meets Insurers on Medical Reports', in *BMJ* 295 (1987) 866; F.T. de Dombal, 'Ethical Considerations Concerning Computers in Medicine in the 1980's', in *JME* 13 (1987) 179-184; Aberdeen Medical Group, 'Drunken Drivers: What Should Doctors do?', in *JME* 12 (1986) 151-155; M. Kottow, 'Medical Confidentiality: An Intransigent and Absolute Obligation', in *JME* 12 (1986) 117-122; J. Havard, 'Medical Confidence', in *JME* 11 (1985) 8-11; Medical Research Council, 'Responsibility in the Use of Personal Medical Information for Research: Principles and Guide to Practice', in *BMJ* 290 (1985) 1120-1124; R. Gillon, 'Confidentiality', in *BMJ* 291 (1985) 1634-1636; Canadian Medical Association, 'Confidentiality, Ownership and Transfer of Medical Records', in *CMAJ* 133 (1985) 142A; A.J. Asbury, 'Confidentiality of Personal Health Information', in *BMJ* 289 (1984) 1559-1565; F.D. Schoeman (ed.), *Philosophical Foundations of Privacy. An Anthology*, Cambridge Univ. Press, Cambridge 1984; S. Bok, 'The Limits of Confidentiality', in *HCR* 13 (1983) no. 1, 24-31.

Chapter 20

Informed consent[1]

This is one of the most complex issues in bioethics and modern medicine. Informed consent is not something new, but it has encountered substantial resistance among health professionals. This has come about as a result of the convergence of a number of factors. These include the sense of freedom that has gradually invaded our social life, the human rights movement, and the development of consumers' rights; other issues are the defensive reaction that has greeted abuses in medical practice and research, changes in the way people see the doctor-patient relationship, and the growing importance of experimentation and research using humans.

Reactions to informed consent are many and various. These include utterly utopian and unreal dreams of freedom and individual dignity, and a belief that it is the enemy of good medicine. The danger of having a naive view of human freedom – let alone of the patient – together with conflicts that can arise between respect for the patient's autonomy and health, must not conceal the fact that this new version of informed consent is pointing in a positive direction.

The right to informed consent extends to the fields of therapeutic and non-therapeutic research and experimentation, and also to clinical care. As far as patients themselves are concerned, these rights range from conscious and unconscious adults to the elderly, and from prisoners and mentally handicapped people to children and foetuses. Informed consent involves two basic demands: informing the patient and obtaining his/her agreement.

20.1 The duty to inform

The objective of informing the patient is to enable him/her to reach a particular decision, but this depends heavily on each individual's autonomy. Keeping the individual in ignorance, or misleading him/her, is in itself an assault on human dignity.

None-the-less, the duty to inform is not an absolute which has to be obeyed unconditionally. The trouble is that there are so many exceptions that they can easily cancel the duty out. Not informing is justified in emergencies, at the patient's request, if the risk is widely known, if the risk is not known to the relevant doctors, and when the doctor exercises what is called 'therapeutic privilege', that is to say when the doctor takes it upon him/herself that it is in the patient's interest not to be told.

The doctor's therapeutic privilege leads us on to a particularly delicate matter: how to define the person's health, the criteria to be used, and the people who have to decide. The patient's views are the most important when it comes to determining that person's health. It is not a question exclusively or primarily for the doctor or the family, although the doctor must say something from a professional point of view. Moreover, it is not just down to members of the family and doctors. The patient has other representatives who sometimes get involved, including ethics committees and judges. Therapeutic privilege can be applied in well-established therapies, rarely in therapeutic experimentation, and never in non-therapeutic experimentation.

The duty to inform is not simply a question of communicating some facts. Steps must be taken to ensure that the information has been understood as well as possible. However, difficulties of all sorts arise when the moment comes to inform the patient, and it is virtually impossible to avoid some of them. For example, there are psycho-dynamic factors which affect the understanding of the information received; these are related to such matters as the patient's intelligence and general situation, the importance of education, age, social class and fear of losing the doctor's attention, and the patient's emotional state. The technical nature of certain information is an added problem, but this can be largely obviated by the use of simple language.

To ensure that the information is properly understood, it can be transmitted both orally and in written form, and the patient must be given the opportunity to ask questions. Then, between the time when the information has been communicated and the point at which consent has to be given, there has to be as long a period as possible to enable the patient to think about it carefully, ask

questions and even consult others. Informing the patient should
not be understood as a one-off, finite duty; it is a continuous
process. The language used, whether it consists of long or short
sentences, also has an influence on the level of comprehension.
One of the most controversial issues concerns which information
to divulge, and I can do no better than refer the reader to the
account of Margaret Somerville:

1. all material or relevant risks must be disclosed as well as
other factors related to the treatment which could influence the
patient's decision to participate, that is, the disclosure must be
complete, accurate and not too complicated;
2. the information should be objective with reference to the
'reasonable patient', with the proviso that this test becomes subjective to the extent that the physician knew, or ought to have
known, that additional information which would not have been
relevant to the 'reasonable patient' was in fact material to his
particular patient or subject in his decision-taking;
3. the test of required comprehension of the disclosure should
be 'apparently subjective', that is, the doctor must take reasonable
steps in relation to the particular patient to ensure that he understood and that objectively, or apparently, he did;
4. care should be taken that the informing process is not
coercive, and possibly in some circumstances an estimation should
be made by a 'disinterested' outside party in this respect and with
respect to the effectiveness to the informing process;
5. in non-therapeutic experimentation there can be no mitiga-
tion of these standards and no waiver of the right to be informed is
allowed;
6. in the therapeutic situation, waiver, 'therapeutic privilege',
and a duty not to inform, may all apply depending on the circumstances, but generally there should be a presumption that they are
inapplicable, with the burden of proof to the contrary on the
person alleging this, and the burden of rebuttal of the presumption
only being upheld when the circumstances clearly indicate it.[2]

The Federal Register of the US Department of Health,
Education and Welfare also contains the essential information
that must be given to the patient (and/or the subject of the experimentation).

The advice is as follows:

– an honest explanation of the nature and objectives of the intervention which is to take place and, above all, some reference to its experimental nature;
– a description of the drawbacks and dangers that might reasonably be anticipated;
– a description of the advantages that might reasonably be expected;
– reference to any other intervention that could be beneficial to the patient;
– an offer to answer any questions relating to the intervention in question;
– a reminder to the patient that he/she is free to withdraw his/her consent and refuse to undergo the treatment or intervention at any time without prejudice.[3]

Different criteria have been employed to define the different kinds of information that need to be given to the patient. At first, a professional criterion was adopted; this was based on medical practice in general, either obtaining in the same or a similar community or locality, or as practised by a reasonable doctor in similar circumstances. Since round about 1971, we have moved on to accept criteria that have originated outside medicine. This came about when some United States courts began to demand that facts which had influenced a patient's decision should be divulged, irrespective of whether it was medical practice. Some people have adopted the criterion of the patient, but even here there are those who talk about the will and wishes of a reasonable patient, while others look at each patient individually.

My view is that we have to aim to care for the patient we have in front of us, with his/her values, view of life, wishes, preferences and so on. This means that we have to try and get to know not only the individual who has been brought in for treatment but also the structural and personal conditions that will enable us to learn all this. If these prerequisite conditions for getting to know the patient fail to materialize, there is nothing else for it but to rely on more objective criteria.

As a general rule, the patient has to be given some information. Often, when the prognosis is pessimistic, there is a tendency to inform the relatives, who are then given the job of telling the patient. We need to keep in the forefront of our minds the basic objective of informing the patient, and we have to accept that the achievement of this objective is more important than the procedures that are ultimately employed. Just the same, it would be a good thing as far as the procedures are concerned if it was not automatic for the family to be told rather than the patient, as that can make it appear as if the patient is being treated like a child. It never ceases to amaze me that so many people will query the rights of the family to decide on behalf of an incompetent member, and yet also allow them to speak and decide for members who have all their faculties.

20.2 Free consent

By demanding a person's consent for biomedical interventions (treatment and both therapeutic and non-therapeutic experimentation) to take place, the doctor is seeking the protection of the patient's personal autonomy and integrity. In this way, the patient is more closely involved in the joint task between him/her and the doctor. This gives the patient more power by correcting the imbalance of the relationship with the doctor, whose job gives him/her considerable power. This has advantages for the health professional over and above the moral meaning of informed consent in that it also offers him/her excellent protection against any claims for damages.

None-the-less, informed consent is a value that must be promoted, given that it stimulates rational and free decisions, avoids dishonesty, deception and coercion, involves the patients in issues that concern them intimately, encourages self-examination among doctors and researchers, and reduces their legal responsibilities and the likelihood of redress in the courts.

Medicine was once characterized by a form of paternalism, which understandably flourished in an era which also encouraged it. Nowadays, it is the practice to try and obtain people's consent on matters that concern them. There can be exceptions to this rule arising out of earlier inertia, the patient's present situation, or because s/he is not well-educated, has inferior social status and so on. However, the type of intervention will give an indication

about the degree of risk. Attempts are being made to establish a
gradual approach, but generally speaking there is less agreement
in research than in clinical work; it should be borne in mind, in
respect of the former, that there is a clear difference between
therapeutic and non-therapeutic research. In the case of emergencies, it is much easier to assume the patient's consent than in
normal circumstances. There can even be times when the public
interest overrides the need to elicit the patient's wishes; an example of this would be if the individual was opposed to a compulsory vaccination. When life and health are at grave risk, there are
many people who consider it to be totally legitimate to act against
the person's wishes because of the broader danger to the public at
large.

The only consent that accords with human dignity is one that
is given freely. However, free consent can be facilitated, encouraged and impeded in all manner of ways. As we have already
seen, information makes it possible, but obfuscation, deceit, dishonesty and mistakes can seriously compromise it.

The disparity existing between doctor and patient is part of the
freedom which the doctor must try and reduce as much as possible. Furthermore, the individual's autonomy is limited by fears of
not being properly looked after if s/he turns down a given intervention, and by other anxieties of being criticized or branded a
bad patient. This is particularly acute when well-disposed patients
receive special treatment. Consent which is obtained gradually
and in stages loses its psychological impact, unlike consents
which are requested and immediately granted. A decision taken
before going into hospital is probably freer.

Consent can be given orally and/or in written form, although
there is a growing tendency in some hospitals in some countries to
register the patient's agreement in writing, and even in the presence of witnesses. However, even written consent must leave
open the possibility of the patient going back on the earlier
decision, so the first option seems to be preferable for the person –
the doctor or a third party – who has to obtain the consent.

Encouragement and respect for the patient's autonomy when
making decisions does not mean leaving the patient to his/her
own devices at such a moment. Members of the family and
doctors are well-placed to provide useful assistance.

What the patient decides is not necessarily what eventually

happens. If the patient asks for things which the doctor's conscience will not permit, the latter has every right to refuse. The patient's request will also need to adapt to what society can offer in order to be accepted; purely individual interests can easily clash with legitimate social demands. In such cases, it is difficult to harmonize the patient's wishes with the doctor's views and the capacity and demands of society.

20.3 People who are not capable of giving consent

The ideal of informed consent sometimes runs up against a particularly awkward and problematic reality. This occurs when consent seems to be out of the question, or there appear to be huge obstacles in the way of eliciting it. Examples of people in such situations include patients close to death, foetuses, young children, people suffering from mental handicap and prisoners.[4]

Incapability. The first step is to establish whether the patient is capable of giving informed consent. This presents no problem in many cases like foetuses, young children, and people who have previously been well capable but whose awareness or capacity is now severely impaired. Minors offer a variety of problems, including not only their age but also their level of maturity. Mentally handicapped people also present a number of difficulties; they range from those who are patently incapable to those who have the ability to take certain decisions – leaving a grey area of cases which are much more problematic.

Determining the degree of incapability from a human point of view, as distinct from a legal standpoint, is sometimes so straightforward that it can be legitimately left to carers and family members. On other occasions, a specialist needs to be involved.

Efforts to decide on a person's capability should not necessarily concentrate on age, or simply the current diagnosis. An attempt needs to be made to find out what might have caused the present situation, and if there is any chance of curing it. Some of the best indicators of capability/incapability are the patient's level of communication with carers, and his/her ability to understand information and weigh up various alternatives.

The subjects of decisions. Once it is established that the person is incapable of giving informed consent, it still has to be decided who is going to take decisions on his/her behalf and the criteria and principles that will inform that decision.

In normal circumstances it will be left to a member of the family, less often to an outsider. This is in line with medical opinion. It is only fair to grant the family special status in matters of this sort, as they are most involved in the patient's health and most likely to know what his/her preferences are. Exceptions to this rule can arise in a variety of circumstances. These include when family members cannot make their minds up, when there is a fundamental disagreement between them, when there are indications of negligence on the part of the family, and if there is substantial conflict of interest between the patient and the family. If there are no family members or legal representatives, health workers may be the best placed to take decisions, but this depends on how important and urgent the issues are.

Also involved in situations of this kind are ethics committees and the courts. The role of the former is dealt with in chapter 24. As far as courts are concerned, the law sometimes obliges judges to be involved; an example of this in certain countries is the sterilization of the mentally ill. Apart from such cases, and those where there are conflicts of interest, recourse to the courts is not ideal. As I have already made clear, there are other solutions which make a lot more sense.

Criteria for decision making. I have alluded to a number of guiding principles and criteria to ensure that decisions taken on another person's behalf are not arbitrary.

One approach is to look into the patient's presumed desires or wishes, in other words into what it is imagined s/he would have done if s/he had been in a position to do so. In the absence of a clear indication of what s/he wants, the decision should be based on the values s/he used to profess, on his/her view of life, and on other relevant indications. Here, it can be difficult to know what to do because of uncertainties about the person's preferences. Such an approach is perfectly reasonable, but it rarely illuminates and is not really practical; it does have the virtue, though, of emphasizing the person's autonomy to the maximum.

According to another school of thought, the main criterion is the patient's health. If there is evidence of the incapable person's assumed or presumed wishes, we need to look at the his/her health according to the most objective and socially shared criteria possible. There are some obvious indicators of the patient's health like relief from suffering, functions to be restored or preserved, and the quality and prolongation of life. Such decisions can be determined jointly by health workers and the patient's representative. If the latter opts for decisions that are professionally unacceptable, doctors can reject any conscientious objections, and even go to court.

Ultimately, whichever approach is adopted, it is often extremely difficult to make the right decision.

20.4 The complexity of informed consent

The positive welcome that such a change in medical practice deserves should not stop us from acknowledging its limitations and the difficulties that surround it. It is worth saying at this stage that there are even some people that manage to find so many problems in this area that they end up thinking that informed consent is not worth the paper it is written on.[5]

I would like to add one more thing to the comments I have made above. Attempts have been made to locate the basis of accepting or rejecting informed consent inside two kinds of culture. One of them is paternal, and focuses more on the achievement of the objectives than on the patient's involvement; the other is maternal, and has more to do with subjectivity and the patient's emotional state. No less influential, in my view, is how the doctor's role is viewed, and there is a preference to see him/her as a clinician or researcher.[6]

It has been said that the theory and practice of informed consent runs the risk of courting individualism. There is also the danger of marginalizing the patient's social awareness; the patient's awareness may not be up to the task at times when there is a shortage of resources with which to deal with growing health needs.

Finally, there are claims that the demand for informed consent can lead to the practice of bad medicine because doctors are held back in their search for the patient's well-being by respect for his/her autonomy. Equally, it can cause conflicts between the patient's wishes and the health worker's conscience, and between the patient's wishes and the demands of the common good.

NOTES

1. R. Gillon, 'Medical Treatment, Medical Research and Informed Consent', in *JME* 15 (1989) 3-5, 11; W.A. Silverman, 'The Myth of Informed Consent: in Daily Practice and Clinical Trials', in *JME* 15 (1989) 6-11; J. Wilson-Barnett, 'Limited Autonomy and Partnership: Professional Relationships in Health Care', in *JME* 15 (1989) 12-16; G.R. Gillett, 'Informed Consent and Moral Integrity', in *JME* 15 (1989) 117-123; H. Brody, 'Transparency: Informed Consent in Primary Care', in *HCR* 19 (1989) no. 5, 5-9; M. Shultz, 'Informed Consent, a Symbol Analyzed', in *HCR* 17 (1987) no. 3, 24-25; J. Wilson, 'Patients' Wants Versus Patients' Interests', in *JME* 12 (1986) 127-130; E. Matthews, 'Can Paternalism Be Modernised?', in *JME* 12 (1986) 133-135; J.W. Warren and others, 'Informed Consent by Proxy', in *NEJM* 315 (1986) 1124-1128; J.F. Drane, 'The Many Faces of Competency', in *HCR* 15 (1985), no. 2, 17-21; D. Brahams, 'Doctor's Duty to Inform Patients of Substantial or Special Risks when Offering Treatment', in *Lancet*, 2 March (1985) 528-530; B.G.B. Weiss, 'Paternalism Modernised', in *JME* 11 (1985) 184-187; R.T. Hull, 'Informed Consent: Patient's Right or Patient's Duty?', in *JMPh* 10 (1985) 182-197; P.T. Hershey, 'A Definition for Paternalism', in *JMPh* 10 (1985) 171-182; R. Gillon, '"Primum non nocere" and the Principle of Non-Maleficence', in *BMJ* 291 (1985) 130-131; Id., 'Paternalism and Medical Ethics', in *BMJ* 290 (1985) 1971-1972; Id., 'Beneficence: Doing Good for Others', in *BMJ* 291 (1985) 44-45; President's Commission for the Study of Ethical Problems in Medicine and Biomedical and Behavioral Research, *Making Health Care Decisions: The Ethical and Legal Implications of Informed Consent in the Patient-Practitioner Relationship*, Government Printing Office, Washington 1982; National Commission for the Protection of Human Subjects of Biomedical and Behavioral Research, *The Belmont Report: Ethical Guidelines for the Protection of Human Subjects of Research*, Government Printing Office, Washington 1979; *Ethical Dilemmas in Obtaining Informed Consent*, in T.A. Shannon (ed.), *Bioethics*, Paulist Press, 1970, 311-373.
2. M.A. Somerville, *Le consentement à l'acte médical*, Commission de réforme du droit du Canada, Ottawa 1980, 27-28.
3. Department of Health, Education and Welfare, Federal Register, 13 March 1975, 40 F.R. 50, 11854.
4. W. Gaylin, 'The Competence of Children: No Longer All or None', in *HCR* 12 (1982) no. 2, 33-38; J. Blustein, 'On Children and Proxy Consent', in *JME* 4 (1978) 138-140; A.G.M. Campbell, 'Infants, Children and Informed Consent', in *BMJ* 268 (1974) 334-338; F. Schoeman, 'Parental Discretion and Children's Rights: Background and Implications for Medical Decision-Making', in *JMPh* 10 (1985) 54-61; P. Ramsey, *The Patient as Person*, Yale Univ. Press, New Haven and London 1976[7], 1-58; 'Consent and Prisons', in *BMJ* 292 (1986) 324; National Commission for the Protection of Human Subjects of Biomedical and Behavioral Research, *Research Involving Prisoners*, US DHEW Publications, Bethesda 1976; N.D. Neveloff, 'Depriving Prisoners of Medical Care: A "Cruel and Unusual Punishment"', in *HCR* 9 (1979) no. 5, 7-10; J.M. Humber, 'The Involuntary Commitment and Treatment of Mentally Ill Persons', in *SSM* 15F (1981) 143-150; D.W. Millard, 'The Treatability Requirement in Psychopathy: A New Ethical Dilemma?', in *JME* 10 (1984) 88-90; R. O'Neil, 'Determining Proxy Consent', in *JMPh* 8 (1983) 389-403.
5. W.A. Silverman, *op.cit.*, 6.
6. A. Filiberti and M. Bellotto, 'Consenso informato: biases psicosociali', in *MM* 40 (1990) 41-59.

Chapter 21

The right to turn down treatment[1]

In the last chapter, we looked at the patient's autonomy from a very specific angle – the demand for informed consent prior to various therapeutic and non-therapeutic interventions. Now, we consider autonomy from another standpoint: the right to reject treatment. Like informed consent, this is something that can give rise to conflicts with doctors.

Traditional medicine did not really consider either of these notions. Only the doctrine of the non-obligatory nature of extraordinary means in both health care and the prolongation of life came anywhere near it. In modern medicine, this request is articulated as an expression of personal autonomy, or as an appeal to religious beliefs – which is at the same time an invocation to freedom.

In principle, every patient must be accorded the right to turn down a given form of treatment by virtue of these very principles. On the other hand, each person is asked to approach this decision, like any other aspect of life, with a level of responsibility that is in keeping with the importance of the decision to be taken. All this requires a reasonable attitude on the part of the individual. The wish itself is not a criterion of morality; it has to be responsible and sensible, and not arbitrary. There are many reasons for rejecting treatment: the fact that it will not serve any purpose, the arduous nature of the intervention, and doubts about the advantages, consequences and repercussions for the patient and for others. However, rejection should not mean avoiding social or family responsibilities, or rejecting important values.

Rejection of treatment can come into conflict with other values and interests of the same person. For example, this can come about when the patient turns down a transfusion when his/her life is in danger. The conflict can also affect the interests of other people, for instance when the treatment endangers the life of

247

another person, such as a child or foetus. The patient's autonomy comes into conflict with society when the latter finds itself obliged to protect someone's life, perhaps by force; this can happen in the case of a prisoner on hunger strike. Finally, conflict can involve health workers who feel obliged to oppose the patient's freedom in order to maintain their ethical integrity as health professionals.

It can also happen that conflict arises between the patient's autonomy and his/her health. The solution to this problem depends on the value that is placed on his/her freedom. In the case of the most striking conflict – that between autonomy and life – there is nowadays a tendency in secular morality for autonomy to triumph over freedom. The standard procedure in the past, however, favoured intervention. It was not simply permitted; it was compulsory, particularly when the patient was not capable of expressing his/her objections.

When rejection of treatment endangers the life or integrity of the foetus, the Christian doctrine still insists on the moral obligation to accept the treatment. However, in a society that is so tolerant of abortion, it is to be expected that large numbers of people will be opposed to compulsory intervention. For this reason, the position adopted by some courts in the USA, which have forced some pregnant women to accept treatment that was considered medically necessary for the foetus's health, has stimulated reactions ranging from approval to outrage.

There is much more agreement when rejection of treatment places the life of a minor in danger. The most common example in this context is that of Jehovah's Witnesses who are opposed to blood transfusions. Other people even defend the rejection of physical and pharmacological treatment as incompatible with the hope placed solely in God.[2]

Jehovah's Witnesses base their position on several extracts from the Bible, including Deut 12:23-25, Gen 9:4 and Lev 17:10-14. The action of bleeding animals that are to be eaten is given a religious foundation which Jehovah's Witnesses then apply to rejecting transfusions. Blood is identified with life in such a way that drinking blood is the same as eating life, and that means an invasion of an area that is divine: God is the sole lord of life. The way that Jehovah's Witnesses interpret these Biblical texts to defend their rejection of blood transfusions lacks any objective basis, but it has turned into a conviction of conscience. This only

made sense when transfusions were not possible, and many believe that it is an anachronism nowadays. Depending on who is
going to turn down the transfusion (e.g. oneself, a minor or a
pregnant woman), the decision should be determined according to
the advice set out above.

NOTES

1. A. Davis, J. Neals and M. Simms, 'Informed Dissent', in *JME* 13 (1987) 53-
   55; G.J. Annas, 'Transferring the Ethical Hot Potato', in *HCR* 17 (1987) no.
   1, 20-21; Id., 'Protecting the Liberty of Pregnant Patients', in *NEJM* 316
   (1987) 1213-1214; V.E.B. Kolder, J. Gallagher and M.T. Parsons, 'Court-
   Ordered Obstetrical Interventions', in *NEJM* 316 (1987) 1192-1196; A.
   Davis, 'Informed Dissent; The View of a Disabled Woman', in *JME* 12
   (1986) 75-76; J.M. Alimbau, 'The sick person can refuse the technology
   needed to prolong his life', in *LH* 191 (1984) 52-53; C.L., 'The Right to
   Refuse Psychotropic Drugs: The Question in the States', in *HCR* 14 (1984)
   no. 2, 2; S. Vinogradov and others, 'If I have AIDS, Then Let Me Die
   Now!', in *HCR* 14 (1984) no. 1, 24-26; P.S. Appelbaum and L.H. Roth,
   'Patients Who Refuse Treatment in Medical Hospitals', in *JAMA* 250 (1983)
   1296-1301; 'Impaired Autonomy and Rejection of Treatment', in *JME* 9
   (1983) 131-132; J.L. Dixon and M.G. Smalley, 'Jehovah's Witnesses', in
   JAMA 246 (1981) 2471-2472; N.C. Drew, 'The Pregnant Jehovah's Witness', in *JME* 7 (1981) 137-139; B.L. Miller, 'Autonomy and the Refusal of
   Life-saving Treatment', in *HCR* 11 (1981) no. 4, 22-28; J.L. Dixon and
   M.G. Smalley, 'Jehovah's Witnesses. The Surgical/Ethical Dilemmas', in
   JAMA 246 (1981) 2471-2472; T.F. Ackerman, 'The Limits of Beneficence:
   Jehovah's Witnesses and Childhood Cancer', in *HCR* 10 (1980) no. 4, 13-
   18; G.J. Annas, 'Refusing Medication in Mental Hospitals', in *HCR* 10
   (1980) no. 1, 21-22.
2. Cf H.Y. Vanderpool, 'Protestantism II. Dominant Health Concerns in Protestantism', in *EB* II, 1377.

Chapter 22
Professional responsibility[1]

22.1 The current situation

In the past, there were very few allegations of errors, medical negligence, omissions or other shortcomings imputable to health workers; the most blatant cases related to breaches of confidentiality and surgical errors. This can be explained in a general sense and also in strictly medical terms. For one thing, there was but scant awareness of the rights of the individual; at the same time, medicine was wrapped in a mysterious, almost religious, aura which protected doctors and made it difficult for patients to lodge complaints. For another, it was difficult to draw a clear line between a doctor's blameworthiness and the limitations of medicine.

Things have changed a lot since then, with a steep rise in the number of negligence claims and in the sums of money paid out in compensation. The situation does vary from one part of the world to another, and there is a notable difference between the United States and other developed western countries. This is due mainly to the types of health system in operation; in the United States health care is based primarily on private insurance, whereas in other parts of the world it relies on social security and direct taxation. Other influences include the legal systems in force and social awareness of patients' rights. Part of the explanation of the increase in negligence claims lies with other factors like the technical and scientific advances which enable medicine to be more aggressive although more fraught with risks, the ever-rising number of medical interventions, which in itself increases the incidence of mistakes and negligence, and the growing tendency of doctors to establish their own version of what rights should be.

There are no studies that give us an exact picture of the

current situation. Virtually the only data we have come from a study carried out in California in 1974 and published in 1977.[2] According to this, no fewer than 4.65 per cent of all people in hospital were suffering from pathological conditions, and of these 17 per cent were down to negligence. On the basis of negligence claims that have been submitted, P.M. Danzon has estimated that around 10 per cent of patients who have had pathological conditions due to negligence proceeded to put in a claim.[3]

Little more is known of the sums of money received by patients who claim compensation, or about the extent to which doctors' fear of being sued encourages them to take more care not to cause injuries.

Unlike injuries suffered by healthy people at work or in road accidents, morbidity in hospital affects people who are already ill. This is a further complication to add to the difficulty of distinguishing between forms of morbidity that have resulted from negligence and other forms that are inevitable because of the limitations of medicine.

This problem of doctors' responsibility for malpractice worries health workers mainly from legal, penal and civil points of view, and people in the United States have quite different degrees of anxiety from people in other Western countries. It appears that the moral dimension of the question is rarely discussed there.

22.2 Indications for the future

I want to make it clear from the outset that there is likely to be a large element of moral responsibility in the way health professionals carry out their jobs, and that this can involve a duty to make good any damage resulting from a morally culpable action. Let us have a look at how the system works, and then see how this duty can be fulfilled.

For moral responsibility to exist, it has to be possible to attribute to someone an element of personal guilt for negligence or errors; these may occur in the performance of the intervention or may result from unjustifiable incompetence. Furthermore, there needs to be a connection between the doctor's action and the harm caused. Lastly, irrespective of this personal responsibility, when the patient has been made worse but the doctor is not to blame, should we not be trying to set up social machinery to enable serious injury to qualify for compensation as a token of social solidarity and coming out of a special insurance policy?

To make sure we do not lose sight of this problem, as is happening in North America, we need to keep the context of modern medicine at the front of our minds. Unlike other professions, medicine incorporates values such as life, health, and physical and mental integrity, and to promote these values, highly aggressive means are used which may cure, or inflict harm. Furthermore, for doctors to carry out their jobs – and this is more true of certain areas of medicine than of others – there is a need for knowledge and skills that not all doctors have and possess to the same degree. We can ask a lot of medicine, but we must not ask the impossible.

Much more complicated than the moral issue is the legal problem of how to deal with the growing number of negligence claims.

Some people think that health workers should not be liable for mistakes and genuine errors, but only for serious, deliberate malpractice. In my view, the concept of legal liability must be maintained on the basis that all people are equal; otherwise, we are acknowledging the power of privilege. Moreover, if we were to reject the idea of responsibility, there would be a danger that immunity would mean less effort was made to acquire the necessary skills, and that in turn would increase the risk of even worse treatment.

Just the same, we have to bear in mind the conditions in which modern medicine is practised, and also educate the public to have common-sense expectations of medicine; after all, medicine is something in which we all have a role to play. Lastly, we need to do something about certain members of society who far too quickly opt for litigation.

What of the various systems that have been suggested as ways of responding to claims? One consists basically of the doctor him/herself responding, once proof has been established of both the harm and the causal connection between his/her action and the injury to the patient. Such an approach can have major financial implications arising out of expensive insurance policies, an increase in financial compensation awarded by the courts, and difficulties in finding insurance. In order to avoid these problems, several new ideas have been put forward, including attempts to limit the amount of compensation, drawing up a list of litigants which is distributed to doctors prior to payment, and taking out less expensive insurance policies.

Finance is not the only problem standing in the way of the practice of proper medicine. One danger is that the patient-doctor relationship, which should be based on confidence, is now built on mistrust. There is also the fear that certain high-risk specialisms such as anaesthetics, surgery and obstetrics will not attract enough young people, and there might not in consequence be enough doctors to meet society's needs. It is felt that some doctors might insist on innumerable and unnecessary investigations, consultations and analyses just to safeguard their positions, and health costs would go up as a result. However, there is not enough hard information even in North America for us to be sure about all this.

As far as the notion of personal responsibility is concerned, even when, in some places, doctors working inside the system are covered by social security or the National Health Service, some people are proposing other schemes that involve objective or automatic responsibility along the lines of insurance policies covering motor accidents.

NOTES

1. M.J. Hatlie, 'Professional Liability', in *JAMA* 261 (1989) 2281-2282; H.H. Hiatt and others, 'A Study of Medical Injury and Medical Practice', in *NEJM* 321 (1989) 480-484; C. Clothier, 'Medical Negligence and No-Fault Liability', in *Lancet*, 18 March (1989) 603-605; K.S. Abraham, 'Medical Liability Reform. A Conceptual Framework', in *JAMA* 260 (1988) 68-72; C.J. Whelan, 'Litigations and Complaints Procedures: Objectives, Effectiveness and Alterations', in *JME* 14 (1988) 70-76; E. Haavi, 'Cost Constraints as a Malpractice Defense', in *HCR* 18 (1988) no. 1, 5-10; K. McK. Norrie, 'Reasonable: the Keystone of Negligence', in *JME* 13 (1987) 92-94; L. Quam, P. Fenn and R. Dingwall, 'Medical Malpractice in Perspective', in *BMJ* 294 (1987) 1529-1531 and 1597-1600; K. McK. Norrie, 'Medical Negligence: Who Sets the Standards?', in *JME* 11 (1985) 135-137; D. Kloss, 'The Duty of Care: Medical Negligence', in *BMJ* 289 (1984) 66-68;

W.J. Curran, 'A Further Solution to the Malpractice Problem: Corporate Liability and Risk Management in Hospitals', in *NEJM* 310 (1984) 704-705; P.J. Connors and W.J. Curran, 'Malpractice and Informed Consent', in *NEJM* 300 (1979) 928-929; M.D. Bayles and A. Caplan, 'Medical Fallibility and Malpractice', in *JAMA* 238 (1977) 861-863; J.F. Childress, 'Compensating Injured Research Subjects: The Moral Argument', in *HCR* 6 (1976) no. 6, 21-28.

2. D.H. Mills (ed.) *Report on the Medical Insurance Feasibility Study*, California Medical Association, San Francisco 1977. A study prepared for the State of New York in 1989: see Hiatt, *op.cit.*

3. P.M. Danzon, *Medical Malpractice: Theory, Evidence and Public Policy*, Harvard Univ. Press, Mass. 1985.

Chapter 23
Strikes in the health sector[1]

23.1 The general teaching on strikes

In a number of authoritative documents, Catholic morality provides us with a brief summary of the Church's doctrine on strikes at work:

> When [...] socio-economic disputes arise, efforts must be made to come to a peaceful settlement. Recourse must always be had above all to sincere discussions between the parties. Even in present-day circumstances, however, the strike can still be a necessary, though ultimate, means for the defence of the workers' own rights and the fulfilment of their just demands. As soon as possible, however, ways should be sought to resume negotiations and the discussion of reconciliation.[2]

Octagesimo Adveniens also reminds us when it is a question of public services, required for the life of an entire nation, it is necessary to be able to assess the limit beyond which the harm caused to society becomes inadmissible.[3]

From a moral standpoint, a strike must meet three conditions for it to be legitimate:

- the cause must be just;
- it must take place as a last resort, there being no other less harmful alternatives available;
- there must be reasonable prospects of success – on balance.

23.2 Strikes in the health sector

I will here reproduce part of a statement issued by the Episcopal Commission for Pastoral Health which deals with all sides of this delicate problem in a succinct and balanced manner:

Going on strike is the right, though not an absolute right, of every citizen. Strikes in the health sector are not comparable to those that take place elsewhere in the economy since they impact directly on the primary and most fundamental of all human rights, the right to life, and therefore also the right to health. Moreover, they can give lead to major problems, and exacerbate the suffering already being undergone by patients and their families.

It follows that a strike in the health sector can only be justified after those involved – organizers, supporters, workers and government – have looked at the consequences with the greatest care. The fact that the consequences can be very serious, and that those who suffer most are the weak and defenceless, means that a strike can only ethically be defended in truly extreme circumstances. Therefore government particularly, but also private individuals and organizations that perform management functions in the health service, must stress the importance of channels of dialogue. They also need to be specially sensitive to the problems faced by staff and health centres, and place patients' well-being and the social good above all other interests. Therefore...

1. We beg all those calling strikes in the health sector, and others with responsibility for their resolution, to weigh up the consequences for patients with the greatest care, and exhaust all possible means of solving the dispute, in such a way that strike action is only used as the last, unavoidable resort.

2. In the event of a strike being called, we beg organizers, government and health workers to guarantee basic health care services, and not only emergency services but also those which, if they were not performed, could cause serious harm to the health of the patients or suffering to them and their families; a strike cannot be ethically justified if these services are not carried out.

3. We also ask those involved to do everything in their power to avoid or overcome any obstacles which block or stand in the way of mutual understanding and an early solution to the dispute; these include excessive enthusiasm, adopting narrow minded and simplistic positions, using the dispute for political purposes, and manipulating the situation by means of incomplete and tendentious information.[4]

NOTES

1. M. Garty, 'Physicians' Strike. Second Thoughts', in *JME* 12 (1986) 104-105; R. Brecher, 'Health Workers' Strikes: A Rejoinder Rejected', in *JME* 12 (1986) 40-42; S.M. Glick, 'Health Workers' Strikes: A Further Rejoinder', in *JME* 12 (1986) 43-44; P.S. Sachden, 'Ethical Issue of a Doctor's Strike', in *JME* 12 (1986) 53; R. Brecher, 'Striking Responsibilities', in *JME* 11 (1985) 66-69; J.L. Muyskens, 'Nurses' Collective Responsibility and the Strike Weapon', in *JMPh* 7 (1982) 101-112; Editorial, 'On the strike of health workers', in *RF* 998 (1981) 454-457; N. Daniels, 'On the Picket Line: Are Doctors' Strikes Ethical?', in *HCR* 8 (1978) no. 1, 24-29; J. Lister, 'Should Doctors Strike?', in *NEJM* 299 (1978) 1056-1060; G. Dworkin, 'Strikes and the National Health Service: Some Legal and Ethical Issues', in *JME* 3 (1977) 76-82.
2. *Gaudium et Spes*, 68.
3. *Octagesimo Adveniens*, 14.
4. *Comunicado de la Comisión Episcopal de Pastoral sanitaria sobre las huelgas sanitarias*, in *Ecclesia* 2126 (21-5-1983) 12; 7.

Chapter 24
Ethics committees[1]

24.1 Background

One of the ways in which the current interest in ethics in biological and medical affairs has manifested itself has been in the setting up and spread of ethics committees. A number of quite different bodies come under this heading, ranging from committees that evaluate research protocols (although the word 'ethics' is not usually applied to them in such circumstances), national-level committees whose job it is to advise Heads of State, legislative bodies and governments, and hospital ethics committees.

The first to be formed were committees which were charged with evaluating research and experimentation projects that involved human beings. Abuses committed by the Nazi regime, and the growing importance of research aimed at scientific advance and people's health, underlined the fact that there was a need for control bodies which sought to guarantee respect for human rights. Hospital ethics committees, which came later, are what I propose to concentrate on here.

Three events in the United States have aroused interest in hospital ethics committees. In the first, which took place in 1976, the Supreme Court of New Jersey recommended that an ethics committee be consulted to confirm the prognosis on a comatose woman, Karen Ann Quinlan, whose family had asked for her artificial breathing apparatus to be turned off. It was the first time a United States court had recommended that an ethics committee be involved in decision making, a field hitherto reserved for doctors, patients and members of the family. Despite the name which the court gave it, the committee in fact had a purely medical function, and did not deal with ethical questions at all. In 1983, a report produced in the United States by the President's Commission for the Study of Ethical Problems in Medicine and Biomedical and Behavioral Research urged doctors and administrators to set up review and consultation machinery to deal with cases that had ethical implications. It was also suggested that ethics committees should be established. In 1984, the Department of Health and Human Services responded to the case in which treatment was not given to 'Baby Doe' by arguing strongly for the setting up of committees to evaluate infant care.

To understand hospital ethics committees and place them accurately in their medical and social contexts, we have to bear in mind the many cultural changes that have taken place in the last few decades – the rise of the civil rights movement, the defence of consumers' interests (where health has also become a consumer commodity), and a certain distrust for public authorities and authority in general. This general climate has had a major impact on people's attitude towards doctors. In the past, doctors made decisions which were automatically accepted without demur, but now they adopt positions which encourage suspicion. The enormous power that technological advances have placed in the hands of biologists and doctors, certain abuses that have been discussed in the media, and the complexity of some decisions are also factors that go some way to explaining the appearance and spread of these ideas. They have constituted a new attempt to give form to ethical thinking with a new inter-disciplinary style, but in line with a society that offered a range of moral options.

These committees are spreading very unevenly. In 1988, 60 per cent of hospitals in the United States with 200 beds or more[2] had an ethics committee, but even there they are still thought to be dormant.[3] They are still at an early stage of development in Europe, too. A meeting held in London in February 1987 found that they were at a formative stage, and were still seeking an identity. In 1988, they existed in only two English psychiatric hospitals.[4]

Many reasons have been put forward to explain the slow introduction of hospital ethics committees elsewhere in Europe. These include some doctors' fears of interference by outsiders in their clinical judgement and relationships with patients, lack of clarity and disagreements about the objectives that the bodies had, financial questions, and the tiny number of claims for negligence against doctors and hospitals by comparison with the United States.

24.2 Functions

A good way of describing hospital ethics committees is to look at their functions. They have accumulated a large number in their short life:

– reviewing prognoses (as recommended by the Supreme Court of New Jersey). As this is not an ethical function, it would be better not to use the word 'ethics' of committees that do nothing but this; such bodies should be known as 'prognosis review committees';
– consultation: for advice of this sort, the committee might be open not only to health workers but also to patients and members of their families;
– education: this kind of work could be aimed at a wide range of people, including health workers and the community;
– drawing up guidelines: this would mean a policy for each specialism, and might include a policy covering non-resuscitation;
– review of decisions taken both by families of people who are not capable of doing so and by doctors;
– decision taking.

These functions can be divided between mandatory (e.g. reviewing medical decisions that have ethical implications, consultation etc.) and optional (education and guidelines); for the most part, committees will reject the opportunity to take decisions which are properly those of the health workers. Questions relating to research and experiments using human beings should, as a matter of principle, be dealt with by committees which look exclusively at these matters. It is also true that hospital ethics committees sometimes take this function on board.

There are many people who still do not have a clear idea of the functions of these committees, and this is scarcely surprising as they continue to grope laboriously for an identity. Some committees operate without formulating their objectives in advance; it has even been suggested that the whole process of formulating objectives could be counter-productive to the smooth functioning of the committees, although this view is not shared by many.

The ethics committee of the Hospital of St John of God in Barcelona, a religious foundation, goes further than the more widely acknowledged committee models. Unusually, the committee there is empowered to take decisions on certain matters. These include decisions where there might be doubts relating to euthanasia, termination of pregnancy, contraception, procedures involving transplantation or donation of organs, and situations where the door could be left open for human experimentation, where the patient's freedom of conscience could be compromised, where ethical values are being taught, and where there is conflict between therapeutic indications and what the family wants.[5] Some of these issues will not come within the province of the committees of non-Catholic hospitals, and in any case they will not be called upon to make a binding decision.

The ethics committee at the Hospital of St John of God can also be asked to perform advisory functions or 'to illuminate a particular problem' where ethical values are involved. Examples of this quoted by the hospital include issues relating to professional action but in addition to those already established, questions of employment contracts, pay and promotion, matters of interprofessional relationships, issues connected to interpersonal and hierarchical relationships, ways of caring for patients in a more humane manner, and anything that could impact on the hospital's image.[6]

24.3 The way ethics committees work. Administrative matters

To round off this picture of ethics committees, I would like to refer to a few headings which might help them to function better:

– composition: the number of people, groups or institutions represented and the number of seats they occupy. Such matters are determined by the functions that are allotted to the committee and by the hospital itself. It is accepted that, because of the makeup of the committee's membership, it must be interdisciplinary. It is also common practice – although there is an element of flexibility here – for there to be representation from doctors, nurses, experts in medical ethics, administrative grades, legal advisers, social workers, psychologists and psychiatrists, and non-professional staff;

– appointment of members: obviously, the hospital's administrators and senior managers must be there but, if the committee is to fulfil its objectives, it is also important to ensure that representation is fair by talking to interested parties and seeing to it that the committee is independent;

– period of membership: members must be replaced in stages; in this way continuity is guaranteed and the committee's work not interrupted;

– immunity: although ethics committees are not courts, it is often necessary for them to be granted complete civil and criminal immunity when making recommendations, as long as they operate within the aims that are laid down and observe established norms. In these circumstances, all responsibility would fall on whoever took the decisions, but these members of the ethics committee would benefit from a presumption of freedom from civil or criminal action as long as their decisions conform with the committee's recommendations;

– detailed workings of the committee: this concerns which people would be allowed to present problems to the committee, the presence of outsiders at meetings or part thereof, taking the minutes, recommendations by majority voting or by consensus, and the transmission and writing up of recommendations;

– low cost of running the committee.

24.4 Evaluation

It can be difficult to keep personal feelings separate from ethics committees, and one's evaluation can therefore be distorted. An example of this is an excessively enthusiastic or naive attitude which imagines the committee will be able to provide magic solutions to the myriad difficult problems that crop up in a hospital every day; another is a fundamental distrust of a newfangled structure.

We simply have to accept that, even in the United States where ethics committees have been going for a lot longer, they have still not got beyond the teething stage, and we therefore do not have much information to go on. The fact that other countries have even less experience means we have a little more leeway. At the same time, a given committee's successes and failures are not in themselves a basis for judgements worldwide.

In so far as they are an expression of moral sensitivity in an era better known for technology and efficiency, we must accord them a positive welcome. They can give useful assistance to health workers, patients and families as they make difficult and complex decisions. They can provide health professionals with support and emotional peace, as well as some form of guarantee against any legal claims. Another positive characteristic is the fact that they are interdisciplinary; this facilitates analysis and study of problems from a number of different angles. This interdisciplinary nature of ethics committees also makes them much better suited to a pluralistic society. What they can bring to the field of ethical training and the drawing up of guidelines is likely to be warmly welcomed. Also, unlike courts, they work quickly, and they are much more likely to provide confidentiality.

There has also been criticism about ethics committees. For some, they do not constitute an observable improvement on procedures currently used for decision taking (i.e. panels covering doctors, patients and family members, and, where appropriate, courts). Many people are also calling for clearer indications of the value that ethics committee recommendations have, by comparison with court decisions. Others believe that decision taking is being made unnecessarily complicated; ethics committees are seen as talking shops, and some see a danger that they could end up doing nothing more than rubber-stamping other people's decisions. As for the issue of confidentiality, it is claimed that ethics committees could fall victim to the tyranny of consensus and steer clear of proper debate and difference of opinion.

I do not deny that hospital ethics committees have their limitations, but I still believe there is plenty to be said in their favour. I have high hopes for them in the future.

NOTES

1. 'Ethics Committees', in *HCR* 20 (1990) no. 2, 29-34; 'Ethics Committees', in *HCR* 19 (1989) no. 5, 21-26; W.J. Curran, 'Legal Immunity for Medical Peer-Review Programs. New Policies Explored', in *NEJM* 320 (1989) 233-235; Monograph of *JMPh* 14 (1989) no. 4; J.E. Fleetwood and others, 'Giving Answers or Raising Questions? The Problematic Role of Institutional Ethics Committees', in *JME* (1989) 137-142; T.A. Brennan, 'Ethics Committees and Decisions to Limit Care', in *JAMA* 260 (1988) 803-807; J.

la Puma and others, 'An Ethics Consultation Service in a Teaching Hospital', in *JAMA* 260 (1988) 808-811; *Comité de ética. Regolamento interno*, Hospital San Juan de Dios, Barcelona 1988; B. Lo, 'Promises and Pitfalls of Ethics Committees', in *NEJM* 317 (1987) 46-49; VV.AA., 'Ethics Committees: How Are They Doing?', in *HCR* 16 (1986) no. 3, 9-24; F. Rosner, 'Hospital Medical Ethics Committees: A Review of Their Development', in *JAMA* 253 (1985) 2693-2697; Judicial Council, 'Guidelines for Ethics Committees in Health Care Institutions', in *JAMA* 253 (1985) 2698-2699; J.S. Happel, 'Advice on Good Practice from the Standards Committee', in *JME* 11 (1985) 39-41; N. Fost and R.E. Cranford, 'Hospital Ethics Committees. Administrative Aspects', in *JAMA* 253 (1985) 2687-2692; J.M. Faccini, P.N. Bennett and J.L. Reid, 'European Ethical Review Committee: The Experience of an International Ethics Committee Reviewing Protocols for Dying Trials', in *BMJ* 289 (1984) 1052-1054; D. Brodeur, 'Toward a Clear Definition of Ethics Committees', in *LQ* 51 (1984) 233-247; F. Abel, 'Ethics Committees', in *LH* 188 (1983) 89-91; P. Allen and W.E. Waters, *Aptitudes to Research Ethical Committees*, in *JME* 9 (1983) 61-65; A.M. Capron and others, 'Looking Back at the President's Commission', in *HCR* 13 (1983) no. 5, 7-12.

2. C.B. Cohen, 'Ethics Committees', in *HCR* 18 (1988) no. 1, 11.
3. Id., 20 (1990) no. 2, 29.
4. A. Lloyd, 'Ethics Committees in England', in *HCR* 18 (1988) no. 5, 2.
5. *Comité de ética. Regolamento interno*, 5.
6. Ibid.

PART V

Medical treatment
and research

Chapter 25

Health and disease

25.1 What we mean by health and disease[1]

We often talk about health and disease as if they were immutable, uniform and easy to understand. In fact, they are enormously complex.

In certain respects, health and disease are the same for all people, but in fact they incorporate a number of issues that go to make up a conception of an entire human being. Furthermore, at different moments in history, the idea of disease has been dominated by different issues including religion, empiricism and social issues.

For many peoples and cultures, health and disease have been closely associated with the world of religion, and usually with magic. In such circumstances, there has been no room for science, although there was very little scientific knowledge available anyway. Disease was thought to be the result of the action of malevolent powers, or of benevolent forces that had turned against humanity for some reason. The treatment of disease consisted of religious rituals which usually involved forms of social participation like bathing, sacrifices, fire and dancing. Less frequently, disease seemed to be connected to some ethical shortcoming.

In a large number of primitive societies, the social dimension of disease was in many ways far removed from ours, but it was none-the-less extremely powerful – as one would expect from the strong sense of community that characterized these groups. It was for this reason that these societies underlined the role of interpersonal relations in caring for sick people.

The increased importance given to a rational and scientific interpretation of disease has slowly led to a decline in the importance of a religious view. However, this displacement of religion from the world of disease has proceeded unevenly, as there are still well-educated people who retain vestiges of a view of life that incorporates religious and magic elements. In the mysterious

world of life and death, health and disease, and pure rationality
and science, these approaches are never entirely erased.

There have been many attempts to find a scientific explanation
for health and disease, and they have been understood in many
ways, according to the aspects that were highlighted or accentuated. Unlike religious and magic interpretations, modern medicine has accorded decisive importance to biological facts. This
move developed alongside the blossoming of natural sciences,
whose epistemological status medicine was happy to assume.
There is no question about the inroads that medicine made into
the world of natural sciences – in surgery, bacteriology and pharmacology, for instance. However, side by side with these outstanding advances are signs of a weakening of social values: signs
include the marginalizing of the social dimension and personal
importance of disease in favour of other issues that are nowadays
considered to be more important.

Disease is not simply a physical anomaly defined within objective parameters. The most important feature of disease is that it
is a personal experience, and for that reason we cannot go on
thinking of it as something that has nothing to do with us. There is
currently a trend to revive anthropology – it has never appeared in
a form of medicine modelled on natural sciences – and attempts
are being made to give more prominence to the patient's involvement in the history of the disease. This appropriation by the
patient can take many forms:

- information given to the patient;
- respect for his/her decisions;
- patient's co-operation in the entire process;
- the complex issue of assuming responsibility for contracting the disease;
- a personal way of coping with the disease and experiencing it (e.g. feelings and serious questions stimulated by it).

Personal experience of disease is determined and influenced
by the patient's personality and by his/her social and cultural
environment.

The importance of social factors relating to health and disease
began to be acknowledged increasingly in the middle of the
nineteenth century. In other words, health and disease were ceas-

ing to be simply a scientific matter; they now also incorporated social components. Numerous studies have underlined the social dimension of ill health, perhaps the most important contribution coming from the sociologist Talcott Parsons who defined the rights, exemptions and obligations that characterize the patient's social role:

- exoneration from responsibility for catching the disease;
- exemption from a person's normal responsibilities, in keeping with the nature and seriousness of the illness;
- considering the disease as something undesirable;
- the patient's wish to have done with his/her situation;
- looking for assistance when incapable of getting better.

The model proposed by Parsons is useful in that it demonstrates the way in which society controls and institutionalizes illness, although it then confines itself to a particular kind of medicine and certain types of disease. Lack of responsibility for contracting the illness is not absolutely valid as certain diseases carry a stigma. There are several more things I want to say about Parsons' doctrine.

The defining of illness is a skill that society accords to doctors, and doctors use biological information to do this. Professional knowledge acts as a kind of tool which enables the doctor to define disease. Through it, s/he performs a function of social control by drawing a line between normality (health) and deviation (ill health).

It is possible to see from my last few remarks how illness and health are not simply descriptive and scientific words, but terms that incorporate their own evaluative dimension. On the one hand, if we were to get no further than a 'scientific' interpretation, we would completely lose sight of the totality of the person. On the other, we would give the impression of falling into subjectivism: disease and health are what an individual and society identify as such. What we need to do is synthesize naturalist and humanist knowledge.

Furthermore, we have to recognize, like Steudler, that illness only makes sense as a function of a man or woman taken as a whole – a biological, psychological and social being.[2] After rejecting a number of narrow interpretations, the World Health

Organization (WHO) has produced what is now a widely accepted definition of health: 'a state of complete physical, mental and social well-being and not merely the absence of disease or infirmity'. If we take that definition literally, nobody has been, is, or ever will be healthy, and the job of medicine to restore and preserve health will be impossible.

Even if we talk of 'reasonable', 'adequate' or 'moderate' well-being, instead of 'complete' well-being, many people still believe that it is too broad. Like the WHO, we must look upon it as an ideal to aim for, not as something that really exists.

Social sensitivity towards health has developed dramatically in more advanced societies. Scientific and technical progress, improved hygienic conditions and improvements in diet have led to standards of health that were previously unheard of. The growing human rights movement has also moved into the health field, and there is now talk of a right to health or, more accurately, a right to health care. At the same time, there has been a growing awareness of health as a political and social issue. Health has now identified far too closely with health professions; this has led to an obscuring of personal responsibility for health care, but there may be a solution to this in what is referred to as health education.

25.2 Health care[3]

For centuries, health was basically a private matter, and each person took personal responsibility for it. That meant that the rich could get health care from a doctor whom they paid. There was no collective awareness of a general interest in everyone's health, and no one was aware of the scientific and technical potential for the setting up of a health service. The poor were left to suffer in agony; at best, they were admitted to hospital, although for a long time hospital care did not have any therapeutic objectives.

The concept of human rights began to take off in the nineteenth century. These rights included the right to health, or to health care, which has slowly established itself throughout the twentieth century. Interest in people's health also has a financial component, as the aim is to cure the sick person as quickly as possible so that s/he can get back to work. However, people slowly began to acknowledge that health care was linked to well-being, the dignity of the person and his/her quality of life, irrespective of economic considerations.

Currently, there are many models for health services in the western world, but they are not unrelated to the particular forms of society in which they exist. E. Telfor describes four kinds of health service, although none of them exists in a strict form:

– the *laissez-faire* system: this is a typically liberal form of health service. Under it, medical treatment is available to those who can pay for it; those who cannot have to rely on charity;
– the humanitarian liberal system: private health care is available to those who can pay for it; everybody else is looked after by the State;
– the pure Socialist system: here, everyone is theoretically the same; the State provides equal treatment for all, irrespective of their financial circumstances;
– the liberal Socialist system: this scheme looks after everybody, but it leaves the door open for extra health care on a private basis.[4]

I should make it clear from the outset that these schemes are not ends but means, and they should therefore be assessed on the basis of the service that they actually offer people, especially the most needy. All the systems tread a difficult path between freedom and solidarity. In the Western world, the shortcomings of the systems which have underlined solidarity provide an excuse for various forces to defend systems that give precedence to freedom. These forces are not always prepared to take public responsibility for their actions. My view is that, for any system to be fair, it must leave freedom to one side and prioritize a reasonable standard of care for the most needy. Anything else makes the inequalities and injustices even worse, and it is always the poor that come off worst. There is no shortage of formulas that try to harmonize solidarity and freedom. However, they are none of them definitive and perfect; they all have their advantages and disadvantages. For that reason, the situation will always appear temporary. It is not disputed that a large number of people are dissatisfied with the health care they receive – which is not to say that there are not plenty of others who are very pleased.

At all events, there is no question that health services are facing a series of complex challenges. On the one hand, there is the problem of steep increases in expenditure and costs both in themselves and as a proportion of the GNP (Gross National Product). The resources that schemes have at their disposal to meet health needs are declining in relation to people's rising expectations and wishes in respect of health. In these circumstances, either resources will have to be increased, an option which attracts very little support as it involves extra personal expenditure, or – and it is also very difficult to imagine this other option – expectations and demands will have to be reduced. The trend worldwide is to get the best services possible for the lowest personal outlay.

Before I put forward some ideas for a fairer health service, I want to emphasize the need for us to take responsibility, in so far as we are able. I agree that a decisive element in maintaining general health standards is in the hands of the public health authorities, but it would be quite wrong to think of health as solely a public responsibility. Each individual has a duty to look after his/her own health as well as that of other people. Moreover, health education and improvements in lifestyle appear to have a much greater impact on health standards than scientific and technical advances. What is more, changes in eating habits, leisure time, physical exercise, and personal satisfaction at work and in the family all contribute much more than medicine to general well-being. These developments are essential if we really want to ease the tensions that affect health in our society. What it comes down to is personal conversion. I have already indicated a basket of rights, one that is perfectly legitimate although still imperfectly developed in many ways. It is important to promote and foster this idea, but it should not be construed that people may make demands for their own benefit and lack all sense of solidarity. Resources to meet growing needs are limited; we therefore need to encourage a sense of rationality and solidarity so that we do not demand services that society cannot provide, given current needs and resources. This will often mean that people will have to hold back, however unpopular that may prove to be in our consumer society. Solidarity must always function in support of the poor and the needy, both nationally and supranationally, and educating people to accept this is a profoundly humane thing to do, despite the tough resistance that such an approach will encounter these days.

We need to practise constant vigilance over our health services if we are to correct the dysfunctions that currently threaten them, such as the excessive power exerted by the medical profession over people with no medical training, the absence of humanity in medical practice, bureaucratization, inequality, and unfairness in the setting of priorities.

If there are to be changes in health policies, members of the community must be involved as broadly as possible in the fixing of objectives and the control of services. As J.A. Moreno Ruiz has commented in a comparative study of health service models in the USA, Switzerland, the United Kingdom, Sweden, the former West Germany and Spain,

> When we analyse the organization and structure of the various health models, and gradually come to know the different planning systems, we get the feeling that these models, systems and structures have been designed to enable health professionals to do their jobs, solve professional problems and move medicine forwards. It also seems as if the promotion of health and health care is dominated by consumerism above all other considerations concerning the patient. Decisions relating to medical objectives and programmes are taken by committees and structures where you never meet ordinary people, the real or potential users. Health professionals, that is to say the people who sit on these committees and take these decisions, feel they are better equipped to solve their own problems than those of the user. We frequently almost forget that there is no point to health care if there are no patients. The same goes for health and ordinary people.[5]

Any health policy incorporates certain options for all of society, and not just for health workers and public authorities. At times, we may be forgiven for wondering whether health planning is responding to the needs of the majority of the population – or to party political interests, the benefit of medical coteries or the financial advantage of certain groups.

For example, evidence for discrimination is to be found in the unequal geographical distribution of hospitals and health workers, whereby rural areas tend to be poorly provided for.

Another challenge for health services is the need to make them

more humane;[6] this can only come about through health workers
developing better personal attitudes, and through major reforms
in health structures.

25.3 A Christian view of health and disease[7]

The attitudes of Christianity to health, disease and curing have
varied over the centuries, and they have also responded in different ways to various influences. Some of these influences have
been religious, such as readings from the Bible and, in particular,
the way in which Jesus is portrayed; others have owed their
existence both to developments in medical knowledge and technology and to the sort of society that prevailed at the time.

Illness rarely appears in the Bible as a medical reality. Like the
rest of human existence, disease was viewed in a religious setting.
The Bible completely ignored the nature of this human situation,
and how it developed and could be treated, although there are
references to certain therapeutic practices. The Old Testament
condemns magic and other practices related to idolatrous worship, but still does not prohibit recourse to them. Hope of a cure
comes basically either from God, a healing God, or from his
representatives – priests and prophets.[8]

For men and women in the Bible, disease is a sign of a
relationship with God; it therefore has a religious significance.
Sometimes it appears to be a more or less direct sign of sin, while
health is like a grace and blessing of God. However, it is rare for
there to be any explicit relationship between disease and punishment.[9] Christ does not accept discussion as to whether there is, or
is not, an express connection between illness and personal responsibility.[10]

The struggle against disease held an important place in Jesus's
life, and was part of his role as Saviour; furthermore, in his flesh
he suffered the depths of human pain. In a way, this dual attitude
of Jesus' is reflected in a text that has two different interpretations: Isaiah 53:4 says that the suffering servant 'carried our
diseases' whereas in Mt 8:17 Jesus 'took our infirmities'.

Christ's mission of teaching and curing the sick is described
briefly in several passages of the New Testament.[11] A parallel
development of this dual mission has been claimed for the struc-

ture of Mark's gospel: chapters 5-7 include a small collection of teachings while chapters 8-9 include a number of cures. These cures are more to do with the doctrine of salvation than apologetics; they are a sign of new times, an expression of a new order in which evil will not exist, and they draw attention to the reality of the kingdom of God.

The image of Jesus as the suffering servant, the just one who suffers, breaks with the image which links suffering and sin. This process of emptying himself culminates in the passion and the crucifixion. However, it is possible to make various theologies even out of this experience of Jesus: the cross as glorification, the pain-associated vision of the cross as an expression of the greatest suffering, the cross resulting from the injustices and sins of men and women, or as a sign of love. An interpretation of Christ's cross that taught redemption through sacrifice, and was associated with medicine's then meagre potential, encouraged an attitude of resignation in the face of illness.

These two ways of comprehending the person and mission of Christ have, together with a number of other elements, helped to produce two Christian attitudes to illness: one of them is belligerent and sees illness as evil, while the other accords it a welcome and views it as an angel come from God. For many centuries, Christian morality did not concern itself with the implications of disease. For the most part, it contented itself with considering how the state of being ill affected acts of worship – mass, fasting, and more minor matters. The subject was rarely touched on, outside ascetic spiritual literature.

Writings and preaching of this type have encouraged an attitude of resignation. However, it is difficult to draw a clear distinction. It is also difficult to be sure whether this passivity is caused by an accentuation of Christian beliefs, or by the scant resources of medicine at the time which encouraged people to be fatalistic. One aspect of Christianity which might have encouraged people to feel resigned is the interpretation of Christ's passion and death as redemption through suffering; this connection between sin (original and personal) and illness was definitely overdone. No less influential is the contribution made by the heritage of Greek culture which was quickly assimilated by Christianity – the Platonic conception of the body as the prison of the soul, and the distrust of pleasure which had been inherited from Stoicism. This led to a spiritual view of infirmity as a vocation or apostolate that found a resonant echo within the Christian tradition. Piety was a much more effective transmitter of this current than theology.[12]

Christian ethics acknowledges the autonomy that derives from health and disease, and nowadays proposes a model of behaviour that integrates aspects of a religious vision.

a. Life is a gift that has to be lived to the full, and health is a component of this wholeness and healing. As S. Spinsanti has pointed out, 'From this angle, disease is presented to us as something that contradicts, diminishes, impedes or paralyses the desire to live.'[13] In this way, the ethical duty to try and shake off illness and enjoy optimum health extends to become a sign (which is neither infallible nor automatic) of embracing life fully. It follows that health is an essential part of a humanizing process.

b. The struggle against illness need not be Promethean or slip into idolatry. Health is a good, but not a supreme good, in the hierarchy of values. The fight against illness must take many issues into account – including the limitations of science and technology, the limits of the body's strength, the patient's autonomy, and solidarity with other people – so as to avoid selfish, pointless demands for resources that are needed by others. Sometimes health can only be correctly assessed if it is put in danger. B. Häring has approached the problem in another way: he says that anyone who is not prepared to expose his/her fragile, earthly security and health to pain and danger – within reason, of course – with a view to enjoying a greater union with God and a more generous giving of disinterested fraternal love, will never succeed in being holy nor in achieving truly human and redeemed health.[14]

c. Disease is a constituent element of humanity; it is a manifestation of its fragility and mortality. The acceptance of disease is therefore sometimes the same as admitting one's condition and not escaping into a fantasy world.

d. The fight against illness has to take place within a narrow perspective; a clear-minded and universal attitude includes working to eliminate appalling living conditions, the breeding ground of so many illnesses.

e. In a way, there is a legitimate link between illness and sin, but not so much on an individual plane (although that cannot be totally excluded) as in collective situations of sin. Häring accepts that in many cases there is a fairly clear relationship between illness and sin in one dimension or another, although he is absolutely opposed to any exaggerated generalization. Illness cannot be automatically related to personal guilt. For Häring, this is sin in its existential sense, as both a divider of the spiritual unity of men and women and something that acts against the conscience. He also refers to the consequences of sin which engraves wrong 'information' on the cerebral cortex, in the depths of the psyche, in the total being of humanity, and in an increasingly disturbed world.[15]

f. If it turns out to be impossible to cure a disease despite using all the reasonable means available, the Christian must not adopt an attitude of rebellion against, or criticism of, God, but one of hope. Contemplating the figure of Christ can help one comprehend depressing issues, and do so in a positive way.

Illness limits the development of certain facets of a human being and of Christian vocation, but it is not the same as a crisis at the most profound level of being. Illness can also be made into a factor of humanization and Christian life, which thereby boosts aspects of personality and faith.

If illness is not to be the basis for depersonalization or a crisis of faith, but for an encounter with oneself, with other people and with God, it will largely depend on the way in which other people can display solidarity of a respectful, and not infantilizing, type. When life is lived at superficial levels, disease can be a precious, if painful, aid to eliminating the obstacles that obstruct the most profound strata of existence. A. Auer deals with this question as follows:

Illness is all to do with truth. If a man or woman confronts an illness, one of the consequences is that s/he revises his/her scale of values. The pre-eminence that ordinary objects have enjoyed in day-to-day life because of their monotonous presence suddenly lacks legitimacy. What is truly genuine now makes its own demands and claims due respect, so that human beings may move from appearance to reality, from illusion and lies to truth.[16]

NOTES

1. R.M. Hare, 'Health', in *JME* 12 (1986) 174-181; D. Páez, 'El sentido social de la enfermedad', in *RO* 47 (1985) 103-114; M.R. Gillick, 'Common-Sense Models of Health and Disease', in *NEJM* 313 (1985) 700-703; S. Sontag, *Illness and its metaphors*, Muchnik, Barcelona 1980; S. Kelman, 'Social Organization and the Meaning of Health', in *JMPh* 5 (1980) 133-144; VV.AA., 'Social and Cultural Perspectives on Disease', in *JMPh* 5 (1980) no. 2; M. Sendrail, *Historia cultural de la enfermedad*, Espasa-Calpe, Madrid 1983.
2. F. Steudler, *Sociologie médicale*, A. Colin, Paris 1972.
3. R. Gillon, 'Funding and Efficiency in the National Health Services', in *JME* 15 (1989) 111-116, 128.
4. E. Telfor, 'Justice, Welfare and Heath Care', in *JME* 2 (1976), 107-111.
5. Cf J.A. Moreno Ruiz, *Comparative analysis of models and systems for health care*, in VV.AA., *Spanish Health*, 682-683, study of the US, Swiss, British, Swedish, former Republic of Germany and Spanish Models.
6. John Paul II, 'The challenge to humanize medicine', in *Ecclesia* 2350 (19-12-1987) 27-29; John Paul II, 'The Humanization of Medicine is in Everyone's Interest', in *LH* 199 (1986) 29-31.
7. VV.AA., 'Religion, Health and Healing', in *SC* 34 (1987) no. 4; B. Häring, 'Freedom and cure', in *LH* 19 (1987) 174-177; Canadian Bishops' Conference, 'Pour une espérance nouvelle dans le Christ: une vision chrétienne de la maladie et de la guérison', in *MM* 34 (1984) 543-558.
8. Ex 15:26.
9. Num 12:10; 2 Chron 21:11-15.
10. Jn 9:25.
11. Mt 4:23-24; 9:35; Lk 6:17-19.
12. Hans Urs von Balthasar, 'The Elegy and the Cross', in *Concilium* 38 (1968) 430-443; 'Suffering and Christian Faith', in *Concilium* 119 (1976), Monograph.
13. S. Spinsanti, 'Enfermedad', in *DETM* 296.
14. B. Häring, *Medical Ethics,* St Paul Publications, Slough 1972, 153.
15. Ibid., 155 and 156.
16. A. Auer, in VV.AA., *Ethics and Medicine,* Guadarrama, Madrid 1972, 67.

Chapter 26

Transplants[1]

Organ transplantation has become a fairly common medical practice these days, and the fact that there is not a lot more of it is due mainly to a shortage of donors. However, shortage is not the only problem. As far as some organs are concerned, there are still quite a number of major technical and medical difficulties which, it is hoped, will be solved with time.

The problems are not even all medical, though; there are also legal issues that need to be considered. There are many countries that have laws governing transplantation which are favourable to the development of human solidarity at the same time as protecting donors' rights.

There is also a socio-cultural issue here that cannot be ignored; this is that transplantation of organs from dead bodies offends many profoundly deep-rooted beliefs.

In the following pages, I will basically confine myself to the moral dimension of transplants. There are no fundamental problems in Christian morality at the moment about demands put forward from a medical point of view. Morally speaking, this issue has roused little controversy, and a number of books on bioethics do not even touch on it. The moral view of transplants has developed impressively in only a few decades: the reactions and vacillations of a few years ago have been replaced by a basic acceptance, although this is accompanied by criticism of certain details which mainly concern the conditions in which the transplants are carried out. The suspicious and negative reactions of some moralists in the early days of transplants were deflected by a number of factors: they included a very limited concept of the control that human beings have over the body, the limitations and dangers inherent in an experimental intervention, religious beliefs and socio-cultural ideas.

26.1 Types of transplantation and medical issues

Classifications of transplantation depend on the criteria adopted. The two most important deal with the relationship between donor and recipient and to the type of organ transplanted. Transplantation that takes place within the same body (e.g. skin, cartilages, tendons and bones) is referred to as autografting, and a further distinction is drawn between orthotopic and heterotopic transplants, that is to say whether the organ is placed in the same place or a different place in the same body.

Transplantation involving a donor and a different recipient is called heterograft, and in this case the donor and recipient may belong to the same or different species. If they are different, the transplant is called xenograft, and if they are the same, the transplant is referred to as allograft. An important element concerning the human donor is whether s/he is alive or dead. Certain personal circumstances pose a number of specific problems relating, for instance, to the transplantation of organs or tissue of foetuses, children, mentally handicapped adults, and prisoners condemned to death. It is also necessary to distinguish between vital and non-vital, and single and paired, organs because of the nature of the transplanted organs themselves and the consequences for the donor.

Several questions covering donor and recipient have to be settled before a transplant can take place. As far as the donor is concerned, there is one area in which both medicine and morality have an important contribution. This deals with criteria for accepting or rejecting a candidate; these criteria may be both general and particular, and depend on the type of transplant. As for the recipient, s/he is asked similar questions on medical, social and psychological matters.

For the operation to be successful, there has to be excellent coordination between the various medical teams, well-preserved organs, good histocompatibility of tissue, the availability of immunosuppressive techniques, a high standard of surgical skill – and a well-prepared recipient.

After the transplant has been carried out, it is common for there to be unexpected problems and other difficulties.

I have said that good histocompatibility of tissue between donor and recipient is a *sine qua non* of a successful operation, and research into liver transplants surprisingly suggests that this can sometimes be a problem.[2]

There is a wide range of tissue and organs that can be transplanted, including the heart, kidney, cornea, liver, lung, pancreas, ovaries, testicles, blood, skin, bones, tendons and cartilages. There have also been successful multiple transplants such as pancreas and kidney or liver, heart and kidney, heart and lung, and heart, lung and kidney. Moreover, there have been conventional operations one following the other on the same patient, and using the same anaesthetic and the same donor. There have even been cases of grafting viscera without separating them. The most ambitious of all operations consists of transplanting all the abdominal viscera including the gastrointestinal tract all the way from the stomach to the colon. The maximum survival period is six months.[3]

26.2 Moral issues

a. Transplants in the same body

There is no moral problem surrounding transplants within the same body as long as the aim is reasonable and there is an acceptable balance between risks and advantages. Subordination of part of the body for the good of the whole is legitimate when the objective is sensible and not arbitrary. It is not usually necessary for there to be very serious reasons for interventions of this kind to take place, as long as the level of risk is properly understood. Moreover, without getting too involved in the business of personal appearance, aesthetic reasons on their own can be quite sufficient.

b. Transplants from an animal to a human being[4]

For most people, transplants from animals to human beings present no insuperable problem as long as we concentrate solely on where the organ comes from, and nothing else. However, there are certain extreme opinions put forward by those who support animal rights.[5]

The fact that this type of transplant is basically acceptable does not mean to say that we should not discuss the matter, or even reject the idea as far as certain organs are concerned. For instance, on 14 May 1956, Pope Pius XII came out strongly against a practice that is surely hypothetical – that of transplanting an animal's sex organs onto a man.[6]

The most animated debate has arisen over the Baby Fae case. Baby Fae was born in the United States in 1984 with hypoplasia of the left ventricle of her heart; the left-hand side of her heart was much smaller than the right-hand side, and it was not able to pump enough blood to keep her alive for more than a few weeks. This condition occurs in approximately one in every 12,000 live births, and it is thought that 25 per cent of newborn babies who die do so of cardiac arrest. In these circumstances, there was nothing for it but to let the little girl die, or transplant a human heart or an animal's heart.

Baby Fae was operated on at Loma Linda Hospital, California, on 26 October, and her own defective heart was removed and replaced by a baboon's heart. She died on 25 November as a result of complications that developed when she showed signs of rejecting the transplanted heart. It was not the first known case as in 1964 a Dr Hardy had carried out a similar transplant of a chimpanzee's heart into a human being; the recipient lived for only two hours.

Leaving to one side the particular circumstances surrounding the Baby Fae case – many aspects of the case were heavily criticized, and apparently with good reason – what interests us is the general hypothesis of transplanting from an animal to a human being. The normal medical criteria used for many other medical interventions should be applied here: these are the free and informed consent of the parents, highly skilled doctors to perform the operation, the absence of a better alternative solution, an analysis of the patient's general condition, and proper consideration of the advantages and dangers given that the patient's good (his/her survival and general health) is the overall aim. The issue of the socio-cultural significance of the heart as a symbol does not present any problems that are ethically relevant. What is unquestionably important is that there should be a fair distribution of resources.

Sometimes the intervention does not provide the recipient of the transplant with any identifiable benefit, and all it can offer is a contribution to the advancement of science. In these circumstances, there are many people who rule out the intervention completely for children, while others say it is acceptable as long as it brings with it no additional dangers and is a responsible exercise in solidarity. Significantly, this type of non-therapeutic experimentation is viewed as admissible or otherwise according to whether or not the parents' informed consent is accepted as valid.

c. Transplants from a dead body

One of the basic assumptions about transplants from a human body is that the person is dead; this is something I deal with elsewhere in this book (Chapter 14.2). As long as this condition is fulfilled, there are no major moral obstacles to using a dead person's organs for transplantation or research. The stoutest resistance has come from religious organizations and from particular attitudes to be found in certain cultures. Even today, there are Christians who have strong reservations about what they see as mutilation of the corpse, and they base this on their faith in the resurrection. In fact, theology reveals there is a lack of consistency in the ideas and fears of those opposed to transplants; this opposition is based on alleged Christian assumptions. On the contrary, the demands of charity and a sense of solidarity are much better expressed if the organs of dead people are available to help others who are still alive. Lastly, the dead body must not, as happens in many cultures, be compared to that of an animal.

From a moral point of view, there is no absolute need to have the consent of the patient or of his/her family in order to use organs for a transplant, although it is, of course, normal and sensible to involve those who are most closely related. For that reason, those laws that permit transplants when there is no express opposition from the dead donor do not infringe any moral demand, and are an expression of broadly accepted solidarity. When the moment comes to decide on the moral appropriateness of transplanting from a dead body, the fundamental issue to consider is the impact on the sick person's well-being; this is done by comparing the current situation with predictions for the future and using the various alternatives.

d. *Transplants between living human beings*

Transplanting organs from dead people to living people does not present significant moral objections, and the same has always gone for live donors. In this respect, an era of very restrictive positions has given way to one of much more open ones.

In the early days of transplants, there were many people who were resolutely opposed to the idea of transplants when the individuals involved were both still alive. The main reason for condemning this kind of intervention was the intrinsic wickedness of direct mutilation. However, taking out an infected organ for the general good of the whole body was felt to be legitimate by virtue of the subordination of the part for the whole; however, removal of a healthy organ for the good of someone else's body was rejected on the grounds that it involved direct mutilation. An article by Pius XI has been wrongly quoted by way of support:

> Christian doctrine establishes, and the light of human reason demonstrates, that individuals have no power over the parts of their bodies other than the power that relates to the ends of their lives. They are not free to destroy or mutilate their bodies or in any way make them unusable for their natural functions except when the good of the whole body cannot be cared for in any other way.[7]

This principle was formulated by Pius XI to prohibit eugenic sterilization, but it has also been wrongly extended by eminent and distinguished scholars of moral theology to reject transplants of this type as well. Statements originally made in all seriousness and in good faith strike us now as quite surprising. For instance, M. Zalba wrote in 1956,

> We cannot seriously believe that one of the possible natural purposes of Peter's eyes is for them to be inserted into Andrew's empty sockets. Nature ordains that Peter's eyes should perform their normal task in Peter's body. Medicine may ordain that they serve John, but only by distorting the natural function they once had. Anyway, this sort of mutilation, which is fairly futile as it only enables the other person to see partially, obviously does not serve the good of the whole body, as the Pope demands.[8]

Such an approach, however respectable and understandable it may have been at the time, is not compatible with a correct view of Christian morality. A narrow version of nature and of respect for nature has only served to dash outstanding acts of Christian personal kindness.

Nowadays, the removal of a healthy organ from a living person in order to transplant it in another presents no moral problem as long as we only consider it in isolation. The legitimacy of transplants will depend fundamentally on the following factors: the relative importance of the organ to be given away, informed and free consent, and any damage caused by the removal. As far as the recipient is concerned, the main issues are that his/her consent must be given and his/her well-being is the objective.

A delicate problem relating to donors is the question of minors as donors, and their ability to give organs. Some people say it cannot be legitimate because of the problems of eliciting a sufficiently free and clear consent; others say that it cannot be legitimate in any circumstances.

e. Artificial hearts[9]

It has been a long-standing ambition of human beings to be able to replace used organs with new ones. When French troops under General de Bourmont landed in Algeria in 1830, they were almost immediately struck down by malaria, and the following year the General wrote that he was quite convinced that the day would come when men could be kept alive thanks to science. 'Hearts of steel will beat in their breasts, and livers of copper and granite will be inserted into their stomachs', he wrote, and as a result, his men would be 'tough and invincible'.[10]

It has been known for some time what had to be done, but the first attempts at total replacement of a natural organ by an artificial organ have only taken place in recent times. The first implantation of an artificial heart was carried out in the United States in 1969 by Dr Cooley; the patient only survived for 64 hours, and Dr Cooley was severely reprimanded because of the illegal nature of the intervention. The first legal implantation of an artificial heart occurred in the United States in 1982 under a surgical team headed by De Vries and R. Jarvik.

An artificial heart has normally been looked upon as a temporary measure; otherwise, it has been implanted in an emergency when there was no human heart available or one was being awaited. At all events, there have been plans to construct permanent artificial hearts. However, after the initial phase of enthusiasm, this idea has recently lost momentum in popular and scientific circles, and among those who draft public policies. This is not because of fundamental moral reservations but because, given other pressing needs, they are not seen to be compatible with a fair distribution of available resources.

NOTES

1. M. Evans, 'Organ Donations Should Not Be Restricted to Relatives', in *JME* 15 (1989) 17-20; E.-H.W. Kluge, 'Designated Organ Donation: Private Choice in Social Context', in *HCR* 19 (1989) no. 5, 10-16; H.E. Emson, 'The Ethics of Human Cadaver Organ Transplantation: A Biologist's View', in *JME* 13 (1987) 124-126; T.H. Murray, 'Gifts of the Body and the Need of Strangers', in *HCR* 17 (1987) no. 2, 30-38; R. Manna and A. Migliora, 'La terapia immunosoppressiva: osservazioni metodologiche ed etiche', in *MM* 37 (1987) 633-654; C. Levine and others, 'The Community Blood Supply and Patients' Choice', in *HCR* 17 (1987) no. 2, 5-10; J. Dausset, 'People, personalities, and organ transplants', in *FH* 24 (1986) 73-96; J.B., 'Organs for Sale: From Marketplace to Jungle', in *HCR* 16 (1986) no. 1, 3-4; L.B. Andrews, 'My Body, My Property', in *HCR* 16 (1986) no. 5, 28-38; W.F. May, 'Religious Justifications for Donating Body Parts', in *HCR* 15 (1985) no. 1, 38-42; L.R. Kass, 'Thinking About the Body', in *HCR* 15 (1985) no. 1, 20-30; VV.AA., 'Organ Donation: Is Voluntarism Still Valid?', in *HCR* 15 (1985) no. 5, 6-12; J. Feinberg, 'The Mistreatment of Dead Bodies', in *HCR* 15 (1985) no. 1, 31-37; Pastoral Commission of the Spanish Bishops' Conference, 'Exhortación sobre la donación de órganos', in *Ecclesia* 2195 (3-11-1984) 15; A.L. Caplan, 'Organ Transplants: The Costs of Success,' in *HCR* 13 (1983) no. 6, 23-32.
2. T.E. Starzl, 'Transplantation', in *JAMA* 261 (1989) 2894-2895.
3. T.E. Starzl and others, 'Transplantation of Multiple Abdominal Viscera', in *JAMA* 261 (1989) 1449-1457.
4. Th. Kuehner and R. Belliotti, 'Baby Fae: A Beastly Business', in *JME* 11 (1985) 178-183; C. Levine and others, 'The Subject is Baby Fae', in *HCR* 15 (1985) no. 1, 8-16; G.J. Annas, 'Baby Fae: The "Anything Goes" School of Human Experimentation', in *HCR* 15 (1985) no. 1, 15-17.
5. A publication which pays great attention to animal rights is the journal of *Environmental Ethics*, published since 1979.
6. *AAS* 48 (1956) 464.
7. Pope Pius XI, in *AAS* 22 (1930) 565.

8. M. Zalba, 'La mutilación y el trasplante de órganos a la luz del magisterío eclesiástico', in *RF* 153 (1956) 539.
9. G. Gil, 'The Artificial Heart Juggernaut', in *HCR* 19 (1989) no. 2, 24-31; A.R. Jonsen, 'The Artificial Heart's Threat to Others', in *HCR* 16 (1986) no. 1, 9-11; C. Lenfant, 'The Process of Evaluating the Artificial Heart', in *HCR* 16 (1986) no. 6, 27-28; H.P. Green and others, 'Allocation of Resources: The Artificial Heart', in *HCR* 14 (1984) no. 5, 13-17; G.J. Annas, 'Consent to the Artificial Heart: The Lion and the Crocodiles', in *HCR* 13 (1983) no. 2, 20-22; R.W. Evans, 'Donor Availability as the Primary Determinant of the Future of Heart Transplantation', in *JAMA* 255 (1986) 1892-1898; F. Ross, 'Ethical Issues in the Implantation of the Total Artificial Heart', in *NEJM* 310 (1984) 292-296; M.J. Strauss, 'The Political History of the Artificial Heart', in *NEJM* 310 (1984) 332-336.
10. F.R. Cerruti, 'Les organes artificiels: étude des aspects éthiques et juridiques', in *Supp* 152 (1985) 142.

Chapter 27

AIDS

Infection with the Human Immunodeficiency Virus (HIV), the terminal stage of which is AIDS, has a wide range of psychological, social, legal, economic and moral implications both at national and international levels. The major part of this chapter is devoted to moral issues, but this is preceded by a brief medical explanation.

27.1 Medical background[1]

The acronym AIDS stands for Acquired Immunodeficiency Syndrome. A syndrome is a range of manifestations and symptoms which characterize an illness and which, in this case, include a serious weakening of the immune system. It is called 'acquired', because it is not hereditary, but the product of an acquired virus.

There are numerous germs in the atmosphere that are frequently dangerous to health; they include viruses, bacteria, microscopic fungi and parasites. To deal with these potential enemies, the body has a defence system called the immune system whose job it is to destroy these invaders and prevent the formation of cancers. Lymphocytes, similar to white corpuscles in the blood, play a key role in this immune system, and of particular importance is the role carried out by the T4 cells which direct the body's defence operations against these invading organisms. When germs penetrate into the body, the T4 lymphocytes detect them and mobilize T and B lymphocytes to respond to the invasion. The terrifying aspect of HIV is that the virus targets the T4 lymphocytes and, as a result, the body's immunological defences are destroyed. A defenceless body with its immune system seriously weakened is at the mercy of attacking germs. What happens is similar to what occurs when the officers of an army are put out of action, or the conductor of an orchestra is taken ill, and this suddenly prevents him/her from being in control of the players.

When HIV penetrates the blood stream, catastrophe is not immediate. It can stay there for varying lengths of time as if dormant, without giving any indication that it is there. The person is none-the-less infected; s/he presents no symptoms, but can infect others. If HIV is active, it replicates and may attack a large number of T4 cells, and it is at this stage that symptoms of AIDS appear. This is a serious phase of the infection which is character-ized by various non-specific symptoms. The first of these are the so-called opportunistic infections, that is to say symptoms that are produced by various germs which take advantage of the weakness of the immune system. The second type consists of various kinds of cancer. The clinical picture varies a lot according to the organs that have been infected; the most frequently affected parts of the body are the lungs, the digestive system, the skin and the brain.

Generally speaking, the principal way of transmitting HIV is through sex, both heterosexual and homosexual. The next most common way is through blood-to-blood contact or through the use of contaminated instruments; the latter is particularly preva-lent among injecting drug addicts, and also arises from the use of unsterilized transfusion equipment in countries with poor medical facilities. Lastly, it can also be transmitted from mother to child. Otherwise, transmission of HIV is very difficult, and for that reason there are no grounds for unjustified alarm concerning transmission by everyday actions and situations.

As no vaccination or effective treatment for HIV exists for the time being, the only way of stopping it from spreading is by prevention and control. Preventing infection is the responsibility of the whole of society, although the various tasks and activities for individual members of society vary in importance. Given the ways in which HIV is transmitted, aware people have decisive roles as far as sexual behaviour and use of drugs go. However, responsible behaviour in these two areas cannot, and must not, be thought of as the personal decisions of private individuals. All of society has an important job to perform in encouraging, stimulat-ing and supporting responsible behaviour through information, training, provision of voluntary tests, counselling and a variety of social services. Political leaders, doctors, teachers, the mass me-dia, Churches and families must also collaborate in the common task in the best way they can. Moreover, public authorities and health professionals have a unique responsibility in respect of transfusions, transplants and other medical activities.

We do not know the origin of HIV, although it is accepted that HIV 1 is the most widespread. How it differs from HIV 2 and viruses found in monkeys throws considerable doubt on the notion that it attacks by a process of mutation. It is thought that the virus has existed for a long time in groups that are immune to it, but this hypothesis has not been confirmed. It seems that HIV 2 is quite close to viruses found in monkeys in Africa, and this has led to speculation that the virus has been transmitted to humans who had no natural immunity to it. As for the timing, we may be forgiven for wondering why it made its appearance when it did at the beginning of the 1980s. We must rule out the suggestion that HIV was manufactured in a laboratory. Factors that have aided its spread include sexual permissiveness, the mobility of populations through migrations to the cities in African countries, journeys from one country to another, the widespread availability of unscreened transfusions, and an increase in the number of intravenous drug users.

27.2 AIDS and morality. An overview

HIV is inspiring plenty of writing on the moral implications of the infection, although it is alarming to note how little Christian reflection this writing contains compared with the amount of scientific and medical information.[2] An indication of the political importance of this dimension of HIV is Recommendation No. R (89) 14 'On the ethical issues of HIV infection in the health care and social settings' adopted on 24 October 1989 by the Committee of Ministers of the Council of Europe.

With so many moral lessons to be learned, here are a few structures to help order this wealth of material. Let us take as our point of departure the concept of an epidemic, and the resulting conflict between the right of society to protect itself and the rights of those affected. On this basis, we can organize the moral issues under two headings. Firstly, let us make a moral assessment of the measures that seek to protect all members of society, ranging from the most coercive to the most liberal:

- quarantine/isolation of sufferers;
- discriminatory measures against certain groups;
- lack of confidentiality;
- application of the law;
- AIDS tests;
- compulsory notification and registration of known cases;
- scrupulous care taken of donated blood and other donated material;
- research into medication and vaccinations;
- information and education.

The second heading examines measures that aim to protect the individual:

- patients' rights: confidentiality; information; treatment;
- fundamental rights of the individual: free movement; education; work; free choice; privacy; no discrimination.

We might also include here the rights of the healthy – for example doctors and people who have had transfusions – to be protected from infection.

Another possible criterion for defining the problem might be based on the people and organizations involved in the problem. These might include political parties, doctors, researchers, the media, schools and colleges, companies, religious organizations and private civil organizations. One of the disadvantages that such a scheme would have is that it would go over the same ground needlessly, because a given activity would involve various people, all with different responsibilities.

Yet another focus consists of the various kinds of action to be taken against AIDS. As HIV is a health problem, it is only to be expected that some of the moral issues concern health, or more precisely health care. As there is no therapy or vaccine in existence, the best barrier to infection for the moment is prevention and control. Another area is research. A fourth area relates to attitudes and social behaviour, since it is possible up to a point to speak of a social epidemic linked to a health epidemic. As a result, the political area would open up completely and incorporate all the areas; a possible problem is that they intertwine in such a way that it might not be possible to distinguish between them satisfactorily.

I have decided to deal next with the issues which I consider to be of greatest interest. The most important are those which are most closely connected to health in terms of welfare or policy:

- a call for solidarity;
- a duty to care for HIV/AIDS sufferers;
- the AIDS test;
- confidentiality and AIDS;
- AIDS and sexual morality;
- isolation and quarantine for HIV/AIDS sufferers.

27.3 A call for solidarity[3]

There is a real danger that our views can become seriously fragmented as we attempt to deal with the many aspects of HIV. For that reason, it seems to me to be appropriate to start off by recommending the need for solidarity, something that may well be much more urgent here than in other health issues.

HIV is not just a health problem, with implications that are enormous, but which are more or less normal and common to other diseases. Even if we look at HIV from this angle, we are already asking for solidarity from everybody. It may be that no other illness in recent times has transcended the world of health so decisively, unleashing such a wave of social reactions (both attitudes and behaviour) that it seems more like a social epidemic. Many people make gestures of closeness and solidarity, it is true; some of them are truly even heroic gestures. Opposed to them, however, is a proliferation of collective attitudes which, according to circumstances, more or less openly express feelings of, intolerance, marginalization, discrimination, violence, fear and fatalism.

Whatever social attitudes might mean in a moral context, they are important in terms of health. Signs of an absence of solidarity with sufferers and with people involved in dangerous activities are a way of encouraging the spread of HIV; they also affect the way the disease develops, and compromise the effectiveness of preventive programmes. Solidarity is not just a way of giving help to sufferers; it is also a way of preventing the disease in the first place. Gestures demonstrating a lack of solidarity originate in a number of quite different sources including public authorities, health professionals, companies, schools and colleges, and tenants' associations. I emphasize the absolute need for solidarity, and denounce the phenomenon of unjust discrimination in all its manifestations.

a. *The people most under threat*

The individuals and groups most under threat from attitudes and gestures lacking in solidarity can be divided into four groups:

– known HIV sufferers at whatever stage of infection. It may be that there are more cases at the HIV-positive stage than when the disease has been established and the individual has to be admitted to hospital;
– people suspected of having HIV. Although strong suspicion of infection never justifies a person being rejected, it none-the-less happens that people who are victims of discriminatory measures are indeed rejected by reason of groundless suspicions, and almost invariably the poorest people and groups are most vulnerable;
– the families of sufferers and of people suspected of having HIV;
– clinics and individuals that specialize in caring for sufferers. The threat here is less than in the above three categories. Nevertheless, there have been cases in the United States of discrimination against clinics, hospitals and doctors simply because they have taken sufferers in and looked after them.

b. *Areas and forms of discrimination*

There are many areas of life where attitudes lacking in solidarity take shape, thereby placing obstacles in the way of people's basic rights. These are:

– medical treatment;
– housing: difficulties that sufferers encounter in renting accommodation, and being thrown out of their homes by force or as a result of popular pressure;

    – public and private schools and colleges which expel students, and sack teachers, who are infected;

    – employment: no job offers made simply because the applicant is infected; AIDS tests insisted on as a condition of employment; and dismissal once infection has been established;

    – the armed services;

    – public transport: sufferers prevented from flying with certain airlines;

    – insurance;

    – frontier restrictions: especially for migrant workers and students from certain countries, particularly poor ones;

    – communal eating areas;

    – undertakers who refuse people who have died of AIDS;

    – prisons.

c. The root of antisocial behaviour

Inaccurate information, ignorance and fear give plenty of sustenance to discrimination, as the desire to protect ourselves from infection leads us to erect barriers against anyone who might be carrying HIV. To get rid of these props of injustice, it is not enough to provide accurate information, although that is very important. So as to be able to fight irrational fear, it is vital to get to know the obscure ways in which it works.

The most common circumstances in which people are infected, homosexuality and drug addiction, help to promote a social setting that is favourable to intolerance. However, that does not justify stigmatizing attitudes towards individuals who are neither homosexuals nor drug addicts, but who lose their human dignity just the same.

There is also in circulation a religious interpretation of AIDS, that has been criticized heavily by the Church but which still serves to reinforce some people's prejudices. It has been appropriated by some sufferers, and has been adopted by many healthy people and the bizarre religious leaders of certain sects. According to this interpretation, AIDS is a scourge of God, and a divine punishment for the sins of homosexuality, promiscuity and drug addiction.

It is absurd from a medical standpoint to look at the world in this way. AIDS does not only affect alleged sinners, but innocent people as well like haemophiliacs, children and individuals infected in the course of their employment. It is also unacceptable from a Christian standpoint. I do not pretend that there is not a link between infection and certain behaviour which Christian morality does not condone, but that is not to say that it is legitimate to link HIV with God. The almost sadistic and vengeful image of God that is associated with this is not compatible with the image given by Jesus. Besides, why should God take pleasure in punishing these forms of behaviour and not others? And why start punishing them at the beginning of the 1980s and not earlier?

This punitive interpretation of events conceals the latent, but absurd, notion that Providence takes no account of cause and effect in nature. There are scientific explanations for AIDS although some of the details are still obscure – but it is neither necessary nor reasonable to involve God so directly.

When Christ met a sick person or a social outcast, he did not wonder whether it was his/her fault or why the individual had got into this situation; he did not pass judgement on the person but infused him/her with hope. It is important not to wonder if a sin has been committed; what really matter are people's sufferings and needs. In his time, Christ welcomed the sick and the outcasts, not to mention sinners, lepers and prostitutes, and he overcame the social fears that people had in those days of the sick.

Sometimes we hear a secular version of punishment, although then it is not God but nature taking revenge on sexual and drug-related abuse in our society. This interpretation will be further discredited as soon as science and technology find a vaccine or a form of therapy to counter AIDS.

27.4 A duty to care for HIV/AIDS sufferers[4]

a. A problem that is both old and new

The question whether health professionals have a duty to care for HIV sufferers re-opens an old, discarded problem. At one time, this kind of problem was dealt with under the same heading as the plagues and epidemics that once periodically laid waste whole countries and cities. The modern generation of doctors was quite unaccustomed to thinking about exposing themselves to a serious occupational risk that endangered their health and lives, as antiseptics and antibiotics had always provided good protection against infection or worse.

HIV has wrecked this 'antibiotic peace'. It has destroyed doctors' aura of invulnerability to the risk of infection by lethal diseases, and it has forced them to acknowledge much more carefully how dangerous their job is. The possibility of HIV infection raises abruptly – and in a new context – the old problem of the relationship between medical risk and professional duty. Perhaps the relative peace of the last few decades has meant the shock has been all the greater, and encouraged an unwarranted and distorted perception of the danger threatening them. This situation poses questions about the extent to which health professionals are obliged to care for HIV sufferers. At what price? How much of a risk should they take? And does the duty apply not only to health professionals, but to society and every one of us?

b. The general rule is that there is a duty to look after HIV sufferers

There is impressive continuity on this issue between the ethical tradition of medicine on the one hand, and statements issued by distinguished medical and political bodies of the present day on the other. Unfortunately, they do not all see with equal clarity the force of the historical argument concerning obligation.

When countries like Great Britain and the United States began to recognize how serious the situation really was, a number of bodies came out in favour of professional obligation. Apparently, the situation was worrying not because there were too many doctors rejecting these patients, but because there was concern that people might jump to the erroneous conclusion that that was what was going on.

The norm covering the duty to care appears in a document produced by the Council of Europe; it states that 'all health care workers have an obligation to care for people infected with HIV and AIDS patients.'[5] Similar pronouncements have come from eminent bodies in Britain such as the Royal College of Nursing (1986) and the General Medical Council (1987), and the Ameri-

can College of Physicians and the Infectious Disease Society of
America in the United States. The American Medical Association
takes the same line, but there is an element of ambiguity in its
view that, as not all doctors are emotionally up to treating AIDS
patients, they need to find ways of observing the norms which the
AMA has laid down for duty of care.[6]

Many articles by moralists recall that there is an ethical obligation to treat patients even when there is a risk to the doctor's life,
and that members of the medical professional have been much
more exposed to danger in the past than now.

There is a majority in favour of obligation, although there are
still isolated instances of doctors and dentists refusing. However,
the majority view is now under pressure as there is a growing
corpus of arguments opposed to professional obligation. These
are based on issues such as the contractual notion of the medical
profession, the doctor's freedom to choose his/her patients, the
more important obligations that the doctor has to him/herself and
family, emotional incapacity to deal with sufferers in such situations, and the danger that treatment given under duress may
jeopardize the quality.

Underlying this debate is a conception of the medical profession as it exists within our particular society. These days, our
view of medicine is that it is less vocational and mystical than it
used to be, and in consequence it is acquiring a more functional
role, like all other public services. Our society has also lost its
enthusiastic, sometimes heroic, sensitivity for great causes and
great ideals. As a result of improved standards of living, a sense
of sacrifice no longer enjoys the popularity it had in harsher
times.

All these factors make it difficult to reach a theoretical and
experienced solution to the problem; finding a solution that contains an ethical demand is, as E.D. Pellegrino has said, 'an urgent
obligation of the whole profession if its moral integrity is to be
preserved'.[7] This fundamental problem is still to be solved, and as
a result no time is being allocated to the consideration of other
highly important issues raised by Pellegrino. These include his
claim that there are at least two aspects specific to medicine that
both impose an obligation on doctors to downgrade their professional interest and distinguish medicine from other professions.
The first of these issues consists of the nature of disease in itself,

which places the patient in a situation of unusual dependency, anxiety, vulnerability and exploitability. This situation of need places a moral demand on anyone who is in a position to give help. The second question deals with the non-proprietary nature of knowledge that the doctor picks up in the course of his/her training. Members of the medical profession form part of a kind of collective alliance. It is received correct behaviour that this knowledge should not be used for personal gain in terms of money, prestige or power. This alliance receives a public endorsement when its members qualify and take their oaths; all medical oaths say something about setting aside one's own interest. I could say a lot of things about these fascinating reflections; one is that they arouse little enthusiasm amongst those who are dominated by certain aspects of our culture.

27.5 AIDS tests[8]

The best way of fighting the HIV infection is prevention, since there is no cure or vaccine in existence for the time being. However, the effectiveness of preventive work depends on a number of measures. The most important of these are information, which should be as widespread as possible, and the use made by people involved in high-risk behaviour of consultation and counselling services and screening for antibodies to HIV. That is what I will be dealing with in this section. Leaving to one side certain scientific, technical and organizational matters, the most important question is whether the tests should be voluntary or compulsory.

a. Classification of the tests

AIDS tests can be classified according to a number of criteria including effectiveness, cost, who they are aimed at, whether they are tests in the first instance or confirmatory, and whether they are voluntary or mandatory. Here, I want to look at the latter category.

V. Bolto Massarelli distinguishes between three types of test: compulsory, voluntary and routine. The routine test is really compulsory, not because the individual's personal behaviour is dangerous but because it forms part of a health audit carried out in association with activities like going to university, into the armed forces, into the labour market or into hospital.[9]

P. Cattorini combines various criteria such as voluntary/compulsory, duration and anonymous/named, and refers to five types. There is the universal test, which appears to be compulsory for all, the test that is compulsory periodically in life (e.g. joining the armed forces, going into hospital and getting married) and the test that is compulsory for certain types of person (e.g. prostitutes and homosexuals). Those who take the voluntary test are sub-divided into two groups: anonymous (no name given) and named (the individuals give their names but in confidence).[10]

J.F. Childress, on the other hand, bases his approach on two criteria, voluntary and compulsory, and describes four models for testing: universal obligatory, universal voluntary, selective obligatory and selective voluntary.[11] I am going to use this schema, and I am also going to advance the following thesis: in the light of current knowledge, and given that there is no vaccine or therapy in existence, the voluntary test is the most correct measure to adopt for two reasons: because it makes the best contribution to public health, and because it best satisfies legal and moral requirements. If there were to be significant changes in the information available on vaccines, therapy and social attitudes, that thesis could well change.

b. The universal obligatory test

The small number of people who believe in such coercive and wide-ranging measures believe that this is the only way of ensuring that public health is effectively protected. Identification of all HIV carriers would, in their view, provide a solid basis for a preventive policy, and for making sure that everyone behaved responsibly at all times. They also think that, if the frontiers of the infection were clearly marked, society would cease to be alarmed and most of those who were not infected would then feel less anxious. If there were a mandatory test for everyone, groups that were most involved in high-risk behaviour would have fewer grounds for feeling discriminated against. Furthermore, the test that is obligatory for all is the only one that guarantees that people who are difficult to contact could in fact be reached.

Rejection of the obligatory test is based as much on the practical impossibility of carrying it out as on moral reservations. In practice, it is impossible to reach the entire population. Moreover, given the way in which HIV spreads, the test would have to be repeated periodically, and at least every six or twelve months, and health budgets of even developed countries would find the financial burden intolerable.

It is also likely that there would be a substantial percentage of mistakes stemming equally from incorrect positive tests, which would cause unjustified fears, and from incorrect negative tests, which would give some people a false sense of security. Even if all carriers could be correctly identified it would be impossible to avoid isolating large numbers of people – the only thing we can do for the time being is to trust that infected people will be responsible in their sexual behaviour and drug taking. It is complete fantasy to imagine that the obligatory test will make public health completely safe.

Anyway, such a massive invasion of people's autonomy and privacy, with its inevitably random results, would be repugnant to moral sensitivity. Furthermore, there is the not entirely groundless fear that there would be breaches of confidentiality, and a consequent chain reaction of discriminatory reactions against sufferers.

Lastly, we might add that this kind of test is quite unnecessary as there are other ways of protecting public health that are almost as effective, and cost less in terms of financial and human resources. I am talking of selective obligatory and totally voluntary tests which can be accompanied by appropriate information and counselling services.

c. The universal voluntary test

This test is recommended for all, but is not imposed on anyone, thereby side-stepping the moral reservations felt about the universal obligatory test with its unacceptable invasion of privacy. However, it is not a sensible measure.

Any idea that it is possible to reach out to everyone through the information media, and by recommendations and invitations, is quite illusory. It implies that there is comprehensive information and a range of consultation and counselling services available; however, this is something that we cannot seriously imagine in even the best organized health service. Anyway, the cost of setting up this infrastructure and the test itself is out of proportion to the results, particularly if we bear in mind that scarce resources have to cover all health and other needs.

I feel that public health can be effectively protected, and the infection prevented from developing further, by other means; an example of this is the selective voluntary test.

d. The selective obligatory test

Let me start off by summarizing a few proposals that have come from different parts of the world. Some of them have become law in a small number of countries, and others are practised in even fewer places although, for the most part, they have not moved on from being simple proposals. Indeed, some of them hardly make any sense at all. The targets of the selective obligatory test include homosexuals, bisexuals, intravenous drug addicts, prostitutes, prisoners, foreign workers in certain countries, students in the same countries, State functionaries, members of the armed forces, students entering university, workers at the commencement of their employment, everybody about to get married, women of child-bearing age, pregnant women, people who handle fast food, people who have been admitted to hospital, and donors of blood, organs, tissue, cells and semen.

Simply reading this list, with its mixture of sensible and ludicrous ideas, must raise a few eyebrows. If we then look at it more carefully, we find that two criteria are being used in justification. The first is the dangerous nature of certain behaviour because of possible contact with HIV; the second consists of the stages that many people go through in life at one point or another – such as starting a job, going to university, entering the armed forces, getting married, and going into hospital – although none of these necessarily has anything to do with behaviour associated with HIV.

Leaving to one side for a moment the groups to which it would be applied, the main reason put forward for this kind of test is the protection of public health together with improved treatment for sufferers. And by comparison with the routine test, it appears to have a number of advantages. One is the fact that, as it is not based on alleged risky behaviour, it does not lead to any stigmatization. There is no psychological pressure attached to it, and in this way it becomes commonplace and attracts no attention. The costs involved would be absorbed by cancelling other tests, and the feeling is that a lot of people would take the test voluntarily.

However, although the invasion of personal autonomy and privacy, which is inevitable in a mandatory test, may not be a decisive element in itself, it will undoubtedly meet with moral resistance from the outset. There is also the danger of unfairly discriminating against a given individual by including him/her in a high-risk group. The very imposition of a test on certain groups seems to imply that there are some highly dubious ideas at work. The mandatory carrying out of tests on members of the armed forces, prisoners, State functionaries and so on might suggest that these people merited less autonomy, or that public authorities had certain rights over them. Moreover, it would be necessary to work out the cost as part of a fair distribution of available resources. It is widely thought that an obligatory test would frighten off a lot of people who are involved in high-risk behaviour, and who would fear breaches of confidentiality and discriminatory practices. If this were the case, the main aim of protecting public health would be severely compromised.

I think it is possible to give concrete advice on this matter without going to all the trouble of carefully analysing the numerous proposals, some of which have been endorsed by law. The imposition of the test prior to all donations (blood, organs, tissue, cells and semen) is morally justified as long as the norms of free consent, confidentiality and counselling are abided by.

It is clear that imposing the test on certain groups just because of their risky behaviour is, as I have written elsewhere, 'unethical, ineffective, disrespectful of private life, discriminatory, and in some cases pernicious', given that there is no treatment available and that it is not feasible to force people to change their behaviour or introduce restrictive measures.[12] It is particularly important not to impose tests on 'captive' populations such as prisoners, immigrants and army recruits.

The Council of Ministers' Recommendation referred to above states clearly that a test compulsorily imposed on various groups simply because of their risky behaviour is 'unethical, ineffective, unnecessarily intrusive, discriminatory and counterproductive'. This is true, given the absence of curative treatment, and in view of the impossibility of imposing behaviour modification and the impracticability of restrictive measures. The Recommendation goes on to say that particular care has to be taken to ensure that compulsory screening was not introduced for 'captive' populations, for example prisoners, immigrants and military recruits.[13]

The same document also says that the systematic (or routine) test is 'unethical and contrary to the rights of individuals' if carried out automatically on population groups without informed consent; as it overrides the principles of autonomy and physical integrity, it 'is likely to have serious psychological, social and financial consequences for the individual'.[14]

However, as I have already stated, any changes in how HIV is perceived could result in new ethical positions. Examples of this might be the disappearance of an inevitable link between HIV and dying, and the disappearance or softening of anti-social attitudes and behaviour towards sufferers or people involved in high-risk behaviour.

e. The selective voluntary test

In this model, the test is only recommended for groups and people involved in high-risk behaviour, although this would not exclude the possibility of testing anyone who asked for it out of personal anxiety or for any other reason.

Recommending the test to certain groups and individuals always assumes that they will undergo the test voluntarily, that they will be given relevant information and that they will receive proper consultation and counselling services in full confidence.

In this way, all reservations about universal and targeted compulsion disappear. Furthermore, this system seems to involve the best use of available resources and, all things considered, is likely to be the most effective method of protecting public health.

To conclude, as I have said earlier, this view might change if factors associated with HIV were to change.

27.6 Confidentiality and AIDS[15]

Confidentiality is one of the most frequently discussed issues in the context of HIV. Elsewhere in this book, I have dealt more generally with respect for privacy and confidentiality; here, I wish to confine my remarks to questions specifically related to AIDS. The whole subject is treated to a lively debate involving a large number of different positions ranging from rigid, unwavering defenders of confidentiality to those who view it as an obstacle to public health and a pernicious residuum that should be got rid of at all costs. Between these two extremes lie some more measured approaches.

a. The context of confidentiality surrounding AIDS

HIV is highly complex and involves a wide range of factors which, if taken together rather than examined separately, ensure that the issue of confidentiality needs to be seen in something of a new light.

The threat of dying. At the moment there is a very close link between HIV and death. This, and other factors which I will deal with shortly, affect both the way in which society reacts and professional respect for confidentiality. On the surface, there seems to be no reason why AIDS, like any other fatal disease, should be treated any differently as far as confidentiality is concerned. In fact, AIDS is enormously different. When, at some point in the future, AIDS ceases to be life-threatening through the availability of effective vaccines or therapy – even if other characteristics of the infection do not go away – the whole issue of confidentiality will change overnight. As soon as the link with mortality begins to get blurred, the really defensive attitudes of healthy people who want to know the names of those who are infected will also lose ground, and confidentiality will cease to be a matter for controversy.

Ways of becoming infected. Two ways of becoming infected, homosexuality and drug addiction, have a high profile in western society, and they have also acquired an evil image because of their close association with death from AIDS. There are many in our society who would like to stigmatize and isolate such people even further, but the effect is that those under threat seek protection behind the barrier of confidentiality.

Reactions stemming from a lack of solidarity. There are several issues that flow from unsupportive social attitudes towards HIV sufferers, individuals with high-risk behaviour and their families. People who live under this threat see confidentiality as a helping hand to defend them from such reactions.

Forms of prevention and control. The absence of a vaccine or therapy means we have to prioritize prevention in the fight against HIV. This struggle will lose much of its effectiveness if there are no information and counselling services and no voluntary testing. Research shows that, when confidentiality is not guaranteed, a lot of people with high-risk behaviour do not voluntarily take up these services or even present themselves for the test. This will in turn increase the spread of the infection. At the end of the day, confidentiality is vital to the success of health policies.

It follows that closely guarded professional confidentiality is of immense specific importance to HIV. Besides protecting the individual's autonomy, identity, privacy and image, it also serves in this instance as a defence against unjust social reactions, and represents a positive contribution in support of public health. Failure to observe the rules of confidentiality can occasionally protect the health of identified third parties. It is scarcely surprising, therefore, that we sometimes encounter situations in which there is a conflict of values. Such situations involve the values of sufferers, of known third parties and of society in general.

b. *Situations involving large numbers of people*

The problem of whether or not to observe confidentiality can lose focus if we do not examine certain situations with particular care. I am referring to people who might or might not be told that a given person is infected. They include health authorities, the family GP, surgeons, gynaecologists and obstetricians, staff working in laboratories and dialysis units and blood and organ banks, doctors treating the patient, emergency workers, first aiders, dentists, chiropodists, funeral directors, and officials who issue death certificates.

There are also a substantial number outside the health field including sexual partners, drug addicts with whom the sufferer shares equipment, and people employed in schools and colleges, at the workplace, and in insurance companies, the media of social communication, the police force and courts.

c. Moral issues

We must steer well clear of two extremist positions: on the one hand, the demand for absolute confidentiality in all circumstances without exception, and on the other a plethora of exceptions which would in practice cancel out the general duty to keep the information secret in the first place.

Basically, the anonymous notification of HIV and AIDS cases to health authorities answers the needs of public health and does not compromise patients' rights. A form of notification that identifies the sufferer can only be justified in very restricted circumstances, such as those where the individual is irresponsible, or is incapable of taking responsible decisions, and might through his/her behaviour contribute to the spread of HIV.

Without doubt, the most hotly debated area concerns information given by the doctor to the patient's spouse or sexual partner. If the doctor is to be obliged, or simply allowed, to disclose the truth, a number of conditions must be met:

– the patient has refused to tell them him/herself despite all attempts to make him/her responsible for doing so;
– the spouse or partner is ignorant of the danger;
– there is a real danger of infection;
– the doctor knows the person who might receive the information.

Assuming that these conditions are met, the question relating to the doctor's attitude is vital. Catholic writers, and also some non-Catholic writers, customarily believe that it is obligatory, or at least legitimate, to inform the spouse or the partner of the sufferer. His or her life is a good that is more important than the patient's privacy, and people who disagree with this have little regard for the doctor's obligation to intervene, let alone the legitimacy of his/her doing so. Those who take this position base their argument on the need for confidentiality to protect public health, something which they consider to be vastly superior to the health of the spouse or partner. The fundamental problem is how to determine the relationship between the patient and society. According to the Catholic tradition, it is not felt to be legitimate to sacrifice one person's will in order to achieve a potential social good; that would be like reducing human beings to the role of cogs in the service of society, and it would also open the door to totalitarianism. People who support this position are not unaware of a person's social dimension, nor do they deny it; they simply believe it is inadmissible that the infection of the spouse should be the price to pay for public health.

Another idea that has generated a substantial literature among health professionals is that of the right to know the identity of patients suffering from HIV, even against their will. Obviously, doctors have to know this if they are treating the patient for the infection. The problem arises whether health workers who are in contact with a patient who is being treated for something else, but who happens to be HIV-positive, may, or even must, be told. It would be necessary to determine exactly how essential or useful this information was for the patient to be treated properly. With that, we come to our first hypothesis.

Ideally, the patient would be quite open about everything, and the doctor would be fully informed. Furthermore, s/he would observe the rules of confidentiality while treating the patient, and would not let the information interfere.

Doctors have a right to know which of the patients they are treating are infected. They have a right to demand that the hospital takes the normal measures and precautions that are recommended in such circumstances by the health authorities to prevent further infection. They must also be informed of the possible risks surrounding them, and have access to facilities and equipment recommended for such a situation like gowns and gloves. They must also be responsible about using them.

As long as all these personal and more general measures have been carried out, it means that everything possible has been done to avoid being infected by the patient. But even then, is it right for doctors to be entitled to know the names of HIV sufferers just because their health might be endangered? In the first place, it is difficult to see how this information gives any protection over and above the general and particular measures that are recommended in such cases; at most, it may encourage people to use the recommended precautions more responsibly. Demanding the right to know which patients are infected is an invasion of their privacy and, given the scant amount of regard there is for confidentiality, a lot of people fear with good reason that the news will get out and that this will lead to segregation and discrimination. However, even if we agree that these ideas make some sort of sense, it would admittedly be extremely difficult in a hospital environment to conceal the fact that someone is HIV-positive if a patient is simply identified as infected but no further information is forthcoming. There is no difficulty about other infectious diseases being known about by doctors caring for the patients concerned. It follows that saying nothing would, to say the least, be an indication of HIV.

Throughout this discussion, there is one detail that has to be borne in mind, and that is the assessment of the real danger of the infection. Scientists talk of a minimal danger, and say that this can be reduced even further if the right precautions are taken; these ideas are usually taken on board by those responsible for determining health policies. The latter, however, do not practise medicine themselves and are far removed from any risk of infection of this type. By contrast, the moment health professionals hear the slightest whisper of danger, they claim that the risk is almost upon them and that their lives are under serious threat, however improbable all that may be in reality. If we are to have a proper dialogue between the two groups, we must ask the former to develop a better understanding of the anxieties of practising professionals, and the latter not to overstate their fears.

One final situation which is less common and less controversial than those discussed above concerns the infected health worker.[16] The question arises whether the patient has the right to know his/her doctor's HIV status. Because of the work they do, many doctors do not imagine that their patients face any risk at all. The question continues to be relevant when the very practice of medicine brings with it a risk of infection. In that case, the strategy to adopt is not to communicate with the patient, but to follow the line recommended by the British General Medical Council. This states that a specialist's advice should be sought to determine whether the individual may continue practising and to what extent. This may mean refraining from working solely on the basis of the individual's own assessment of the risk; alternatively, it may involve following the advice received from the specialist, who may sometimes ask him/her to stop working completely, or at least limit the number of hours spent at work.

These are only a few of the many situations where confidentiality plays a part.

27.7 AIDS and sexual morality[17]

The link between sexual behaviour and HIV infection is well known, although it is established in many different ways.[18] In Africa, promiscuous heterosexual relationships are the predominant source of infection, whereas in the United States homosexuality continues to be the main source although there are fears that heterosexuals will be increasingly infected. In other countries, too, heterosexuality and drugs are decisive. As far as promiscuous relationships are concerned, there are indications that certain sexual practices are particularly likely to lead to infection.

These facts have helped to frame new questions about morality. Some people have seen in the connection between AIDS and certain forms of behaviour an indicator or proof of their immorality. Such an interpretation is incorrect, as enlightenment on the morality of sexual behaviour can only come either in the form of the word of God or as a result of a human global examination of the subject.

Any responsible human being must wish fervently to break the link between sexuality and HIV infection, and the Church shares this concern. Differences emerge as soon as ways of achieving this objective are suggested.

a. Shortcomings of the health approach

There is an approach that seeks to remove the link between sexuality and HIV infection; it is a view that might be described as a health approach. Hopes of achieving this objective are based on people being responsible in sexual matters, and in this context behaviour is described as responsible, not in terms of its sexual content, but in so far as it stops the spread of HIV. This approach is widely known, and is frequently espoused by those responsible for health policies, and by scientists, the media of social communication and other groups.

The guidelines underlying this suggestion are twofold. Firstly, relationships should be avoided with people who are likely to pass on the HIV infection: monogamous relationships with uninfected people are safe; casual and promiscuous relationships are dangerous. Secondly, condoms are recommended; when there is a risk (because one's partner may be infected or his/her life style is unknown), condoms still provide protection and allow what is often referred to as 'safe sex'.

Leaving Christian moral assessments to one side, this approach suffers from a number of purely scientific doubts about the alleged effectiveness of condoms to prevent HIV infection. There are grounds for accepting that this method gives quite good protection against infection, bearing in mind the ways in which HIV is transmitted; however, it does not provide complete protection and it is misleading to describe it as 'safe sex'.

Another criticism is the coyness with which monogamous relationships are discussed as a means of prevention. This criticism is now seen as part of a health approach, given its effectiveness at putting the brake on the spread of epidemic. It is to be condemned, though, from the point of view of preventive medicine for making no mention of sexual restraint as an effective means of limiting the spread.

The reason for this approach's reticence about monogamous relationships and sexual restraint is that the whole idea is based on fantasy, given the sexual mores of present-day society. Moreover, the insistence on condoms suggests that, in a culture dominated by technology, we are in danger of resorting too swiftly to technical solutions instead of facing up to what is at the root of this kind of behaviour.

The most fundamental criticism, however, of this approach is the outright refusal to take a close look at sexuality in our society. Many people believe that it is possible, even in a pluralistic society, to draw up a series of common values which do not necessarily coincide in every way with Christian values, but values none-the-less that encompass promiscuous behaviour and marital infidelity. As a result, this approach is open to accusations of encouraging sexual behaviour that could easily accelerate the spread of HIV, thereby fundamentally compromising the main objective.

b. *The Church's proposal*

The Catholic Church has put forward a proposal that seeks to combine two values: one that is to do with health (the effective prevention of HIV) and the other to do with morality (in accordance with sexuality experienced from the point of view of human and Christian demands). This Christian proposal is faithful to a conception of sexuality, and concentrates on two measures:

- sexual abstinence for unmarried people;
- fidelity by both partners within a monogamous and indissoluble marriage.

The Church's position in this respect is faithful to its traditional teaching about contraception which is dealt with elsewhere, although the current situation has thrown up new issues.[19] Interest is now centred not on contraceptives in general but on a method, and the main difference is in the objective itself: avoiding HIV infection and not controlling birth. However, in spite of these new issues, the old doctrine is as valid as ever.

I would like to summarize what I have written elsewhere. According to the Church's official doctrine, the use of a condom is in itself immoral. This does not exclude the possibility of using a condom in a way that is subjectively correct if, as I said earlier, a person honestly reaches that conclusion, since according to traditional moral teaching, the conscience is the proximate norm of morality. The conscience, for its part, is obliged to use all means at its disposal to find the truth.

Another problem centres on the moral position of educational and public health programmes which, in a pluralistic society, promote the usefulness of the condom as a way of preventing HIV. North American bishops have analysed this question more thoroughly than anyone else. They feel that in a pluralistic society there is legitimate room for such programmes as long as they meet two conditions, and the programmes are not imposed on society but are offered:

– precise information on how effective condoms are at preventing HIV;

– locating this measure within a vision of sexuality which takes on board all implied values.

This position should not be understood as an invitation or encouragement to use condoms; nor should it be seen as support for campaigns promoting their use. The bishops justify their teaching from the standpoints of social pluralism and the State's mission within a pluralistic society.[20]

27.8 Isolation and quarantine of HIV/AIDS sufferers[21]

Isolation means separating carriers of infectious agents during the period when the virus is active. Quarantine was originally a period of 40 days during which ships arriving from areas known to have contagious diseases were isolated. Nowadays, it refers to restrictions imposed on the movements of healthy people who might have been exposed to the risk of infection. It even covers people in whom no infection can be detected.

To understand the legitimacy of a measure such as this which restricts freedom so radically, we need to take a look at the medical and moral criteria. Obviously, we must acknowledge the importance of medical criteria when we make moral assessments, so when we are examining contagious diseases in general, we have to consider the following issues from a medical point of view:

– the seriousness of the disease;
– the degree of infection;
– the way in which it has been transmitted (by casual contact e.g. from the air, water or food, through normal behaviour, or in specific ways which are personally controllable);
– the extent to which the disease can be prevented (with vaccines or through responsible behaviour);
– the period of time when the disease will remain infectious (for the rest of the sufferer's life, for a long time or recurrently);
– the existence or otherwise of therapy.

None of these criteria is sufficient by itself to give us an answer. At least it can be said of isolation that it is particularly appropriate if the disease is serious, the cure difficult, infection easy, ways of transmitting the disease numerous, other means of prevention less effective, and the period of infection limited.

If, however, we confine our attentions to HIV, we see that there is general[22] agreement among health professionals, those responsible for health policies and moralists that isolation is not acceptable for moral, medical, legal and practical reasons.[23] Further support for this position from an ecclesiastical source comes from bishops in the United States. As there is no basic medical justification at the present time, they say, for indiscriminate quarantine of people suffering from the AIDS virus, they are opposed to the introduction of quarantine legislation. The same goes for other laws that are not backed by medical fact nor supported by experts in public health and medical practice. American civic history contains many examples of extreme care being exercised in the limitation of human and civic rights, and that should serve as a model in this situation and in all others. The American bishops then call on legislators to act sensibly, and not to react hysterically because of latent prejudice.[24] The Council of Europe Recommendation quoted elsewhere in this book also states that public health authorities should 'not resort to coercive measures such as quarantine and isolation for people infected with HIV or those who have developed AIDS'.[25]

Although isolation and quarantine would provide the best protection of public health against the spread of HIV, there are some very powerful reasons for rejecting such restrictive measures. As things stand, isolation would have to last for the sufferer's whole life, and that would be a cruel restriction of freedom. It would also affect a very large number of people – another reason for rejecting such a coercive plan. Lastly, it would not work because it would be impossible to identify who the carriers were, and the economic cost of such measures would be very high and out of proportion. Given the ways in which HIV is spread, there are other ways of protecting public health without the contradictions implied by isolation and quarantine.

There is a lot less difficulty about a modified form of isolation. This could be used particularly on recalcitrant individuals who are aware that they can infect others, but continue with their dangerous practices without telling the people who are thereby threatened and without taking precautionary measures. A similar

situation surrounds infected people who are incapable of understanding what is going on and are involved in behaviour which
endangers others.[26]

NOTES

1. From among the abundant literature that exists on the subject, and given its
   characteristics, I refer only to the December issue of *Scientific American*
   1988.
2. C. Manuel and others, 'The Ethical Approach to AIDS: A Bibliographical
   Review', in *JME* 16 (1990) 14-27.
3. 'AIDS: beyond the scourge', Pastoral Message of the Canadian Bishops'
   Conference, in *DC* 86 (1989) 648-651; Bishops' Conference of USA, 'The
   Many faces of AIDS', in *Moralia* 11 (1989) 117-132; L.O. Gostin, 'Public
   health Strategies for Confronting AIDS', in *JAMA* 261 (1989) 1621-1630;
   W.C. Spohn, 'The Moral Dimensions of AIDS', in *TS* 49 (1988) 89-109;
   R.J. Blendon and K. Donelan, 'Discrimination against People with AIDS.
   The Public's Perspective', in *NEJM* 319 (1988) 1022-1026; G.W. Matthews
   and V.S. Neslund, 'The Initial Impact of AIDS on Public Health Law in the
   US, 1986', in *NEJM* 257 (1987) 344-352; G.S. Searle, 'Knowledge, Attitudes and Behaviour of Health Professionals in Relation to AIDS', in *Lancet*
   3 January (1987) 26-28; 'AIDS and the Christian', in *LV* (1990), Monograph; J. Dominian, *Sexual Integrity. The Answer to AIDS*, DLT, London
   1987; Dennis Altman, *AIDS and the New Puritanism*, Pluto Press, London
   1988; J. Allison, *Catholics and AIDS: Questions and Answers*, CTS, London 1987; V. Cosstick (ed.), *AIDS, Meeting the Community Challenge*, St
   Paul Publications, Slough 1987.
4. J.R. Allen, 'Health Care Workers and the Risk of HIV Transmission', in
   HCR 18 (1988) no. 2, Spec. Supp., 2-5; G.J. Annas, 'Legal Risks and
   Responsibilities of Physicians in the AIDS Epidemic', in *HCR* 18 (1988) no.
   2, Spec. Supp., 26-32; J.D. Arras, 'The Fragile Web of Responsibility: AIDS
   and the Duty to Treat', in *HCR* 18 (1988) no. 2, 10-19; General Medical
   Council, 'The Doctor's Duty Towards AIDS Patients', in *Lancet* 30 May
   (1987) 1274; H.A.F. Dudley and A. Sim, 'AIDS: A Bill of Rights for the
   Surgeon Team?', in *BMJ* 296 (1988) 1449-1450; E.J. Emanuel, 'Do Physicians Have an Obligation to Treat Patients with AIDS?', in *NEJM* 318
   (1988) 1686-1690; D.M. Fox, 'The Politics of Physicians' Responsibilities
   in Epidemics: A Note on History', in *HCR* 18 (1988) no. 2, Spec. Supp., 5-
   10; B. Freedman, 'Health Professions, Codes, and the Right to Refuse to
   Treat HIV-Infection Patients', in *HCR* 18 (1988), no. 2, Spec. Supp., 20-25;
   B. Gerbert and others, 'Why Fear Persists, Health Care Professionals and
   AIDS', in *JAMA* 260 (1988) 3481-3483; R. Gillon, 'Refusal to Treat AIDS
   and HIV Positive Patients', in *BMJ* 294 (1987) 1332-1333; E.D. Pellegrino,
   'Ethics', in *JAMA* 258 (1987) 2298-2300; Id., 'Altruism, Self-Interest and
   Medical Ethics', in *JAMA* 258 (1987) 1939-1940.
5. *Recommendation* (89) 14, 69.

6. W.C. Koff and D.F. Hoth, 'Development and Testing of AIDS Vaccines', in *Science* 241 (1988) 426-432.

7. E.D. Pellegrino, 'Ethics' in *JAMA* 258 (1987), 2299.

8. F.J. Elizari, 'El "test" del SIDA', in *Moralia* 11 (1989) 23-50; F.S. Rhame and D.G. Maki, 'The Case for Wider Use of Testing for HIV Infection', in *NEJM* 320 (1989) 1248-1254; B.S. Turnock and C.J. Kelly, 'Mandatory Premarital Testing for Human Immunodeficiency Virus. The Illinois Experience', in *JAMA* 261 (1989) 3415-3418; W.C. Spohn, 'Moral Dimensions of AIDS', in *TS* 49 (1988) 89-109; J.F. Childress, 'An Ethical Framework for Assessing Policies to Screen for Antibodies to HIV', in *AIDS and Public Policy Journal* 2 (1987) no. 1, 28-31; R. Gillon, 'Testing for HIV without Permission', in *BMJ* 294 (1987) 821-823; R. Bayer, C. Levine and S.M. Wolf, 'HIV Antibody Screening. An Ethical Framework of Evaluating Proposed Programs', in *JAMA* 256 (1986) 1768-1774.

9. V. Bolto Massarelli, *op.cit.*, 137-141.

10. P. Cattorini, *op.cit.*, 276.

11. J.F. Childress, *op.cit.*

12. Cf F.J. Elizari, *op.cit.*, 34-39.

13. *Recommendation* (89) 14, nn. 33-34.

14. Ibid., no. 29.

15. F.J. Elizari, 'SIDA y secreto medico', in *Moralia* 12 (1990) 55-86; C. Manuel and others, 'The Ethical Approach to AIDS, A Bibliographical Review', in *JME* 16 (1990) 14-27; Canadian Medical Association, 'Le syndrome d'immunodéficience acquise', in *CMAJ* 140 (1989) 64C-64D; Ohi and others, 'Notification of HIV Carriers: Possible Effect on Uptake of AIDS Testing', in *Lancet*, 22 October (1988) 947-949; W.C. Spohn, 'Notes on Moral Theology. The Moral Dimensions of AIDS', in *TS* 49 (1988) 89-109; 'General Medical Council Agrees Guidelines on AIDS', in *BMJ* 296 (1988) 1613; B.M. Dickens, 'Legal Limits of AIDS Confidentiality', in *JAMA* 259 (1988) 3449-3451; R. Gillon, 'AIDS and Medical Confidentiality', in *BMJ* 294 (1987) no. 1, 22-23; *Guide to Public Health Practice: AIDS Confidentiality and Anti-Discrimination Principles: An Interim Report,* Association of State and Territorial Health Officials, 1987; D.M. Fox, 'From TB to AIDS: Value Conflicts in Reporting Disease', in *HCR* 16 (1986) no. 6, Spec. Supp., 11-16; C. Marwick, '"Confidentiality" Issues May Cloud Epidemiologic Studies of AIDS', in *JAMA* 250 (1983) 1945-1946.

16. M.W. Adler, 'Patient Safety and Doctor with HIV Infection', in *BMJ* 295 (1987) 1297-1298; D. Brahams, 'Confidentiality for Doctors Who Are HIV Positive', in *Lancet* 21 November (1987) 1221-1222; 'GMC Warns Doctors Infected with HIV or Suffering from AIDS', in *BMJ* 295 (1987) 1500.

17. Bishops' Conference of the United States of America, 'The many faces of AIDS: an evangelical response', in *Moralia* 11 (1989) 117-132; Cardinal Basil Hume, 'Prevention of AIDS and the Moral Question', in *Ecclesia* 2319 (1987) 24-25; Permanent Commission of the Spanish Bishops' Conference, 'Pastoral notes on AIDS: some Christian reflections', in *Ecclesia* 2324 (1987) 9-10; F.J. Elizari, 'Sexual behaviour and AIDS', in *Moralia* 10 (1988) 379-408.

18. Cf J.M. Mann and J. Chin, 'AIDS: A Global Perspective', in *NEJM* 319 (1988) 302-303.

19. Cf pp. 104-111.

20. See 'Los multiples rostros del SIDA', in *Moralia* 11 (1989) 128.
21. C. Manuel, *a.c.*, 16; D. Francis and J. Chin, 'Prevention of AIDS in the United States', in *JAMA* 257 (1987) 1363-1364; L. Gostin and W.J. Curran, 'The Limits of Compulsion in Controlling AIDS', in *HCR* 16 (1986) no. 6, Spec. Suppl., 24-29.
22. Cuba is an exception, see R. Bayer and C. Healton, 'Controlling AIDS in Cuba. The Logic of Quarantine', in *NEJM* 320 (1989) 1022-1024.
23. Swiss Justice and Peace Commission, 'L'AIDS è una sfida per tutti', in *Il Regno* 33 (1988) 224.
24. *The Many Faces of AIDS*, 118.
25. Council of Europe, *Recommendation* (89) 14, 48.
26. See P. Cattorini, *a.c.*, 275.

Chapter 28
Drugs[1]

There is evidence that drugs have been in use since ancient times at various rituals and initiation ceremonies, and with diagnostic, therapeutic and hedonistic objectives. These uses were considered quite normal by the society of the time.

However, the middle of the nineteenth century ushered in a new period during which drugs became much more widely used. This came about for a number of reasons including greater availability of the drugs concerned, improved communications systems, a number of socio-economic factors, emigration, rapid urbanization, changes in social attitudes and values, and exploitation on the part of unscrupulous individuals.

This spread of the drug phenomenon led to the setting up of control mechanisms, and these began to be even more widespread in the 1960s. By this time, drug addiction had begun to be much more worrying, as there was now a steady increase in the number of users of all ages, particularly the young.

28.1 Background

It is not easy to define exactly what we mean by drugs, given the wide range currently available. One possibility is to take them to mean products that have a particular effect in the nervous system, and which are taken to enhance intellectual or physical performance, to achieve new sensations, or reach a more agreeable mental state. What is crucial to bear in mind when we talk about drugs is that it is very easy for people taking them to slip into habitual and harmful use. It may be difficult to determine precisely what drugs are, but they can still be classified in a number of ways.

Two essential features about drugs are dependency and tolerance. Mental or psychological dependency occurs when the taker

317

has a need to take the drug periodically or continually in order to give pleasure or avoid unhappiness. Physical dependency, or neuroadaptation, is a pathological state brought on by the repeated use of drugs.[2] If consumption of drugs stops or is sharply reduced, specific symptoms appear; they are called withdrawal symptoms. Physical dependency greatly reinforces mental dependency. Tolerance is a state of adaptation characterized by decreased response to the same amount of the drug, or by the need for a bigger dose to achieve the same effect.

Drug abuse has numerous harmful effects on both society and the user. Recourse to drugs and the need to obtain them frequently leads to forms of antisocial behaviour, and is the reason for massive financial outlay for many families and society as a whole. Their most obvious effect on users is on their nervous systems, although other organs and systems can also be affected.

Effect of tolerance and dependency of the main types of drug[3]

Drugs	Objective of initial use	Tolerance*	Dependency* Mental	Physical
Morphine, opiates	therapeutic	+++	+	+++
Synthetic analgesics	not therapeutic	+++	+++	+++
Cocaine	therapeutic	–	+/–	–
	not therapeutic	–	++++	–
Amphetamines	therapeutic	++	++	–
	not therapeutic	++	+++	–
Barbiturates and other sedatives	therapeutic	++	+/–	++
	not therapeutic	++	+++	++
LSD and other hallucinogens	not therapeutic	+	+	–
Cannabis or marijuana	not therapeutic	+/–	+	–
Alcohol	not therapeutic	++	++	++
Tobacco	not therapeutic	–	+	–
Caffeine	therapeutic	+	–	–
	not therapeutic	+	+	–

The number of plus signs indicates the intensity of the reaction

28.2 The origins of drug addiction[4]

To answer this question, we need to ask two other questions: Why is there a drug boom in our society? and Why are particular individuals in this society victims of the scourge while others living in similar conditions are free from it?

The causes of drug addiction are varied and complex, and are linked to an interaction of genetic, psychological and environmental factors. Alcohol dependency is closely linked to heredity, but this is less evident for other drugs, although a high proportion of the parents of opium smokers in Asia are dependent on that drug.

As far as psychological factors go, personality studies have identified a number of characteristics of drug abusers including hostile dependency, a blocking of emotional feelings, high anxiety levels in interpersonal relations, poor tolerance of frustration, low self-image and uncontrolled reactions.

The family and social environment also have a major impact on the spread of drug abuse, with many addicts coming from families that are divided or have other problems. During adolescence, the influence of friends is also decisive.

The World Health Organization (WHO) has published a study on the subject of drug abuse called *Young people's health – a challenge for society. Report of a WHO Study Group on Young People and 'Health for All by the Year 2000'*. It lists the following circumstances that encourage the use of drugs:[5]

- unemployment;
- living a long way from one's real home;
- emigration to the city, and city life;
- lack of parental control;
- breaking off contact with the family;
- improper use of medicines;
- early experience of drugs;
- leaving school too early;
- poor upbringing;
- families that are divided or have other problems;
- drug abuse within the family; easy access to places where drugs are sold or manufactured;
- contact with criminal environments;
- existence of gangs that take drugs;

– certain jobs (commerce, tourism, production and sales of drugs, medical and para-medical jobs that provide easy access to drugs).

Report No. 18 of the WHO Expert Committee on Drug Dependence highlighted eight factors that contribute to drug dependency:[6]

– the development of an underlying character disorder;
– the development of delinquent or deviant behaviour;
– examples of self-medication by people who suffer from mental or physical illness and who believe in the special powers of drugs to prevent these illnesses or to stimulate sexual activity; a conviction that drugs provide acceptance in a given subculture;
– the development of permanent or recurrent disturbance of the metabolism due to repeated ingestion of strong doses of drugs;
– a challenge to conventional values in respect of pleasure taking, traditions, success or social status;
– a reaction to traditional education;
– socio-cultural pressures which encourage abuse of various substances, e.g. alcohol.

On the same subject, a pastoral letter from the Basque bishops drew a distinction between the complicities and meanings of drug dependency.

They talk of four complicities of juvenile drug abuse. One of these concerns youngsters who sometimes fall into drug taking, although they have only themselves to blame; they are young people who take refuge in drugs or who are 'enthusiastically' initiated into the world of drugs. Others are personally without blame; they suffer from mental disorders or have been victims of trauma prior to adolescence.

Another important complicity is the drug trade with its multiple networks linking small and large traffickers, some of the latter being substantial commercial undertakings. There is also the associated complicity of governments which have substantial interests in this field.

Lastly, the bishops drew attention to the complicity of the Church for having reacted too late, for not being clear enough about the dissemination of drugs in our society, and for not offering alternative structures.

I would sum up moral reflection on drug matters under three headings:

- the pointlessness of using drugs;
- prevention (this must be the priority ethical challenge);
- caring for people who are dependent on drugs.

28.3 The pointlessness of using drugs

This is not the moment to make drug-dependent people responsible for everything that is going on. There are also two unfair generalizations which have to be avoided here. For a start, it would not be right to blame drug-dependent people for everything; it is not as if they have deliberately set out to create the situation they are in. Nor would it be fair to let society take all the blame, as if we were all simply the unaware playthings of alien forces. I do, however, want to draw attention to the values that are threatened or denied by drug-related behaviour. The whole business of values and drugs is double-edged: on the one hand, the absence or weakening of certain values makes it easier for drugs to establish a base; on the other hand, drugs both express and reinforce the eclipse of these very values.[7]

a. Drugs: the inability to defer the satisfaction of desire

Desire is a powerful force in the make-up of human beings, but it does not act automatically or blindly as a humanizing influence. Hence the need for human reason to be discerning. Apart from the inherent moral ambiguity of desire, there is another issue that has nothing to do with the object of the desire, but concerns the gap between the appearance of the desire and its satisfaction. The greater or lesser distance between those two moments is of no moral significance in itself, but the ability to put space between the emergence of the desire and its satisfaction is unquestionably important for its humanizing value. Ability to do this is a sign of freedom, whereas inability denotes slavery and tyranny. The passage on this subject in the Basque bishops' pastoral letter is of great interest:

> Men and women mature in so far as they learn how to defer the immediate satisfaction of their desires for the sake of some ideals or some more reasonable or more enriching ulterior satisfaction.
>
> In the gap between the emergence of the desire and deferred satisfaction, the desire is prepared, humanized and tamed. The arrogant demand that others should give 'everything – and now' slowly turns into a humble request, and it is this request that takes into account the principle of reality, and prepares to achieve the desired object gradually, and with the collaboration of other people. A desire thus elaborated is prepared in such a way that, when the moment of satisfaction comes, it produces enjoyment and well-being of the highest order.
>
> When satisfaction is always immediate, the desire does not go away. Similarly, satisfaction once obtained is not relished slowly; nor does it do much to calm the human spirit. It is not long before a new desire springs up, one that longs for something even more intensely exciting. The person then finds s/he has to cope with the tension that separates an increasingly tempting desire and chronic dissatisfaction that is becoming increasingly intolerable.
>
> We believe that this weakness in the way people elaborate their desires – desires which have been encouraged by a society that makes a virtue of permissiveness, hedonistic stimuli and the fear of being a failure – is at the root of a lot of drug addiction. Drug use might be the expression of a desire for satisfaction which can neither hope for, nor fashion, nor achieve the object of the desire. Drugs might provide this satisfaction quickly, but it is unreal, and anyway lasts for only a moment. The ecstasy that exhausts the body and the psyche soon gives way to depression and disgust. Before long, the person is thrown back on the starkness of a desire that is forever emerging and forever unsatisfied. The repetition of this cycle sums up the life of the drug addict.[8]

b. Drugs: the inability to deal with an imperfect world

Let us start off with something that is really very obvious: there is a huge chasm between the ideal world that we dream about and the real world in which we live. The distance between the two breeds anxiety and dissatisfaction in us. The mature response to this is to be patient and try and change imperfect reality as much as possible. The immature response is to escape into an artificial paradise; this includes drug taking. Let me quote once again from the Basque bishops' pastoral letter:

> The personal reality surrounding us, however positive it may be, is far from the ideal that we sometimes glimpse. Neither our bodies, nor our characters, nor our families, nor our school, nor our friends, nor society are what we would like them to be. The gap between the reality we live through and the ideal we dream of then begins to produce anxiety.
>
> This anxiety, which characterizes human beings and distinguishes us from animals, can be directed in one of two directions. The first involves accepting reality as it is, and trying to nudge it in the direction of the ideal by altering it. In these circumstances, anxiety turns into a positive influence for the improvement of life.
>
> However, this direction is extremely hard for adolescents and young people who are still unused to recognizing reality's resistance to change, who are too impatient to acknowledge the exasperatingly slow speed at which reality changes, and who are not prepared to put up with the frustration that comes with observing that, after all their efforts, there really is a gap between the ideal and reality.
>
> This gives rise to a temptation to direct the anxiety elsewhere. In these circumstances, the person tries to deny reality and flees towards the imaginary construction of 'a happy world'. Drugs are an ideal vehicle for this imaginary journey. They give the addict a sense of peace which blots out life as it really is, and things are perceived in the imagination as they would be in an ideal world. The most that can be said is that it creates in the person a physical and mental state of pleasure and tranquillity which makes him/her temporarily immune to the harshness of everyday life. This harshness

inevitably reappears at the end of the short 'trip'. Then, there are only two choices left: become reconciled critically to things as they are, or carry on 'tripping' for ever. The drug addict chooses the latter.

The real world may be rejected in the drug-taker's imagination, but it continues to be something fearsome and loathsome for him/her. The addict's main objective is never to face up to the real world as it really is. For this, he/she needs drugs, and drugs thus become the idol of the addict's life. His/her life begins to revolve round drugs, and everything is sacrificed for this new 'god'. For the addict, life without drugs is grey and meaningless. Nothing is of any value except this deified substance. Family and old friends will be used in any way possible to get hold of some drugs. Ideals and moral conscience will be gradually extinguished until the final disaster looms. Living ends up being the same as getting high. This is the desolate and desolating world which a lot of drug addicts are heading for.[9]

28.4 Drugs as a symptom of an inhumane society

The pointlessness of which drugs are partly an effect, an expression and a reinforcement is rife everywhere in our society, and people who take these drugs internalize them to a greater or lesser extent. However, there are other features of the world we live in which can encourage people to take up drugs. These include the contradiction between the values that are recommended on paper and those by which many people live, uncertainty about the future for so many young people, model relationships inside the family both between spouses and between parents and children (frequently characterized by permissiveness and rigidity), and an obscuring of ideals. Let us now return to the pastoral letter of the Basque bishops:

> The face of society that many young people see is strange, hostile and even despicable. It is dominated for the most part by 'values' which are opposed to those which it theoretically professes: possessing instead of sharing, dominating instead of serving, using others instead of being useful to them, and appearances instead of reality.

Side by side the many normal, and even exemplary, families that exist, there are numerous other families which give young addicts unsatisfactory models of married life, or an upbringing based on rigidity or permissiveness. Excessive rigidity frequently stimulates wishes to break laws and, in this context, taking drugs can symbolize lawbreaking and even be the individual's major illegal act. Unrestrained permissiveness, on the other hand, can make people incapable of putting up with life's inevitable frustrations, and therefore more likely to go looking for artificial and harmful solutions like toxic substances.

Academic failure, particularly when it happens early on in life, slowly erodes the enthusiasm of thousands of less talented or less motivated adolescents. It is an experience that leads them to lose their self-esteem and to feel unvalued and not looked up to by other people. This lack of self-esteem is an encouragement to go in for marginal activities – and that includes drugs.

The current and prolonged economic crisis is also feeding young people's uncertainty about the kind of job they are going to get. Work is one of the most important elements in their life plan. As we have already pointed out, the *motives* for living are in short supply, to make matters worse, the *means* for getting on in life have now become uncertain. Not all young people are equipped to deal with this uncertainty without cracking up. It is hardly surprising if so many of them look for imaginary and harmful escape routes in the world of drugs.

To sum up, the shortcomings and contradictions of society – one that is organized as if it were a technical project rather than as a community which builds its history round a shared, meaningful destiny – are clearly reflected in the phenomenon of juvenile drug abuse.[10]

28.5 Prevention as an ethical task

It is the ethical duty of every individual and of society to try and prevent the spread of drugs among both themselves and other people. It is a duty which extends to each and every one of us although people's individual contributions will vary according to circumstances.

Public authorities, educational establishments, workplaces, non-governmental organizations, families, the Church and the media all have a role to play here.

The contribution of the mass media[11] is important because of their widespread impact, although it can be both positive and negative. To give an instance of a negative contribution, there is a UN report that refers to the imprecise or equivocal language that is used when distinguishing between soft and hard drugs. Other issues raised by the UN report include defending the legalization of the use of drugs for non-therapeutic purposes, the reference to drugs in songs, films and other commercial products, the excessive publicity given to the profits that can be obtained from captured drug consignments, and the use of drugs by celebrated and popular figures. All of these issues can alter the way we perceive the drug phenomenon.

There is a danger that the prevention strategy focuses on only part of the problem by concentrating more on the product than on the person or on society, and more on the technicalities of drug taking than on the broader issue of educating and changing people. The UN recommendations do little to emphasize educational work in schools and the family. Nor do they give much prominence to the correction of certain aspects of our society such as the yearning for immediate pleasure, hostility to anything to do with self-control, recourse to technical, quick, and automatic solutions rather than gentle personal change, and an obscuring of big ideals and values.

Some people believe that the best preventive action consists of reducing the supply of drugs, on the grounds that this will lead to a drop in consumption. It is true that supply falls back from time to time when there are cut-backs in the cultivation, production, processing and marketing of drugs, and of course the destruction of illegal crops places further obstacles in the way of illegal trafficking. Others say that the best hope lies in the demand for drugs: if demand drops, the drug problem declines.

Obviously, preventive action must concentrate on both supply and demand. As for limiting supply, there is no question that public authorities have a major role identifying illegal crops, stopping cultivation on the plantations where they grow, and starting to grow other products on them. However, an approach of this type can run into a multiplicity of problems – for instance, it can be difficult to identify illegal drugs in out-of-the-way places. The destruction of illegal plantations is also out of the question as it would sometimes have a harmful impact on other cultivation, and serious repercussions on the families who make a living from this kind of work. Ideally, the growing of these plants will be stopped by voluntary rather than compulsory measures. Two of the obstacles standing in the way of eliminating this form of agriculture are the rugged terrain and the huge financial cost – a matter of considerable significance for poor countries.

There is no question that we need to try and use this land for other purposes, although this is far from easy. The cultivation of these drugs takes place in areas notorious for their poor soil, it does not call for special agricultural techniques nor expensive equipment, transport costs are very small given the product's value and weight, and it brings in bigger profits than anything else. Rich countries are in no position to condemn the growers who are mostly poor and live in conditions of appalling degradation. They must be offered dignified ways of converting their fields to other uses. We also need to be alert to substances that are similar to drugs, and to equipment and chemical products that are used in the processing.

Illegal trafficking is essential to the supply of drugs. If we are unable to make any progress in this direction, the effects of prevention and rehabilitation will be greatly reduced. Pressure should be concentrated not on small dealers but on the big traffickers who often present themselves as large important enterprises, and are completely legal on the surface. This is extremely difficult, partly because there are so few people employed on policing duties, but also because they are easy prey to pressure and bribery and other means at the disposal of those who carry out this deadly work.

An effective struggle against drug trafficking must entail information being shared between the various countries, the tactic of allowing some merchandise to circulate as a way of identifying the nerve centres of distribution, the encouragement of extradition, sometimes allowing small portions of seized merchandise to circulate instead of keeping the whole cache, appropriate levels of punishment, the confiscation of drugs and the equipment used to produce them, and control of frontiers, postal services, money movements and bank accounts.

28.6 Treatment and rehabilitation

One of the most important ethical responsibilities is caring for people who are drug-dependent. The bottom line is to look upon them as sick people who need very considerable care.

Medical treatment is usually necessary, and this is an important way of side-stepping some well-meaning individuals who want to give help that is exclusively spiritual. We live in a world full of short-sighted, ill-thought-out charisms.

Another question is the kind of treatment that will enable the person to rehabilitate after his/her health has been seriously compromised by drug taking. There is a major role here for help from the family, and from counselling and support services, and for assistance from a range of health professionals. Drug-dependent people need help in recovering their self-esteem, establishing proper relationships, integrating values and controlling themselves. One final component of permanent recovery is the attitude of society; much hangs on whether the patient finds a welcome or rejection there.

NOTES

1. M. Segura, 'La droga, una escalada preocupante', in *Proyección* 36 (1989) 3-14; L. Lorenzetti, 'Questione droga', in *RTM* 83 (1989) 93-100; United Nations, 'Raccomandazioni circa l'abuso e il traffico illegale di droghe', in *Il Regno* 33 (1988) 89-127; A. Coppel and J. Fatella, 'Drogue: de nouvelles réponses?', in *Ésprit* 148-149 (1989) 26-35; S. Bignamini and G. Brunetta, 'Fenomeno droga e cooperazione internazionale', in *AS* 40 (1989) 581-598; F. Bueno, 'La droga y los establecimientos penitenciarios', in *RFS* 43 (1988) 139-148; M. Pelletier, 'La drogue, pas de solution miracle', in *Études* 366 (1987) 463-469; *La lutte contre l'abus des drogues,* Dossiers Pro mundi vita (1987) no. 4; A. Berstain, 'Problemas juveniles en el campo de la toxicomanías', in *RS* 41 (1986) 305-312; *El oscuro mondo de la droga juvenil,* Pastoral Letter of the Bishops of Pamplona and Tudela, Bilbao, San Sebastian and Vitoria, November 1984; 'Drogue, famille, sociéte, Propos recueillis par B. Matray auprès de Joâo Fatela', in *Laennec* Decembre

(1986) 14-16; G. Ceirano, 'L'usage de la drogue, signal d'alarme d'une société', in *DC* 82 (1985) 661-662; A. Boado, 'Reseña histórico-antropólogica de las drogas en distintas culturas', in *CRS* 23-24 (1984) 131-152; Swiss Bishops' Conference, 'Les chrétiens face à la toxicomanie', in *DC* 76 (1979) 835-838; B.A.M. Peters, *Drugs and morals*, PS, Madrid 1969. D.M. Warburton (ed.), *Addiction Controversies*, Harwood Academic Press, 1990; M.M. Glatt, *A Guide to Addiction and its Treatment*, John Wiley and Sons, New York 1974; G. Edwards and M. Lader (eds.), *The Nature of Drug Dependence*, OUP, Oxford 1990; G. Edwards, J. Strang and J.H. Jaffe, *Drugs, Alcohol and Tobacco: Making the Science and Policy Connection*, 1993; M. Lader (ed.), *The Psychopharmacology of Addiction*, OUP, Oxford 1988.
2. A working Party formed in August 1981 by the OMS recommends the use of the term 'neuroadaptation' instead of 'physical dependency', and requests that the term 'abuse' be replaced by 'dependency syndrome'. See G. Edwards and A. Arif, *Les problèmes de la drogue dans leur contexte socio-culturel*, OMS, Geneva 1982.
3. Taken from the dossier 'Pro mundi vita', (1987) no. 4, 6.
4. Cf Ibid., 8-12.
5. OMS, *Young People's Health. A Challenge for Society*, Geneva 1986.
6. Cf dossier 'Pro mundi vita', 5.
7. Under this section I recommend the excellent exposition of the charter written by the Basque bishops.
8. III, 1.
9. III, 2.
10. III, 3.
11. United Nations, *a.c.*, nn. 88-105.

Chapter 29

Medical interventions in mental illness and behavioural problems

29.1 Psychopharmacology[1]

Psychopharmacology made its first appearance as a way of treating mental breakdown in the 1950s. Its effect on brain chemistry, and therefore on one's mental state, is achieved through certain chemical substances being ingested into the body. The table below classifies the numerous products that have rapidly proliferated in this field:

CLASSIFICATION OF PSYCHOTROPIC SUBSTANCES[2]

1. *Psychoactive* (which depress mental activity):
   (a) Hypnotic (sleep-inducing);
   (b) Tranquillizer (anxiety-reducing);
   (c) Neuroleptic (calm agitation and delirium)
   (d) Anti-depressants (prevent manic episodes and depression).
2. *Stimulants* (which stimulate mental activity):
   (a) Central nervous system stimulant (psychoactive, anorexiant);
   (b) Mood modifiers (antidepressives).
3. *Psychodysleptic* (which disturb the mental state):
   (a) Hallucinogens;
   (b) Euphoriants;
   (c) Stimulants.

Many radical positions are adopted on this subject, but I do not feel there are any moral reservations about using medication as such. This kind of therapy has substantially reduced the amount of time spent in psychiatric hospitals, and has enabled a lot of people to re-enter society satisfactorily. It has also done much to improve the social image of many mentally ill patients, and has made mental illness less dramatic.

The problem we face is not, therefore, in the use of this medication, but in the way that pharmacology has invaded these illnesses. It is a question that cannot be isolated from characteristics of the society in which the phenomenon occurs. Some people are beginning to wonder whether we might not be relying too much on medicine to treat psychological and related problems. 'Pills' are a solution to personal or social conflicts, but to what extent are they the most humane solution? Are we not slipping into a deterministic and mechanistic conception of life? Can obtaining gratification in itself be considered real therapy? Are we not victims of a predominantly technical view of the world which prioritizes rapid, short-term effectiveness by means of automatic measures over the slow business of changing the person? What I am fundamentally questioning is the way we deal with human problems. To my mind, the spread of psychopharmacology is simply one more manifestation.

What is really worrying is not the use of medicines but the way they are trivialized. I am now thinking of people who are unable to put up with the most minor ailment or deal with the tiniest problem – let alone analyse its causes and try and find a solution for themselves – without reaching for some medicine. A puritanical approach that rejected outright the quick solutions of pharmacology would mean that people could easily remain in pain for a long time; perhaps they would do this out of some loyalty to the idea that people must give more of themselves and make greater efforts. An easy surrender to the temptations of psychopharmacology, on the other hand, invites us to question certain facts that are widespread in our society. Another complex issue is the difference between mental and other forms of illness; this distinction is becoming more and more difficult to determine in our civilization.

29.2 Psychosurgery

Psychosurgery is the treatment of certain illnesses by means of brain surgery; the first major figure in this field was the

Portuguese Egas Moniz in the 1930s. A definition put out by the US Department of Health and Human Services in 1978 appears to introduce the idea of values into the technique; it does this by presenting it as a form of surgery either (a) on the tissue of a normal brain, seeking to change or control behaviour, or (b) on the tissue of a brain that has deteriorated with a view to controlling or altering behavioural problems.

This kind of treatment was frequently used until 1954, and attracted attention for its widespread application and its uncritical acceptance by numerous psychiatrists. Its popularity has fallen dramatically since then with the appearance of psychotropic drugs, and an increase in the amount of criticism relating to possible abuses. These practices were forbidden by law in the former Soviet Union in 1951. In Great Britain, it is estimated that there were 158 operations in 1974, but this number fell to 154 in 1975, 119 in 1976, 70 in 1979, and finally, 37 in 1983. Figures for operations in the United States suggest no more than 400 during the early 1970s, and this in all probability had dropped by the end of the 1980s.

From a moral point of view, the most difficult question is determining how effective the method is. There are many obstacles to an objective assessment, includingt the lack of sufficient follow-up to discover whether the results are long-lasting; other variables are difficulties in measuring these results, and the personal views of doctors convinced of the validity of this procedure. There is also a multitude of psychosurgical and a wide range of illnesses and situations in which they are used. All of these points combine to make it difficult to know for sure whether we are talking about a form of treatment that has been properly tested or one that is still at an experimental stage. If it is the latter, the requirements of all therapeutic research need to be met.

Uncertainties about its effectiveness must not prevent us from admitting quite openly that certain psychiatric problems do respond to psychosurgical treatment.

If there are medical grounds for an intervention of this sort, and if the doctors are sufficiently skilled, there is also a need for the patient's informed consent if s/he can give it personally; if the patient is incapable of doing so, his/her legitimate representatives have to give permission.

There have been risks associated with using these techniques on prisoners with a view to controlling their aggressive behaviour. Two moral issues arise here: the possibility of discriminating against such people because they are in a disadvantaged position when it comes to freedom of consent; and the distinction between therapy on the one hand and social control and manipulation on the other.[3]

29.3 Electroconvulsive therapy[4]

This technique consists of applying electric currents to the brain so as to produce convulsions that can cure mental disorder. The first to use it were Cerletti and Bini in Rome in 1938. Their patient was a schizophrenic who was leading a normal life within two years of the treatment, and was capable of holding down a job quite satisfactorily. In the course of this form of treatment, there is usually a convulsion lasting a few seconds which is similar in appearance to an epileptic fit.

The idea that convulsions could influence people's mental state owes much to a belief prevalent among Greeks that epilepsy was a form of possession by the gods. Nowadays, thanks to muscular relaxants and short-term anaesthetics, electroconvulsive therapy is more reliable and is much less distressing than it used to be. The illness most appropriate to this kind of treatment is severe depression. Depression of this type is resistant to pharmacological therapies and, when the condition is complicated by dehydration, is accompanied by suicide attempts and important bodily changes such as severe weight loss. It is also effective in cases of childhood psychosis. Electroconvulsive therapy has been used less in schizophrenia since the arrival of neuroleptic drugs, but many studies have demonstrated its effectiveness in psychotic depression; indeed, its clinical value in this field is undisputed.

It is not known exactly how electroconvulsive therapy works. There are very few absolute contra indications to its use, although one of them is high intercranial pressure. It is also contraindicated in patients with elevated systolic blood pressure, and when there is a history of cerebro-vascular illness, aneurism of the brain or aorta, or recent cardiac arrest. A general anaesthetic can add complications in the case of serious cardio-respiratory illness. Secondary effects are well documented, and include mental confusion, headaches and poor memory, but they are benign for the most part and transitory. As for loss of memory, most studies have concluded that loss is not permanent.

There is, however, considerable resistance to electro-convulsive therapy among health professionals and even more so among outsiders. For many people, its image is very negative, and it is associated with executions, medieval witchcraft and inhumane punishment. Others see it as a method of punishment and social control applied mainly to people who have been committed to psychiatric hospitals, but also to radical and minority groups. In 1982, the citizens of Berkeley voted to prohibit its use in local hospitals, although this decision was later overturned by a judicial ruling which declared it was unconstitutional to deprive patients of treatment; this ruling was later confirmed on appeal. There are now other therapies available for mental illness, and it seems that electroconvulsive treatment is rarely used these days.

From a moral point of view, there are no objections to this technique providing its effectiveness is well documented – as it is, for example, with severe depressions – and there are no other more benign treatments available. The other essential condition is the patient's consent, if s/he is able to give it; otherwise the consent of the patient's legitimate representatives is necessary.

29.4 Psychotherapy[5]

Under this heading come a number of therapies which have very different bases and techniques, and which are used with both groups and individuals. Of the individual dynamic therapies, the four most important are classical psychoanalysis, interpersonal therapies or personal effectiveness therapies as postulated by Jung and Adler, and which Erikson and Fromm placed in a social context, a form of therapy which seeks to get rid of neuromuscular rigidity through counselling, and client-centred therapy, whose most celebrated practitioner is Carl Rogers.

Normal therapeutic technique in individual dynamic psychotherapy is the transference, or counter-transference, between therapist and patient. It is based on the assumption that disorder is manifested in actions whose motives are unconscious; the patient represses the motives out of anxiety, and does so by means of defensive manoeuvres. Therapy consists fundamentally of making these motives conscious and placing them under the patient's control.

As it is not possible to give a detailed analysis here of the many questions raised by the various psychotherapeutic procedures, I shall confine myself to some general remarks.

The effectiveness of psychotherapy is sometimes questioned. There do not appear to be any scientific, empirical proofs of the validity and effectiveness of this kind of treatment. It has been pointed out that the peculiar characteristics of this therapy mean that the results cannot be verified solely from observed behaviour because psychotherapy incorporates many important, but invisible, elements. Therapy of this kind bears a closer resemblance to friendship, upbringing or a sexual relationship.

However, the most fundamental question refers to the values which we need to use in order to assess results, and this leads us on to more global conceptions of human beings. When the client's demands and wishes do not respond to those held by the therapist, what can therapy do? Let us take an example: if a woman feels her self-respect is crushed by her husband's infidelities, and the reason for this is that she does not want to jeopardize her marriage, what should she do? Should she inure herself to a situation that she knows is not right, or should she be allowed to remain in painful circumstances which will only make her more miserable?

Another problem is the proliferation of psychotherapists, many of whom do not appear to have any qualifications of competence. Moreover, there is an element of ambiguity in the psychotherapist's function. On the one hand, s/he is the patient's doctor; on the other, the work has a social and political component in the sense that the psychotherapist can encourage attitudes of rebelliousness or accommodation towards the system and social values. Observations which Häring has made on psychoanalysis may be valid, at least in part, to other techniques. For one thing, psychoanalysis often affirms its independence from all other value systems, although even this position itself involves taking a view which includes making an assessment. The second danger is manipulation of the patient who does not respect his/her autonomy. A criticism made of certain psychoanalytical methods is their individualistic conception of the person. When dealing with patients who have a tendency to evade things, psychoanalysis may encourage them to flee from their own responsibilities.[6]

29.5 Behavioural therapy[7]

Behavioural therapy has been enormously popular in Britain since the late 1950s, and is now making inroads into other schools of therapy. Very gradually, it is gaining ground at the expense of traditional psychotherapy of a more psychoanalytical persuasion.

According to the various theories within this group, mental disorder and behavioural disorders are not caused by complexes, but are the result of a mislearning. These disorders often stop spontaneously, but sometimes, when they fail to do so, it is necessary to have recourse to a therapy which, by means of relearning, eliminates the reactions which are causing the person so much suffering. It is in this way that conditioned responses are produced.

There are two types of conditioning, Classical Conditioning (Pavlov) and Operant Conditioning (Skinner). Pavlov carried out an experiment with a dog in which a bell was rung several times a few moments before it was given food; in the end, the dog began to salivate at the sound of the bell even when food did not arrive. Operant Conditioning tends to create a response, but through a positive action. For example, an animal is placed in a box in which it can move about, and on one of the walls there is a small item (perhaps a lever or a button) which, when pressed, allows the animal to obtain some food. The animal experiments and performs different actions, until at last it presses the lever or button and gets some food. In Operant Conditioning the subject collaborates actively, while in Classical Conditioning it remains passive.

The three most common techniques of Classical Conditioning are desensitivization, flooding and modelling. Desensitivization consists of associating other responses with a stimulus which produces a reaction. These other responses slowly eliminate or reduce the reaction which is considered to be anomalous. For instance, if someone responds with fear to a given object like a cat, an attempt is made to associate the object with other responses, e.g. happiness, relaxation or tranquillity.

Flooding, or Implosive Therapy, seeks to make the subject live the anomalous situation with as much intensity as possible. For example, if someone needs to wash his/her hands continually no matter what object s/he has touched, she is made to touch dirty objects so as to be able to get rid of the obsession.

In modelling, the patient follows the therapist who acts as an example and stimulus in the performance of certain actions. If the subject does not dare to touch a dog, s/he is made to see by example how touching it does not produce the effects that were feared.

Sometimes, use is made of aversion therapy, the form of therapy most hotly criticized by its opponents. Its use is concentrated on behaviour that is socially disapproved of, like alcoholism and homosexuality. Stimuli which cause reactions considered to be anti-social are linked to responses that are disagreeable to the subject; this is done with a view to creating aversion to earlier behaviour. We have an example of this in the film *A Clockwork Orange*.

It is true that some defenders of these therapies believe that they can be applied to any behaviour and to all symptoms. A more objective view sees otherwise. Results with psychosis are very disappointing; they are positive or very positive with certain symptoms like phobias, tics, and sexual and social inhibitions, but less successful in the treatment of obsessions and hysteria.

There is quite a substantial body of criticism of behavioural therapy, and particularly of Operant Conditioning, from both a scientific and an ethical point of view. There are those who believe that it is not only debatable in terms of effectiveness, but dangerous and unacceptable in respect of its principles and philosophy. Others do not share this negative view.

According to its critics, aversion therapy encourages a disinterest in, or disregard for, the subject as such. The person's essential experiences are of no interest; only his/her observable behaviour is. The patient's view of the world and him/herself is not taken into account, and the relationship between the patient and therapist is mechanized and depersonalized. The causes of the disorder are not attacked, just the symptoms. The assumption that all behavioural disorder is due to mislearning, when understood in absolute terms, is questioned, as many anomalous phenomena appear to be due to the subject's biological mechanisms or personality.

It is said that these therapies are an assault on people's freedoms because they attempt to change the illness by mechanical means, and this reveals a deterministic concept of human beings. However, a more profound examination of what happens shows that this type of control sometimes tries to eliminate types of behaviour that have great power over the patient. This criticism may be generally true, but it cannot be said to be valid in all circumstances.

Another criticism is the complicity of social conformism in forms of therapy aimed at anti-social behaviour like homosexuality and alcoholism. Behavioural therapy inspires a whole series of questions. They include: Who exercises control of the behaviour? Over whom? With what right? In whose interests? What other approaches are available? What kind of person do we want? Unfortunately, behavioural therapy is not equipped to deal with them.

Therapy of this kind provides a solution to a conflict that often arises between the right to a tolerable life, which is not threatened with continuous suffering, and the right to enjoy the dignity and freedom of a human being.

NOTES

1. E. López Azpitarte, 'Psicofarmacología y control de la persona. Aspectos éticas', in *Jano* 723 (1986) 84-92; H.N. Wagner, 'Probing the Chemistry of the Mind', in *NEJM* 312 (1985) 44-46; R. Gfeller, 'Médicaments psychotropes et relation médecin-malade', in *Mhyg* 38 (1980) 2486-2493; G.L. Klerman and J.E. Izen, 'Psychopharmacology', in *EB* III, 1378-1386.
2. Reproduced from the *Enciclopedia de la psicologia y pedagogía*, III, Sedmay, Madrid 1979, 456.
3. S. Bloch, 'Whatever Happened to Psychosurgery', in *HCR* 16 (1986) no. 6, 24-26; R. Neville, 'Psychosurgery', in *EB* III, 1387-1391; 'Hostility to Psychosurgery' (editorial), in *Lancet*, 17 February (1979) 367-368; G. Perico, 'Lobotomy', in *AS* 29 (1978) 227-232; G.J. Annas, 'Psychosurgery: Procedural Safeguards', in *HCR* 7 (1977) no. 2, 11-13; L.O. Gostin, 'Ethical Considerations of Pyschosurgery: the Unhappy Legacy of the Pre-Frontal Lobotomy', in *JME* 6 (1980) 149-154.
4. A. Linington and B. Harris, 'Fifty Years of Electroconvulsive Therapy. Value Undoubted, Mode of Action Unknown', in *BMJ* 297 (1988) 1354; B.F. Hoffman, 'The Impact of New Ethics and Laws on Electroconvulsive Therapy', in *CMAS* 132 (1985) 1366-1368; R.R. Crowe, 'Electroconvulsive Therapy. A current Perspective', in *NEJM* 311 (1984) 163-167; 'Effects of Electric Convulsive Therapy' (editorial), in *BMJ* 281 (1980) 1588; R.M. Restak, 'Electroconvulsive Therapy', in *EB* I, 359-361.

5. S. Pattison and P. Armitage, 'An Ethical Analysis of the Policies of British Community and Hospital Care for Mentally Ill People', in *JME* 12 (1986) 136-142; R.B. Edwards, 'Mental Health as Rational Autonomy', in *JMPh* 6 (1981) 309-322; P.A. Trafford and S. Spencer, 'Psychiatres et patients. Aspects éthiques', in *MH* 152 (1987) 20-23.

6. B. Häring, *Medical Ethics*, St Paul Publications, Slough 1972, Madrid 1972, 171-173.

7. E. Dalton, 'Ethical Issues in Behaviour Control: A Preliminary Investigation', in *ManM* 2 (1976-1977) 1-40; G. Dworkin, 'Autonomy and Behaviour Control', in *HCR* 6 (1976) no. 1, 23-28.

Chapter 30

Research using human beings[1]

30.1 Background

If we want a precise definition of the notion of research using human beings, we need to refer back to therapy. Therapy is understood to mean any intervention which seeks exclusively to benefit the patient, and it can take a variety of forms including treatment to cure an illness, diagnosis, and a range of preventive measures. Research, by contrast, aims to contribute to the general advance of knowledge and obtain generalizable results; it is normally divided into therapeutic and non-therapeutic.

Therapeutic research incorporates elements of both research and therapy. As research, it involves the search for general information that can be used in other contexts and on other patients. As therapy, it seeks to make the patient well. In therapeutic research, the patient's health is the primary concern, while finding generalizable results is important but not essential. Non-therapeutic research does not consider the patient's health; it is concerned solely with scientific goals.

The conceptual distinction between therapy and research, and between therapeutic and non-therapeutic research, is far from clear in practice. Even the most familiar forms of treatment can run up against unforeseen factors and produce unexpected results. That is why health professionals should be always asking themselves whether, in the light of things that they observe in the course of their work, they feel obliged, or feel under any pressure, to make changes in the way they practise their profession.

30.2 Research and ethics

There has been no moral consideration for many centuries on the subject of research using human beings; the only related principle for a long time was the requirement to look after the patient's health and not to do him/her any harm. This absence of any further consideration is understandable because there used to be no such thing as research as we know it today – an approximate definition might be a project to discover new information, and which is carried out according to scientific procedures and methods. Even when there has been a method, research using human beings has had to transfer to real projects. An important spur to an ethical awareness of the need to have a moral framework governing human research was provided by the abuses carried out by the Nazi regime. After World War II, ethical guidelines were issued by a large number of civil bodies and religious groups; they all referred to human research. Some of the most important civil contributions were the Nuremberg Code (1946), Helsinki I (the World Medical Association's Declaration of Helsinki, adopted in 1962 and revised in 1964), Helsinki II (the name sometimes given to the Declaration of Tokyo, adopted in 1975), a statement on 'Responsibility in Investigations on Human Subjects' (Medical Research Council of Great Britain, 1963), 'Experimental Research on Human Beings' (British Medical Association, 1963), 'Ethical Guidelines for Clinical Investigation' (American Medical Association, 1966), 'U.S. Guidelines on Human Experimentation' (United States Department of Health, Education and Well-being, 1971), and 'Avis sur les essais de nouveaux traitements chez l'homme' (Note on experimental new treatment on human beings) (National Consultative Ethical Committee for Life and Health Sciences, France 1984).

Important Papal pronouncements have included Pius XII's address of 14 September to the 1st International Congress on the Histopathology of the Nervous System, a radio message of 11 September 1956 to the 7th International Congress of Catholic Doctors, a speech on 10 April 1958 to participants at the 13th International Congress of Applied Psychology, and an address on 9 September 1958 to members of the International College of Neuropsychopharmacology. There have also been three important speeches made by Pope John Paul II to members of the Congress of Italian Associations of Medicine and General Surgery (27 October 1980), to the Congress of Catholic Doctors (23 October 1982) and to delegates to the World Medical Association (29 October 1983).

30.3 Ethical considerations

– *The legitimacy of research.* Biomedical research is essential for scientific progress and, indeed, for the well-being of humanity. Its moral legitimacy is assured as long as a number of conditions are met, as we shall now see.

– *The human being must not be reduced to being a means for doing research.* The person's dignity must be respected, and one of the fundamental consequences is that the patient's basic interests must not be subordinated to those of science or society.[2]

– *A sense of solidarity.* At the same time, there needs to be stimulated in each human being a voluntary willingness to collaborate for the well-being of humanity, always bearing in mind his/her freedom and respect for his/her convictions of conscience and any other legitimate interests.

– *Fairness* whereby research shares out the risks and benefits equally among different peoples and social groups, steering clear of any discrimination which might result in some people suffering the risks and others enjoying the benefits.

– *Informed and free consent.* This ethical demand, which has been dealt with elsewhere in this book, must be observed in therapy as well as in research.

Research using human beings assumes, in the first place, that there is sufficient information on 'the objectives, methods, hoped for benefits and potential risks of the study and the problems that could arise from it'.[3] Certain people, like children, patients in a coma and mentally handicapped individuals present specific problems for this demand to be met. There is a debate as to whether moral imperatives always demand that this norm is observed in the case of adults who are competent; there is no shortage of arguments supporting the view that, in particular cases, there is no insuperable moral reservation about concealing information. Indeed, in certain situations, it seems to be reasonable for patients, and even the doctors involved, not to know who is receiving well-tried treatment, and who is getting experimental treatment or a placebo.

As far as consent is concerned, the patient must have the right to take part freely in the experiment, and also withdraw just as freely without fear of any recriminations. Special measures need to be taken to deal with freedom of consent when it applies to people who are dependants; in the event of mental or legal incompetence, consent has to be given by the next of kin or legal guardian.

As I have already indicated, there are questions here about whether the need for consent is an absolute norm, or whether it might be ethically done away with in certain circumstances. This problem arises particularly when the distribution of patients between the two groups is random.

– *Assessment of benefits and damage.* This question can be examined from two angles: on the one hand, the benefits to science and society and any harm that may befall the patients that have taken part in the research, and on the other, the benefits and risks to the patients involved.

As for the first of these assessments, we should remember what was said earlier on: the patient's basic interests must always prevail over those of science and society. Research of great social interest that places the individual in danger loses legitimacy unless s/he agrees to take part as a token of solidarity. If the research involves minor risks for the patient, there are no moral reservations as long as s/he accepts them.

A much harder problem surrounds the assessment of the benefits and risks to the patient taking part in the experiment. Here, the person's integrity and private life must be respected. However, the situation varies according to whether the research is being carried out on healthy people (with no therapeutic objective) or on sick people. In the latter case, there needs to be an assessment of the risks as well as the benefits that can be predicted in the various scenarios (not being treated, and being treated with well-tried and new forms of treatment). These risks and benefits have to be assessed in terms of degree (e.g. large and small) and likelihood of success (minimal, small or strong). If all these elements are put together, it becomes more difficult to produce practical norms.

Steps taken prior to carrying out research on human beings. No matter how well organized research on human beings is, the unexpected can never be ruled out. The ethical position is that the margin of unpredictability must be reduced as far as possible, hence the need for prior research in laboratories and the use of animals, always assuming that this is practicable.

Scientific rigour. The need for scientific rigour in the project is based on two issues. They are the respect due to the patients on which the experiment will be carried out, and the invalidity of the intervention's conclusions if it has not been planned scrupulously. There is a lot to be said for submitting projects to an ethics committee; from a moral standpoint this is not absolutely essential, but it is certainly recommended as good practice. On the surface, the ethics committee's function appears to be the scientific verification of the experiment's scientific rigour, but it could also include an element of ethical responsibility.

This is an issue that benefits from further detailed study of the content of the afore-mentioned civil and papal pronouncements. Inter-disciplinary commissions could well throw more light on the subject as well, although we have to face the fact that there will always be grey areas. In order to mitigate the lack of more concrete interpretations, we need to train people to know how to reach a moral judgement and at the same time share views with others.

NOTES

1. M. Angell, 'Ethics in International Collaborative Clinical Research', in
    NEJM 319 (1988) 1081-1083; A. Hersheimer, 'The Rights of the Patient in
    Clinical Research', in *Lancet* 12 November (1988) 1128-1130; Ch. Marviick,
    'Philosophy on Trial: Examining Ethics of Clinical Investigations', in *JAMA*
    260 (1988) 749-751; D. Marquis, 'When Research is Best Therapy', in *HCR*
    18 (1988) no. 2, 24-26; D.J. Rothman, 'Ethics and Human Experimenta-
    tion', in *NEJM* 317 (1987) 1195-1199; B. Freedman, 'Equipoise and the
    Ethics of Clinical Research', in *NEJM* 317 (1987) 141-145; C. Levine and
    others, 'False Date and the Therapeutic Misconception: Two Urgent Prob-
    lems in Research Ethics', in *HCR* 17 (1987) no. 2, 16-24; P. Arpaillange, S.
    Dion and G. Mathe, 'Proposal for Ethical Standards in Therapeutic Trials',
    in *BMJ* 291 (1985) 887-889; 'Guidelines to Aid Ethical Committees Consid-
    ering Research Involving Children', in *BMJ*, January 26 (1980) 229-231.
2. Tokyo Declaration 1975, Basic Principle, no. 5.
3. Tokyo Declaration 1975, Basic Principle, no. 9.

Chapter 31

Interventions on animals[1]

The question of animal rights has been with us now for several years. The most important question in the context of this book relates to research and experimentation, but other issues include the use of animals for teaching and leisure activities and the rearing of animals in captivity.

Concern for animal rights is widespread among certain circles in developed countries, although respect for animals is well-established in other cultures for a variety of religious and philosophical reasons. Discussion on the subject is frequently emotional. Some people consider an interest in animal rights to be an impeccable sign of spiritual purity and an indication of living in a culture liberated from the more humdrum human problems. Others see it as one of the luxuries of the well-off, leisured classes, an outrageous piece of provocation, or else an example of moral incoherence resulting from giving the wrong priority to humans and animals.

This question is closely linked to a number of socio-cultural factors, and we shall examine it by looking at the status attributed to the animal world and the theme of suffering.

31.1 The 'moral status' of animal life[2]

It is difficult to introduce any order into the huge range of opinions that people have on this subject. However, most views may be grouped around two main currents, with shades of opinion inside each of them. The first is the liberationist/progressive school which includes those who defend animal rights or people's duties towards animals, and who fight for the well-being and rights of animals; the second is the speciesist and egalitarian group. Some people also talk of a middle way.

345

I have already referred to the shortage of philosophical background necessary to tackle this question, and also how the lack of agreement on certain abstract points does not prevent a convergence on a number of issues.

a. The speciesist theory

Speciesism allocates more importance to the rights and interests of humans than to those of animals, on the simple grounds that human beings form part of a superior species. According to his school of thought, there is a qualitative difference between human beings and animals. The most radical variant of this approach reduces animals to the status of things with neither rights nor interests, and towards which humans have no duties. In these circumstances, the way in which human beings make use of animals is of no moral significance.

Another form of speciesism does not recognize the rights of animals, but does acknowledge their interests. According to this view, animals' interests are so subordinate to those of human beings that even the interests of nature are lower than human, non-vital interests. A major factor supporting speciesism is its mechanistic view of modern science and the importance granted to Cartesian thinking.

b. Egalitarianism

This current, too, contains a radical wing that rejects all reference to other species; the sole criterion for both human beings and animals should be the degree of vitality of the interest in question. There is also so-called two-factor egalitarianism according to which, in the event of a conflict, priority must be given to the organism that is best equipped mentally, that is to say the one most capable of a painful, conscious decision. According to this principle, an aware adult stands above any animal, although an animal would have preference over a human being in a coma, or a foetus incapable of feeling pain.

31.2 Suffering

Some people marginalize the question of animals' moral status, and focus their attention on suffering as a vehicle for reaching a conclusion covering this whole issue.

The American Veterinary Medical Association has tried to produce a precise definition of the adverse effects that can befall animals; they are pain, distress, discomfort, anxiety and fear.[3]

As with all other experiences, there is a problem assessing the suffering undergone by animals. It does not, however, prevent us from understanding something through various modes of expression such as gestures and behaviour, although generalizations of this can only go so far. Another problem is the difference between humans and animals. Moreover, we put animals to many different uses, and some of the resulting situations can be very dangerous for them; these include painful tests, and the unsatisfactory conditions in which animals are kept when in captivity or as pets.

In a society that takes so much pride in pleasurable matters, it is hardly surprising to find that a stubborn response has developed towards suffering, and this has been extended to animals. It is not easy to say whether this desire to spare animals suffering should be described as moral or not; at all events, it is a sensible, reasonable and humanitarian attitude and worthy of being encouraged.

31.3 Research and experimentation

Of the various uses that are made of animal research and experimentation to benefit humanity, I am going to concentrate on two: research and experimentation. I will deal with them in this section, together with the use of animals for patenting.

In the field of research and experimentation, animals constitute only one of the many potential groups used. They are inanimate equipment like computers and mechanical models, plants, human beings, and various culture systems including microbes and organic tissue.

In the last 100 years, animals have played a vital role in the understanding, treatment and sometimes elimination of diseases that had previously been killing large numbers of humans, and even other animals. Examples of success in this area include the production of various vaccines for polio and insulin therapy/ treatment for diabetes.[4] There are also hopes that experimentation with animals will play an important role in future in the treatment of such conditions as heart disease, nervous illnesses and cancer.

In principle, the use of animals for the benefit of human beings presents no insuperable moral reservations, and the moral rejection of all research and experimentation with animals does not seem to be either sensible or sustainable. It is, however, legitimate to insist on certain conditions being met.

All research and experimentation must start off on the basis of an investigative project that is as precise as possible. Components might include a specific question, an outline of the kind of response, familiarity with current literature on the part of the researchers, the objectives, other approaches (using animals or otherwise) to achieve the aims, and the pros and cons of these other approaches. In this context, one issue that needs to be looked at very closely is the choice of the subjects to be researched or experimented on; various criteria are involved here, including scientific questions, social attitudes and financial implications. When it is settled that an animal might be used, one of the questions that needs to be asked is the number that will be needed and the number of the species available.

31.4 Patenting living organisms[5]

The last issue deals with the patenting of living microorganisms which have been created artificially in the laboratory by genetic engineering. Other scientific developments are related to attempted and successful hybrids, such as the tiger-lion, the zebra-horse, the sheep-donkey and the hen-quail, through artificial fertilization or the creation of chimeras. This is also linked to the production of animals with unusual characteristics through genetic engineering, like cows which produce exceptional quantities of milk, and giant rats.

Let us first take a look at the legal aspects before moving on to moral issues. An important milestone in this context is a finding of the United States Supreme Court on 16 June 1980; by five votes to four, the Supreme Court established the principle that the criterion of patentability was not the distinction between living being and non-living being, but between existing in nature or invented by humans. This decision was applied to single-cell beings like bacteria, and was extended by the Patents and Trade Marks Office on 3 April 1987 to multicellular organisms.[6]

Social reaction to this new situation was divided. Some people were alarmed by the negative impact on humanity in the future, and by possible anthropological and social repercussions. Others gave it a warm welcome, seeing it as an incentive for the development of the biotechnology industry, and the forerunner of financial profit and social benefits.

Reactions have also been based on religious and ethical beliefs. At a meeting held in Airlie House on the outskirts of Washington DC, the Human Society of the United States together with representatives of six religious groups called for a moratorium on animal patenting. The declaration, which was published in July 1988, first recalls certain principles and ideas of a general nature, and then moves on to a judgement of the whole issue;

> This states that humankind and all of nature live in a relationship of interdependence and interaction in an alliance with the Creator. Participants at the meeting recognized that the human species does not have a correct relationship with the rest of creation. Our sinfulness, they said, was rooted in our continual abuse of creation and desire to refashion it in our own image – and, what is more, solely as a means of satisfying needs. Redemption does not just mean personal salvation, but also the restoration of the natural world and the establishment of a protective relationship towards all creation. The ethical, environmental, socio-economic and teleological ramifications of genetic engineering and patenting life are immense. They are leading, the declaration goes on, to even greater danger for the integrity and future of creation if the new genetic influences over life are not used carefully and also seek to restore the alliance of saving the earth and ourselves.[7]

The whole question of patenting forms of life that have been artificially created by human beings does not in itself present unacceptable moral problems. It must not be seen, however, as a necessarily dangerous desecration of living beings or of life. It could be part of the promotion of financial interests of more self-centred individuals, and even be the instigator of a new form of economic colonialism, particularly in poorer countries. There are those who fear that this measure is symptomatic of the slow, gradual emergence of a social attitude that permits indiscriminate and unjustified experiments on genetic material.

31.5 Theological and ethical considerations

In the course of the last few decades, ecology has stimulated much debate on the relationship between Christianity and nature. If we confine ourselves here to the issue of animal life, we know from reading the Bible that it has often been said that Christian theology has defended the arbitrary and cruel use of animals. The most telling passage comes from Genesis: 'Fill the earth and subdue it; and have domination over the fish of the sea and over the birds of the air and over every living thing that moves upon the earth.'[8] There are many and varied references to the animal world in the Bible, but it is not easy to find a single theme running through them. Just the same, there is no point in trying to extract specific material norms from the Bible to solve our problem. The most we can hope for is a new way of looking at the relationship between human beings and nature, based on God's covenant with all living beings created by him; it is a covenant compromised by sin, but is initially restored by Christ as the final hours approach.[9]

From a moral point of view, a common feeling places human beings in a privileged position in relationship to animal life. Using animals for the benefit of humanity is a criterion of correct behaviour; however, this is no basis for making animals into sacred beings or thinking of them as untouchable. Just the same, humanity's interest has to be global and must heed a variety of issues. For that reason, we need to question an ideology that is consumerist, one that seeks purely financial or immediate advantages. If austerity and sobriety more aptly characterize the human race, that ought to provide good protection against the many abuses suffered by animals. The interconnection and interdependence of the various forms of life are often forgotten as well, and give way to half-baked objectives. A sense of mercy will encourage people to avoid unnecessary suffering. There are abuses that reveal a certain absence of solidarity both towards future generations and between peoples at loggerheads with one another. The two fundamental indicators of human behaviour towards animals are service and responsibility, along the lines of what I have written above.

NOTES

1. S. Donnelley, 'Speculative Philosophy, the Troubled Middle, and the Ethics of Animal Experimentation', in *HCR* 19 (1989), no. 2, 15-21; Council of Scientific Affairs, 'Animals in Research', in *JAMA* 261 (1989) 3602-3606; 'Animals in Research', in *JMPh* 13 (1988) no. 2; J.A. Thomas and others, 'Animal Research at Stanford University. Principles, Policies and Practices', in *NEJM* 318 (1988) 1630-1632; C. Cohen, 'The Case for the use of Animals in Biomedical Research', in *NEJM* 315 (1986) 865-870; Canadian Medical Association, 'L'utilisation d'animaux d'expérimentation en recherche biomédicale', in *CMAJ* 135 (1986) 928B; J. Tannerbaum and A.N.O. Rowan, 'Rethinking the Morality of Animal Research', in *HCR* 15 (1985) no. 5, 32-34; J.K. Iglehart, 'The Use of Animals in Research', in *NEJM* 313 (1985) 395-400; R.G. Frey, 'Vivisection, Morals and Medicine', in *JME* 9 (1983) 94-97; see also 98-104; R.E. Leake, 'Live Animal Studies', in *S.A.M.*; McLean, *Legal Issues in Medicine*, Gower, Guildford 1981, 53-66; W. Lane-Petter, 'The Ethics of Animal Experimentation', in *JME* 2 (1976) 118-126; US Congress Office of Technology Assessment, *Alternatives to Animal Use in Research, Testing and Education*, US Government Printing Office, Washington DC 1986; US Department of Health and Human Services, Public Health Service, National Institutes of Health, *Guide for the Care and Use of Laboratory Animals*, NIH Publication, 85-23 (1985) 81-83; T. Regan, *The Case for Animal Rights,* Univ. of California, Berkeley 1983; P. Singer, *Animal Liberation,* Avon Books, New York 1975.
2. For a good summary of the position, refer to A. Bondolfi, 'The "rights" of animals and experiments on animals', in *Concilium* 223 (1984) 495-507.
3. 'Panel Report on the Colloquium on the Recognition and Alleviation of Animal Pain and Distress', in *Journal of the American Veterinary Medical Association* 191 (1987) 1186-1191
4. A detailed picture of the animal contribution can be found in Council of Scientific Affairs, *op.cit.*
5. E. Brovedani, 'Il brevetto di organismi viventi ottenuti con l'ingegneria genetica. Aspetti scientifici, giuridici ed etici', in *AS* 39 (1988) 245-257 (this article provides a valuable perspective on the various issues, and I have based part of my argument on it); 'Religious Groups Call for Animal Patenting Moratorium', in *Church and Society Newsletter* 10 (July 1988) 4; J.E. Densberger, 'Patents for Life Forms: An Inappropriate Response to Biotechnological Advancement', in *Journal of Bioethics* 5 (1984) no. 2, 91-115; A. Cooper, 'Patentability of Genetically Engineered Microorganisms', in *JAMA* 249 (1983) 1553-1554; Office of Technology Assessment (OTA),

Impacts of Applied Genetics, Patenting Living Organisms, Washington DC 1981; G.J. Annas, 'Patenting Life', in *HCR* 9 (1979) no. 6, 49; I. Hotzman, 'Patenting Certain Forms of Life: A Moral Justification', in *HCR* 9 (1979) no. 3, 9-11.
6. F.K. Beier, R.S. Crespi and J. Straus, *Biotechnologie et protection par brevet. Une analyse internationale*, OCD, Paris 1985.
7. 'Call for Animal Patenting Moratorium', in *Church and Society Newsletter* 10 (July 1988) Religious Groups, 4.
8. Gen 1:28.
9. A. Bondolfi, 'Rapporto uomo-animale. Storia del pensiero filosofico e teologico', in *RTM* 82 (1989) 57-77.